Current Clinical Psychiatry

Series editor

Jerrold F. Rosenbaum
Boston, MA, USA

For further volumes:
http://www.springer.com/series/7634

Ranna Parekh • Ed W. Childs
Editors

Stigma and Prejudice

Touchstones in Understanding Diversity
in Healthcare

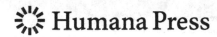 Humana Press

Editors
Ranna Parekh
Massachusetts General Hospital
Boston, MA
USA

Ed W. Childs
Morehouse School of Medicine
Atlanta, GA
USA

Current Clinical Psychiatry
ISBN 978-3-319-80176-6   ISBN 978-3-319-27580-2   (eBook)
DOI 10.1007/978-3-319-27580-2

Printed on acid-free paper

This Humana Press imprint is published by Springer Nature
The registered company is Springer International Publishing AG Switzerland

"It is never too late to give up our prejudices."

Henry David Thoreau

Foreword

Mental Health: A Report of the Surgeon General was released in November 1999. The report – the first-ever Surgeon General's report to address mental health – had both bad news and good news. The good news was that recent developments in research showed that 90 % of mental disorders were treatable and that these people were capable of living productive lives and having positive relationships with others. The bad news was that fewer than one half of people with mental disorders were accessing treatment. Stigma – real or perceived negative attitudes toward mental disorders and people living with mental disorders – was one of the major barriers to accessing treatment.

This report noted a number of different ways that stigma affects society. First, stigma impacts the individual with the mental disorder, and fear of being ostracized keeps that person from seeking treatment. Stigma oftentimes was what prevented parents of children needing therapy from seeking care for them. Many of them feared that their child might have difficulty accessing college or jobs later on in life were they to be diagnosed with a mental disorder. Unfortunately, negative attitudes toward people with mental disorders mean that there is some truth to the parents' concerns. Nevertheless, the needs of the children should still take priority.

Providers of care can easily include questions in their exams that could reveal the risk for or presence of a mental disorder. Sadly, stigma also impacts these providers, and as a result they often ignore ripe opportunities to diagnose and intervene with mental disorders early on. Society is impacted by stigma around mental disorders, creating an environment of skepticism and shame. That stigma and shame within society become a burden for individuals, families, and the healthcare system.

What was also very clear when we released our report was the tremendous impact of stigma on health policy as it related to mental disorders. In fact, the report called for major policy change such that equity of access to mental health services would become a reality. Even though our report was released in 1999, it was not until 2008 that the Parity of Access to Mental Health and Substance Addiction Treatment Act was passed by Congress under President George W. Bush and not until 2010 with the Affordable Care Act under President Barack Obama that provisions to access were included in most health insurance plans.

Because we noticed that stigma seems to vary among different groups of persons and seems to be related to culture, we followed up our first report with a supplemental report in 2001, *Mental Health: Culture, Race, and Ethnicity*. African Americans, for example, are much less likely to seek outpatient treatment for mental disorders than the general population. Asian Americans are even less likely to seek treatment. Neglecting the problem can lead to illness becoming too severe to manage with outpatient treatment. Thus, groups like African Americans, Asian Americans, and American Indians are often overrepresented among those admitted to inpatient care.

So what can we do to counter the stigma associated with mental illness? Most would agree that education of patients and community is the best approach to stigma reduction. The most important educational message is that we can in fact treat people with mental disorders and return them to productive lives and positive relationships. In short, the most important educational message is that recovery is possible. Believing that recovery is possible enhances health-seeking behaviors and the outcome of healthcare interventions.

Stigma surrounding mental illness persists in part because of the belief that mental illness is someone else's problem. *Mental Health: A Report of the Surgeon General* attempted to place this issue in a broader perspective by defining mental health in such a way that it is clear that none of us can take our mental health for granted. The report defined mental health as *a state of successful performance of mental function, resulting in productive activities, fulfilling relationships with other people, and the ability to adapt to change and to cope with adversity*. None of us can take our mental health for granted.

Environment and life experiences can impact mental health. After hurricane Katrina, I was asked to work to help redevelop the healthcare infrastructure of New Orleans and Baton Rouge, Louisiana. In screening and evaluating people who lived through the disaster, we noticed that depression increased between 10 and 30 %. It is evident then that one can be mentally healthy 1 day and mentally ill the next. That knowledge alone should lead each one of us to not only be sympathetic but actively assured that people with mental disorders are treated with respect and dignity and have the opportunity to access quality healthcare. As mental health is and can be impacted by life experience, we must work to promote the mental health of all people. There is no shame in that.

October 5, 2015

David Satcher, MD, PhD
Founding Director and Senior Advisor,
The Satcher Health Leadership Institute,
16th Surgeon General of the United States,
Atlanta, GA, USA

Preface

Prejudice is ubiquitous. In healthcare, it can lead to adverse consequences for patients. This textbook provides a thoughtful review of populations not primarily viewed as stigmatized patients. It also provides innovative ways to understand and bridge differences. The authors who are also healthcare professionals share their insights about bias in medicine. They show how stigma and prejudice may be hidden and how they affect care, interpersonal relationships among providers, patients, and families. Each chapter highlights the importance of cultural sensitivity when working with people whose "minority" status makes them vulnerable patients.

This textbook is divided into two parts: "Specific Patient Populations" and "Innovative Ways to Bridge Differences." Chapters in Part I describe 13 patient groups: immigrants, veterans, VIPs, the obese, sexually trafficked minors, religious minorities, the homeless, the poor and economically vulnerable, as well as persons with disabilities, borderline personality disorder, substance use disorders, breast cancer, and HIV/AIDS. Each population is unique and heterogenic. Collectively, they share the experience of being stigmatized and discriminated by society including healthcare providers. The authors critically review the literature as they describe these populations and their histories. In addition, they detail how the population is stigmatized and how this prejudice impacts the quality of healthcare rendered. Using their collective clinical expertise, the authors discuss future directions for improved treatment. Readers are left with best practice recommendations including culturally sensitive medical assessments and treatment.

Part II provides requisite reading for those working with minority and vulnerable populations. Each of the seven chapters offers unique strategies. Leveraging information technology and using trained medical interpreters enable healthcare professionals to provide equitable care for all. Increasing diversity in the medical workforce and in clinical patient research studies is discussed in context to rapidly changing US demographics. Also, the authors in this part describe how expanding existing diversity initiatives at academic institutions – incubators of the next generation of healthcare professionals – are critical for future patients. Finally, this part explores the role of introspection and precision medicine including pharmacology and genetics in expanding healthcare providers' knowledge about diversity.

The editors believe this textbook will provoke discussion. Recognizing prejudice and stigma in healthcare is challenging. Not noticing, however, can lead to decreased quality of health for our patients. We hope this textbook will be a useful reference for *all* health professionals and advocates of vulnerable patient populations.

Boston, MA, USA   Ranna Parekh, MD, MPH
Atlanta, GA, USA   Ed W. Childs, MD

Acknowledgments

The editors would like to acknowledge all the supporters of this textbook. We are grateful to the chapters' authors for their expertise and commitment in bringing this project to fruition. In addition, we thank Joseph Quatela, Nadina Persaud, and Richard Lansing, the publishers at Springer for their tireless support and efforts.

The inspiration for this book comes from our patients and their families. The authors hope this book stimulates thought and encourages dialogue about a difficult topic in medicine; it is essential in order to provide equitable healthcare for all and especially the vulnerable.

Finally, we would like to thank our family, friends, and loved ones. We dedicate this textbook to you.

Ranna Parekh, MD, MPH
Ed W. Childs, MD

Contents

Contributors

Bijay Acharya, MD Harvard Medical School, Boston, MA, USA

Edward P. Lawrence Center for Quality and Safety, Boston, MA, USA

Department of Medicine, Massachusetts General Hospital, Boston, MA, USA

Blaise Aguirre, MD 3East DBT Continuum, 3Eat Mclean Hospital, Belmont, MA, USA

Shirin N. Ali, MD Department of Psychiatry, New York state Psychiatric institute, New York, NY, USA

Jonathan Avery, MD Department of Psychiatry, Weill Cornell Medical College, New York, NY, USA

Miri Bar-Halpern, PsyD Adolescent Acute Residential Program, McLean Hospital, Boston, MA, USA

Harvard Medical School, Boston, MA, USA

Derrick J. Beech, MD, FACS Department of Surgery, Morehouse School of Medicine, Atlanta, GA, USA

Maged N. Kamel Boulos, MD, PhD The Alexander Graham Bell Centre for Digital Health, University of the Highlands and Islands, Inverness, UK

Christina Brezing, MD Division on Substance Abuse, Columbia Department of Psychiatry, Columbia University Medical Center, New York State Psychiatric Institute, New York, NY, USA

W. Scott Butsch, MD, MSc MGH Weight Center, Massachusetts General Hospital, Boston, MA, USA

Department of Medicine, Harvard Medical School, Boston, MA, USA

Katia M. Canenguez, PhD, EdM Department of Child and Adolescent
Psychiatry, Massachusetts General Hospital, Yawkey Center for Outpatient Care,
Boston, MA, USA

Ed W. Childs, MD Department of Surgery, Morehouse School of Medicine,
Atlanta, GA, USA

Clarence E. Clark, III Section of Colon and Rectal Surgery, Department
of Surgery, Morehouse School of Medicine, Atlanta, GA, USA

Omar K. Danner, MD, FACS Department of Surgery, Morehouse School
of Medicine, Atlanta, GA, USA

Denise De Las Nueces, MD, MPH Boston Health Care for the Homeless
Program, Boston, MA, USA

Department of Medicine, Boston University Medical Center, Boston University
School of Medicine, Boston, MA, USA

Eunice Malavé de León, EdD, LCSW Behavioral Health Department, Southside
Medical Center, Atlanta, GA, USA

Louise Dixon, BA Department of Psychology, University of California Los
Angeles, Los Angeles, CA, USA

Daleela G. Dodge, MD, FACS Department of Surgery, Lancaster General
Hospital, Lancaster, PA, USA

LG Health Breast Service, Ann B Barshinger Cancer Center, Lancaster,
PA, USA

Anne Emmerich, MD, MA Department of Psychiatry, Massachusetts General
Hospital, Boston, MA, USA

Harvard Medical School, Boston, MA, USA

Anthony Fatalo, RPh, MS, BCPS Department of Pharmacy, Massachusetts
General Hospital, Boston, MA, USA

Lior Givon, PhD, MD Cambridge Health Alliance, Cambridge, MA, USA

Harvard Medical School, Boston, MA, USA

Elizabeth M. Goetter, PhD Department of Psychiatry, Harvard Medical School,
Red Sox Foundation and Massachusetts General Hospital Home Base Program,
Boston, MA, USA

Mark J. Gorman, PhD MGH Weight Center, Massachusetts General Hospital,
Boston, MA, USA

Department of Psychiatry, Harvard Medical School, Boston, MA, USA

Schuyler W. Henderson Child and Adolescent Psychiatry, Bellevue Hospital,
New York, NY, USA

Department of Child and Adolescent Psychiatry, New York University, New York, NY, USA

Celsie M. Hiraldo-Lebrón, PhD Behavioral Health Department, NYU Lutheran Medical Center, Brooklyn, NY, USA

Lisa I. Iezzoni, MD, MSc Department of Medicine, Harvard Medical School, Mongan Institute for Health Policy, Massachusetts General Hospital, Boston, MA, USA

Andrew M. Jarowenko Tufts University, Boston, MA, USA

Aida L. Jiménez, PhD Department of Psychiatry, Vanderbilt University, Nashville, TN, USA

Daniel Knoepflmacher, MD Department of Psychiatry, Weill Cornell Medical College, New York, NY, USA

Hermioni N. Lokko, MD, MPP MGH/McLean Adult Psychiatry Residency Training Program, Harvard Medical School, Massachusetts General Hospital, Boston, MA, USA

McLean Hospital, Belmont, MA, USA

Wendy Macias-Konstantopoulos, MD, MPH Division of Global Health and Human Rights, Department of Emergency Medicine, Massachusetts General Hospital, Boston, MA, USA

Harvard Medical School, Boston, MA, USA

David Marcovitz, MD Department of Psychiatry, Massachusetts General Hospital, Harvard Medical School, Boston, MA, USA

Luana Marques, PhD Department of Psychiatry, Massachusetts General Hospital, Boston, MA, USA

Department of Psychiatry, Harvard Medical School, Boston, MA, USA

Sophia L. Maurasse, MD Department of Psychiatry, McLean Hospital, Belmont, MA, USA

Neel Mehta, MD Department of Pain Medicine, Weill Cornell Medical College, New York, NY, USA

Anabela M. Nunes, MBA Interpreter Services, Massachusetts General Hospital, Boston, MA, USA

Joel Okoli, MD Morehouse School of Medicine, Atlanta, GA, USA

Julie Penzner, MD Department of Psychiatry, Weill Cornell Medical College, New York, NY, USA

Janey Pratt, MD MGH Weight Center, Massachusetts General Hospital, Boston, MA, USA

Department of Surgery, Harvard Medical School, Boston, MA, USA

Noreen A. Reilly-Harrington, PhD MGH Weight Center, Massachusetts General Hospital, Boston, MA, USA

Department of Psychiatry, Harvard Medical School, Boston, MA, USA

Lauren K. Richards, PhD Department of Psychiatry, Harvard Medical School, Red Sox Foundation and Massachusetts General Hospital Home Base Program, Boston, MA, USA

Manisha Salinas, MA Department of Psychiatry, Massachusetts General Hospital, Boston, MA, USA

Department of Public Health, Texas A&M Health Science Center, School of Public Health, Round Rock, TX, USA

Naomi M. Simon, MD, MSc Department of Psychiatry, Harvard Medical School, Red Sox Foundation and Massachusetts General Hospital Home Base Program, Boston, MA, USA

Ginette Sims, BA Department of Psychiatry, Massachusetts General Hospital Psychiatry, Center for Diversity, McLean Hospital, Belmont, MA, USA

Phillip J. Small, MA Department of Psychology, Arizona State University, Tempe, AZ, USA

Stephanie Sogg, PhD MGH Weight Center, Massachusetts General Hospital, Boston, MA, USA

Department of Psychiatry, Harvard Medical School, Boston, MA, USA

Valerie E. Stone, MD, MPH Department of Medicine, Mount Auburn Hospital, Cambridge, MA, USA

Charles S. Davidson Professor of Medicine, Harvard Medical School, Boston, MA, USA

Magdalena Wojtowicz, PhD Department of Psychiatry, Harvard Medical School, Red Sox Foundation and Massachusetts General Hospital Home Base Program, Boston, MA, USA

Part I
Specific Patient Populations

Chapter 1
Stigma and Persons with Disabilities

Lisa I. Iezzoni

Introduction

Anyone can become disabled in an instant, and across the life span, almost everyone spends some time living with disability. According to the World Health Organization (WHO), disability is "a continuum, relevant to the lives of all people to different degrees and at different times in their lives," virtually a "universal phenomenon" and "natural feature of the human condition" [1]. Indeed, as the Institute of Medicine observed:

> If one considers people who now have disabilities …, people who are likely to develop disabilities in the future, and people who are or will be affected by the disabilities of family members or others close to them, then disability affects today or will affect tomorrow the lives of most Americans. Clearly, disability is not a minority issue. [2]

Given this near universality, why does disability continue to be so stigmatized? Certainly in the USA, the acceptance and inclusion of persons with disabilities has improved significantly since the mid-twentieth century. Perhaps the seminal event occurred on July 26, 1990, when President George H. W. Bush signed the Americans with Disabilities Act (ADA) and proclaimed, "Let the shameful wall of exclusion finally come tumbling down." Bush's remarks acknowledged millennia of discrimination against persons with disabilities, which this landmark civil rights law aimed to reverse. However, although persons with disabilities have made critical gains since then, significant barriers remain to achieving the full participation of persons with disabilities in community life. Compared with nondisabled

L.I. Iezzoni, MD, MSc
Department of Medicine, Harvard Medical School,
Mongan Institute for Health Policy, Massachusetts General Hospital,
50 Staniford Street, Room 901B, Boston, MA 02114, USA
e-mail: liezzoni@mgh.harvard.edu

© Springer International Publishing Switzerland 2016
R. Parekh, Ed W. Childs (eds.), *Stigma and Prejudice: Touchstones in Understanding Diversity in Healthcare*, Current Clinical Psychiatry,
DOI 10.1007/978-3-319-27580-2_1

persons, individuals with disabilities have greater disadvantages in education, employment, income, housing, transportation, and other eco-social determinants of health. They also often experience disparities in their health-care services.

Conceptualizing Disability

Disabilities are diverse. Nonetheless, they share one common element: persons with disabilities perform basic human functions – such as seeing, hearing, speaking, moving, thinking, and emoting – in different ways than do other persons. In the public's mind, these basic functions crystallize the essence of what it means to be "human," distinguishing Homo sapiens from other creatures. Thus, these differences distance persons with disabilities from the normative human, implicitly raising questions about their core humanity.

Although basically a biomechanical function, the ability to walk encapsulates this complex perspective. "Walking is not merely a physical activity which enables individuals to get from place A to place B. … It is also culturally symbolic …" [3]. Bipedal locomotion, not expanded intellect, differentiated the first human ancestors from other species. America's national ethos demands citizens moving freely at will, acting independently, assuming control and responsibility, and avoiding burdening others. Bipedal imagery suffuses American aphorisms – "standing on your own two feet," "standing up for yourself," "standing your ground," "walking tall," "climbing the ladder of success," and "one small step for a man, one giant leap for mankind." After seriously injuring his left leg, neurologist Oliver Sacks observed, "Erectness is moral, existential, no less than physical" [3].

However, disability also carries intensely practical implications, such as defraying the costs of acquiring assistive technologies to accommodate functional impairments (e.g., obtaining a wheelchair, which can cost over $40,000 depending on specific technologic capabilities). For meeting such practical needs, such as income support through the Social Security Administration or entitlement to public health insurance, defining disability assumes a different imperative. Thus, no single definition serves all societal, governmental, or individual purposes (Table 1.1) [4].

Human societies have struggled with defining disability since their earliest days. Wherever people gathered for communal subsistence, some individuals could not hunt, gather, labor, or fulfill expected social roles because of physical, sensory, cognitive, or mental health impairments. To survive, these people needed help, which societies provided. However, as pressures on charitable coffers grew, so too did demands to determine eligibility for societal largesse. Documents from Medieval Europe indicate that some supplicants feigned disability to claim alms or other benefits [5]. Fourteenth-century English laws held that "honest beggars" – persons deserving alms – were forced involuntarily into their plights by circumstances beyond their control. Detecting disability deception preoccupied charitable authorities centuries ago and continues today.

Table 1.1 Examples of disability definitions

Source	Definition of disability
World Health Organization, *International Classification of Functioning, Disability and Health*, 2001	"Umbrella term for impairments, activity limitations or participation restrictions," conceiving "a person's functioning and disability … as a dynamic interaction between health conditions (diseases, disorders, injuries, traumas, etc.) and contextual factors," including the social, attitudinal, and physical environments and personal attributes. Impairments are "problems in body function or structure such as a significant deviation or loss."
Americans with Disabilities Act (ADA), P.L. 101–336, 1990	Sec. 3(2) "The term 'disability' means, with respect to an individual — (A) a physical or mental impairment that substantially limits one or more of the major life activities of such individual; (B) a record of such an impairment; or (C) being regarded as having such an impairment."
ADA Amendments Act (ADAAA), P.L. 110–325, 2008	Retains the ADA's definition of disability but broadens the definition by:
	Expands "major life activity" definition to include not only activities but also major bodily functions
	Major life activities include, but are not limited to, caring for oneself, performing manual tasks, seeing, hearing, eating, sleeping, walking, standing, lifting, bending, speaking, breathing, learning, reading, concentrating, thinking, communicating, and working
	Major bodily functions include, but are not limited to, functions of the immune system, normal cell growth, digestive, bowel, bladder, neurological, brain, respiratory, circulatory, endocrine, and reproductive functions
	Specifies that impairments that are episodic or in remission would qualify as disability if, when active, they substantially limit a major life activity
	With one exception (ordinary eyeglasses or contact lenses), prohibits the consideration of the benefits of "mitigating measures" when considering whether an impairment substantially limits a major life activity
Social Security Administration	"Inability to engage in any substantial gainful activity by reason of any medically determinable physical or mental impairment(s) which can be expected to result in death or which has lasted or can be expected to last for a continuous period of not less than 12 months." Medically determinable impairment is "an impairment that results from anatomical, physiological, or psychological abnormalities which can be shown by medically acceptable clinical and laboratory diagnostic techniques." Impairments "must be established by medical evidence consisting of signs, symptoms, and laboratory findings – not only by the individual's statement of symptoms."

In the nineteenth century, a wave of new diagnostic instruments gave medicine an aura of scientific objectivity [5]. This began in 1819 with René Laënnec's invention of the stethoscope, followed by development of the microscope, ophthalmoscope, spirometer, x-rays, and other diagnostic instruments. With each new technology, proponents extolled its ability to detect disease without relying on persons' subjective reports and thus its usefulness for distinguishing legitimate and thus meritorious disability. Furthermore, these new diagnostic instruments provided insights into biological causes of functional impairments and cemented the primacy of physicians in treating disability. Thus, by the end of the 1800s, the "medical model" of disability prevailed.

> The *medical model* views disability as a problem of the person, directly caused by disease, trauma or other health condition, which requires medical care provided in the form of individual treatment by professionals. Management of the disability is aimed at cure or the individual's adjustment and behaviour change. Medical care is viewed as the main issue, and at the political level the principal response is that of modifying or reforming health care policy. [6]

Two beliefs thus support the medical model [4]. First, guided by health-care professionals, persons should strive individually to overcome their impairments. Second, doctors know what is best for their patients. If impairments are not cured, persons must accept their losses and adapt, preferably cheerfully, to reduced circumstances.

By the late 1960s as described below, perceptions of disability began changing radically. A new paradigm emerged, holding that disability is caused by environmental factors – physical barriers, negative societal attitudes, and inadequate public policies – that fail to accommodate difference, thus isolating persons and excluding them from full participation in community life.

> The *social model* of disability … sees the issue mainly as a socially created problem, and basically as a matter of the full integration of individuals into society. Disability is not an attribute of an individual, but rather a complex collection of conditions, many of which are created by the social environment. Hence the management of the problem requires social action, and it is a collective responsibility of society at large to make the environmental modifications necessary for the full participation of people with disabilities in all areas of social life. The issue is therefore an attitudinal or ideological one requiring social change, which at the political level becomes a question of human rights. For this model disability is a political issue. [6]

In its disability classification scheme, the *International Classification of Functioning, Disability and Health* (ICF), WHO melds the medical and social models of disability (Table 1.1) [6]. ICF links biological, individual, and social perspectives into a comprehensive view of health. It explicitly recognizes that external forces – such as physical environments, social structures, governmental policies, and societal attitudes – contribute to or mitigate disability.

Disability Stigmatization

Stigmatization of disability has a long history, reaching back millennia and paralleling evolution of the conceptualization of disability described above. Throughout early history, persons with disabilities were shadowy figures living on the fringes of society or explicitly isolated (e.g., in "leper colonies," "madhouses," "insane asylums"). "Normals" feared contamination or taint from interacting with disabled persons. The implied moral culpability of persons with disabilities for their impairments compounded this isolation. For instance, Leviticus (16:18–20) in the Old Testament catalogued "blemishes" that precluded persons from joining religious ceremonies: "a man blind or lame, or one who has a mutilated face or a limb too long, or a man who has an injured foot or an injured hand, or a hunchback, or a dwarf …"

Jumping forward to seventeenth-century America, the demands of settling this rugged country "meant that early colonists put a premium on physical stamina" [7]. The initial settlers opposed immigration of individuals requiring community support and sometimes deported persons with physical or mental impairments [8]. These attitudes eased somewhat by Revolutionary War time, although most disabled people remained behind closed doors. In 1781, Thomas Jefferson observed that Virginians without "strength to labour" were "boarded in the houses of good farmers" funded by local parish tithes [9]. Throughout nineteenth-century America, persons with disabilities generally were hidden within homes or increasingly placed in institutions founded to house (warehouse) disabled individuals, especially persons with severe mental illness or developmental disabilities.

The eugenics movement in late nineteenth- and early twentieth-century America explicitly questioned the humanity and value of disabled persons. In particular, eugenics proponents stoked fears about women with disabilities having babies, inflaming public views that disabled women are unfit to bear or raise children. Thirty states legalized the forced sterilization of disabled women, many states banned them from marrying, and some laws mandated compulsory contraception [10, 11]. These policies applied particularly to women with intellectual or mental health disabilities. In the 1927 *Buck v. Bell* decision, the US Supreme Court ruled that the Commonwealth of Virginia could forcibly sterilize Carrie Buck, an institutionalized woman described as "feebleminded" and daughter of a "feebleminded" mother living in the same facility, after she became pregnant following being raped. In concluding the court's decision, Justice Oliver Wendell Holmes, Jr, observed, "Three generations of imbeciles are enough" [11]. Under these state laws, an estimated 65,000 Americans with disabilities and other "social inadequacies" were sterilized by 1970. Although the eugenics fervor eventually abated in the USA, some credit American eugenics proponents with inspiring German Nazi programs involving forced sterilization and extermination of tens of thousands of persons with disabilities.

The most famous disabled person of the twentieth century – Franklin Delano Roosevelt – left a complicated disability legacy. In August 1921 at his Campobello resort, Roosevelt (age 39 years) contracted polio, and he never took another true step. Knowing the public would not elect a man who could not walk, Roosevelt crafted a fiction, aiming to "stand easily enough in front of people so that they'll forget I'm a cripple" [12]. Through arduous practice, he learned how to appear to walk while being carried forward by his bent arm and cane. The public accepted FDR's elaborate deception, believing that Roosevelt was simply a little lame. Even privately, as Eleanor Roosevelt conceded, Roosevelt "never admitted he cannot walk" [13]. His attitude exemplified the prevailing national ethos: "stiff upper lip, good soldier to the last" [13]. From his unseen wheelchair, Roosevelt led the nation through some of its darkest days and is widely acclaimed as one of America's greatest presidents.

Roosevelt's silence meant a "teachable moment" was lost – the public never understood their generally exalted leader was disabled. Societal attitudes about disability changed little for two decades. In 1963, sociologist Erving Goffman published his classic book on stigma, asserting that being "lame," "crippled," or "multiple sclerotic" qualified as stigmatized attributes (along with minority race and religion), tainting, discounting, or discrediting people in their own and society's eyes [14]. However, within several years, the disability civil rights movement began its early tentative steps, spurred by the independent living movement, consumer self-help initiatives, deinstitutionalization, and civil rights advocacy for racial and ethnic minorities and for women. It is beyond my scope here to chronicle its progress and ultimate achievement – passage of the ADA, which defined disability broadly (Table 1.1). Today, more than two decades later, persons with all sorts of disabilities are prominent on the public stage, as government officials, actors, artists, athletes, academics, advocates, and attorneys, and serving in many other roles. Many people proudly wear their disability identity as they participate fully in community life. Nonetheless, as described below, the goal of the ADA – ensuring equal rights and opportunities to Americans with disabilities – remains a work in progress.

Disability Civil Rights

The demands of disability civil rights differ in fundamental ways from those achieved by racial and ethnic minorities. For example, on December 1, 1955 in Montgomery, Alabama, Rosa Parks refused to give up her seat on a bus to a White passenger. Years later, Parks knew she had achieved equal rights when she could board any bus and take any seat. Observers might notice the color of her skin, but being Black no longer dictated where – or if – she could sit on the bus.

In contrast, for me – a wheelchair user – to even get onto a bus, the bus must be specifically configured to allow me to board, typically by having a ramp or lift. The bus driver must notice my stigmatized attribute (i.e., my disability) and must proactively deploy either the ramp or lift to allow me to board. For safety, local rules require that drivers secure wheelchair passengers in the allocated wheelchair space, a process that requires several minutes. When I leave the bus, this procedure happens in reverse. During this process, I am not independent: I must rely on the driver's actions. I also must hope that the ramps or lifts are functioning properly (which is not always the case). And finally, the time elapsed in this process might inconvenience other passengers, especially persons in a hurry to reach their destinations. It is impossible not to be aware of their annoyed glances or stares.

Thus, because persons with disabilities perform basic human functions in different ways, accommodating these differences – and providing equal rights, access, and opportunities – requires proactive modifications in the way these actions are performed, such as a different method for boarding a bus or making the environment more accessible.

The ADA is unique in the context of civil rights legislation because it requires that businesses and government do more than just cease discriminatory actions. They must also take proactive steps to offer equal opportunity to persons with disabilities ... [15]

This requirement for proactive action contributed to difficulties in passing the ADA, as some business leaders argued that providing disability accommodations would cost too much [7]. In fact, studies showed that many disability accommodations cost nothing or at most up to several hundred dollars. To address the cost concern, however, the ADA put strictures on the reach of disability accommodations, requiring that they be "reasonable" and "readily achievable" within the resources available to an organization. In early rulings, the US Supreme Court ratcheted back who qualified as disabled under the ADA, forcing Congress to pass the ADA Amendments Act in 2008 to reinstate the intended inclusive definition of disability (Table 1.1).

Nonetheless, certain disability accommodations inevitably affect nondisabled persons in particular ways, sometimes igniting discord. For example, in my city, Boston, historical preservationists have objected to replacing the irregular bricks paving sidewalks and to installing sidewalk curb cuts that do not meet their aesthetic criteria, arguing that these changes detract from the nineteenth-century charm of certain neighborhoods. However, these modifications are essential for me to roll safely and comfortably throughout the city. Furthermore, even though these initiatives aim to assure equal access for persons with disabilities, the changes will likely assist other people as well, such as parents pushing children in strollers or travelers pulling their rollaboard suitcases. This notion of "universal design" – making changes that benefit many people – is a core recommendation for moving forward, as described in concluding this chapter.

Population Prevalence and Demographics

Worldwide, an estimated one billion persons live with disabilities [16]. Precise population estimates of disability in the USA depend on the data source and how disability is defined. Drawing from 2011 National Health Interview Survey (NHIS) data, an estimated 60.5 million (26.5 %) of the civilian, noninstitutionalized US population ages 18 and older report some type of chronic disability (Table 1.2) [17]. Women are more likely to report functional impairments than are men, although this varies by impairment type. Movement difficulties are the most common chronic disability, affecting 54.0 million (23.3 %) of adult, civilian, noninstitutionalized US residents. This high prevalence of mobility problems is not surprising: according to the Centers for Disease Control and Prevention, arthritis is the most common disabling condition among adult Americans, affecting an estimated 22.2 % of the population (2007–2009 data) [18]. Arthritis is more common in women (24.3 %) than men (18.2 %).

Both the numbers and percentages of US residents with chronic disabilities are rising over time. Analyzing NHIS data across selected years from 1998 through

Table 1.2 Estimated rates and population numbers by chronic disability type: US civilian, noninstitutionalized residents ages 18 and older, 2011

Disability type	Percent of population	Estimated population (millions)
Total US population age ≥18 (millions)	100.0 %	231.4 million
Disability defined by functional impairments (basic action limitations)		
Movement difficulty	23.3	54.0
Sensory difficulty (difficulty seeing or hearing)	7.4	17.1
Emotional difficulty	2.7	6.3
Cognitive difficulty	3.3	7.6
Any chronic disability defined by functional impairment	25.4	58.4
Disability defined by difficulties performing social roles (complex action limitations)		
Limitations in self-care (activities of daily living [ADL] or instrumental ADL limitations)	4.6	10.6
Social limitations (difficulties in going out, participating in social roles, or relaxing)	8.1	18.2
Work limitations	11.4	26.3
Any chronic disability defined by social roles	14.1	32.1
Any chronic disability	26.5	60.5

Adapted from: Iezzoni et al. [17]

2011, the percentage of persons within every disability type increased significantly (*p* < 0.0001) [17]. Other population trends – including rising numbers of elderly individuals and the obesity epidemic – could contribute to these increasing disability rates. However, the growth of disability rates over time generally remains statistically significant even after accounting for these other population trends [17]. Disability rates are also rising among children due to several factors, including survival of extremely premature infants, who often sustain significant functional deficits; new medical therapies saving lives of children with major congenital or acquired health conditions that would previously have been fatal; and the obesity epidemic among children and youth, which is causing earlier onset of disabling conditions such as diabetes and joint diseases.

Disability is strongly associated with sociodemographic attributes that are also stigmatized or disadvantaged, as follows:

• Black persons generally report higher disability rates than do Whites. However, accounting for education, employment status, and poverty attenuates these differences [17]. (Hispanic and Asian individuals report lower disability rates than Whites and Blacks, but these relationships are complicated by extent of acculturation and cultural factors affecting responses to surveys, the data source. Native Americans and Alaskan Natives report the highest disability rates of all races, but their numbers in surveys are generally too small to analyze in detail.)

• In 2012, 34.4 % of persons with disabilities had just a high school (or equivalent) education, compared with 25.5 % of nondisabled persons [19]. Only 12.4 % of disabled persons had a college degree or higher education, compared with 31.7 % of persons without disabilities.

- In 2013, only 17.6 % of persons with disabilities were employed, compared with 64.0 % of other persons [20].
- In 2012, 28.4 % of working-age persons with disabilities lived in poverty compared with 12.4 % of nondisabled persons [19].
- In 2012, the median income of households including any working-age person with disability was $37,300, compared with $60,600 for households without disabled members [19].

Thus, persons with disabilities are much more likely than other persons to experience disadvantages considered to be social determinants of health.

Health and Health Care of Persons with Disabilities

On average, persons with disabilities are much more likely than nondisabled individuals to have worse health and higher health risks and to receive substandard care, although the nature and extent of these disparities varies by disability type.

Health Disparities

Persons with disabilities are much more likely than other persons to report fair or poor health. Among US adults without disability, only 3.4 % report being in fair or poor health. In contrast, the percentage reporting fair or poor health is 37.9 % among persons with movement difficulties, 30.6 % for vision or hearing difficulties, 51.8 % for emotional difficulties, and 63.8 % for cognitive difficulties [21].

Persons with disabilities are also more likely than nondisabled individuals to report behaviors or conditions that heighten risks for other diseases. Notably, while 20.4 % of nondisabled US adults currently smoke, smoking rates are significantly higher among disabled individuals: 23.9 % for movement, 23.3 % for seeing or hearing, 43.0 % for emotional, and 26.7 % for cognitive disabilities [21]. Similarly, 18.7 % of nondisabled persons are obese compared with 33.4 % of persons with movement difficulties, 27.1 % with seeing or hearing, 33.0 % with emotional, and 27.2 % with cognitive difficulties [21]. Persons with disabilities are also significantly less likely to perform leisure time physical activity.

Health-Care Disparities

Persons with disabilities are also much more likely than others to experience substandard health care. The 2013 National Disparities Report from the Agency for Healthcare Research and Quality (AHRQ) included a special focus on persons with disabilities [22]. AHRQ examined the proportion of quality measures that had improved, not changed, or worsened for selected populations, and persons with disabilities did worse than all other groups studied. In 2013, the percent of quality measures that showed improvement by population subgroup were as follows: 59.5 % for all persons, 58.3 % for Hispanics, 57.1 % for Blacks, 56.9 % for Asians, 53.7 % for poor persons, 42.0 % for American Indians and Alaskan Natives, 36.0 % for persons with "basic action limitations" (Table 1.2), and 20.8 % for persons with "complex action limitations" (Table 1.2).

Persons with disabilities often fail to receive important screening and preventive services than are nondisabled individuals. For example, 82.5 % of nondisabled US women received a Pap test in the prior 3 years, compared with 69.3 % of women with movement, 68.6 % with seeing or hearing, 72.4 % with emotional, and 58.3 % with cognitive difficulties [21]. About 74 % of women age 50 and older without disabilities received a mammogram in the previous 2 years, compared with 66.4 % of women over 50 with movement, 62.8 % with seeing or hearing, 58.4 % with emotional, and 52.1 % with cognitive difficulties [21].

Health-Care Experiences of Persons with Disabilities

Many factors might explain health-care disparities for persons with disabilities, including competing health-care priorities given the clinical needs of their underlying health conditions; persons' preferences for care; "magical thinking" or the erroneous belief that having a disability somehow prevents other health problems from occurring; previous difficult or unpleasant experiences getting health care; transportation problems, especially in rural regions and urban areas with poor public transportation; physical barriers to care; faulty or inadequate knowledge of clinicians about the disabling condition; ineffective communication with patients; and stigmatizing attitudes of clinicians, as elsewhere in society [23]. I describe several factors in greater depth below.

Inadequate Knowledge Base

Persons with disabilities are routinely excluded from the clinical trials that researchers conduct to measure the effectiveness of different therapies and develop the scientific evidence base. Therefore, clinicians are frequently unable to give persons with disabilities evidence-based therapeutic recommendations for even common, well-studied conditions (e.g., certain cancers, cardiovascular diseases). This leaves persons with disabilities without adequate information to make fully informed decisions about their care.

Furthermore, many health-care professionals lack knowledge about specific disabling conditions, especially relatively rare disorders. A survey of 344 persons with movement disabilities found that 24.4 % left primary care visits feeling that some of their needs were not met; 36.4 % reported having needed to teach their physician about their disability [24]. Many persons with disabilities become experts in their own conditions, able to work collaboratively with physicians in their care. But as described below, physicians sometimes negate, disregard, or discount the patients' expertise.

Physical Barriers to Care

As with the bus example above, to obtain care persons with disabilities must be physically able to get onto examination tables as well as to enter and navigate around health-care facilities [23]. Even such routine activities as performing complete physical examinations and obtaining accurate weights require specific accommodations for some persons with disabilities. A survey of persons needing assistance with transfers found that 59 % were examined in their wheelchairs by their primary care physicians [24].

Little systematic information is available about how often these physical barriers occur in health-care facilities. A study of California Medicaid providers found that only 8.4 % of providers had a height adjustable examination table, and just 3.6 % had an accessible weight scale [25]. Recently, internist Tara Lagu in western Massachusetts was frustrated by problems finding specialists to see her patients who use wheelchairs. In response, Lagu and colleagues conducted a "secret shopper"-type study, telephoning subspecialty offices ostensibly to make an appointment for a fictional patient described as obese, with hemiparesis, using a wheelchair, and unable to transfer independently from the wheelchair to exam tables [26]. Among 256 practices across four US cities, 56 (22 %) indicated that they could not accommodate the patient; 9 (4 %) said their building was inaccessible and 47 (18 %) reported they could not transfer the patient onto an exam table or chair. Across the eight specialties, gynecology had the worst inaccessibility rate (44 %). Only 22 (9 %) practices indicated they had either a height adjustable examination table or lift device. The refusal of the 22 % of practices to schedule the fictional patient violated the ADA. However, the ready willingness of respondents at these inaccessible practices to explain their reasons for refusing to schedule the patient suggests they failed to appreciate the illegality.

Communication Barriers

Effective communication between health-care professionals and patients is essential to effective care, but numerous communication barriers prevent or compromise these interchanges [23]. Patients may be blind, deaf, hard of hearing, or have low vision, speech impediments, or intellectual disabilities. However, clinical settings and providers often fail to offer communication accommodations, such as Braille, large print, or audio instructional materials; sign language interpreters or communication access real-time translation (CART); closed captioning on educational videos; or pictorial or low literacy explanatory information. Health-care providers cannot charge patients for these communication accommodations, some of which (e.g., sign language interpreters) can occasionally cost more than the visit fee. Busy clinicians often admit that they neither have time nor patience to communicate effectively with patients using augmentative communication devices (e.g., persons with cerebral palsy) or patients with intellectual disabilities. A survey of providers across a range of care settings found that persons with communication impairments were viewed as the most difficult patients with disabilities [27]. It is beyond my scope here to discuss this complex topic in detail, but it is critical to underscore that failures to ensure effective communication are among the most common complaints in ADA lawsuits against health-care providers.

Attitudinal Barriers to Care

Throughout history, health-care professionals have been complicit in egregious discriminatory acts against persons with disabilities, such as performing sterilization procedures during the eugenics frenzy, administering legally imposed injection contraceptives (e.g., Depo-Provera) to unwilling women, and overseeing institutions warehousing persons with intellectual disabilities or serious and persistent mental illness. Especially among persons with disabilities who experienced these injustices, establishing trusting relationships with health-care practitioners can be challenging.

A small body of research has explored the attitudes of clinicians about disability. A seminal article from 1994 reported on attitudes of 233 physicians, nurses, and emergency medical technicians working at 3 Level I trauma centers about treating persons with spinal cord injury (SCI) and compared clinicians' responses with those from a prior survey of individuals with SCI [28]. Among clinicians, 22 % indicated they would not want life-sustaining treatment if they themselves had a SCI; 23 % would want pain relief only; and only 18 % imagined they would be glad to be alive after SCI. In contrast, 92 % of respondents with SCI indicated they were glad to be alive [28]. Most troubling, 41 % of clinicians felt that clinicians in their emergency departments tried "too hard to resuscitate or save" person with new SCIs.

In 2011, researchers conducted a systematic review of publications across health-care disciplines that addressed the attitudes of students and clinicians toward caring for patients with physical disabilities [29]. They identified 22 studies including international research, which in general showed positive attitudes toward persons with disabilities, especially among respondents who had previous experiences with these individuals. Women typically report more positive views of patients with physical disabilities than do men. However, the studies also revealed fear and discomfort in treating persons with disabilities, in particular when respondents lacked knowledge about disability [29].

In a 2014 commentary, physician Leana Wen, who has a significant stutter, summed up her current impression of her colleagues' attitudes:

> ... Patients may have had unnecessary tests ordered because of their disability. Doctors and nurses label such practice with the disparaging term of "veterinary medicine." In other words, just as for an animal that can't speak for itself, they order tests instead of talking to patients who are perceived as being "slow" or "difficult." These patients often receive inadequate care: Either doctors can't see past their disability and attribute all problems to it, or doctors fail to acknowledge the true impact of their impairments. [30]

"Because nearly every provider will take care of substantial numbers of people with disabilities during his or her career," Wen concludes, "health professional education must mandate training focused on recognizing and caring for people with disabilities" [30].

Future Directions

Disability advocates rally under the phrase "nothing about us without us," asserting that persons with disabilities must participate in all decisions – from the personal to policy – that might affect them [31]. This phrase has recently broadened into the more direct exhortation: "nothing without us." This formulation recognizes that disability is, over the life span, virtually universal, and thus, disability is ubiquitous. Therefore, all societal decisions must consider the perspectives of individuals with disabilities.

The concept of "universal design" offers a unifying principle: designers of products, places, programs, policies, and other human initiatives must consider the needs of everyone who will be affected and aim to meet or accommodate their diverse needs to the extent possible. Involving persons with disabilities in the universal design process is essential; otherwise, their views will not be represented fully. This is especially true in health care [23]. As noted above and in the 2011 *World Report on Disability*, the complicated history of persons with disabilities with health-care worldwide and physicians, specifically, has engendered a sense that many doctors "just don't get" important aspects of the lives and expectations of persons with disabilities [16]. Therefore, even within the health-care delivery system, persons with disabilities must be included in making decisions that will affect them.

Reducing stigma and eliminating health and health-care disparities for persons with disabilities will require efforts on many fronts. According to *Healthy People 2020,* which in 2010 set US national public health priorities for the next decade, improving the health of persons with disabilities requires addressing their disadvantaged position in the social determinants of health – such as reducing poverty, improving education, increasing employment, ensuring housing and other supports for independent living, and eliminating physical barriers throughout communities [32]. The *World Report on Disability* provides a comprehensive agenda cutting across societal sectors. This chapter concludes by highlighting several specific concerns.

Language

One starting point is language. Word choices efficiently convey complex perceptions about the agency, respect, and dignity of population groups. As individuals, persons with disabilities refer to themselves according to their personal preferences. For example, writer Nancy Mairs, who has multiple sclerosis and uses a wheelchair, prefers "cripple," seeing it as "a clean word, straightforward and precise" [33]. She admits that sometimes people "wince" when she uses it: "Perhaps I want them to wince. I want them to see me as a tough customer … who can face the brutal truth of her existence squarely. As a cripple, I swagger."

Nonetheless, such words as "crippled," "handicapped," "gimp," "retarded," or "crazy" are no longer considered acceptable in routine public use, and referring to persons as an adjective ("the disabled," "the quad") is disrespectful. A general preference has emerged for so-called "person first" language, followed by a qualifier, i.e., "person with a disability." However, some disability advocates resist this formulation, worried that rigid insistence on "person first" language disparages the disability experience. They recommend phraseology that puts disability first, connoting pride in the disability identity (i.e., "disabled persons") [10]. This chapter has used these two phrases interchangeably. Preferences for global language choices will likely continue evolving along with societal attitudes.

Specific disabilities raise particular language issues, as follows:

- "Intellectual disability" has replaced "mental retardation" even in several federal statutes. In 2010, Congress passed "Rosa's Law," named for Rosa Marcellino, a Maryland girl with Down syndrome whose family objected to her being called "a retard."
- The umbrella phrase "developmental disability" applies to disabilities that are congenital or arise in childhood, encompassing not only intellectual disabilities but also such diverse conditions as autism spectrum disorders and cerebral palsy.
- While the lowercase "deaf" indicates the inability to hear (the audiological condition), the capitalized "Deaf" represents the cultural identity and the linguistic minority, American Sign Language (ASL) speakers.
- "Hard of hearing" typically applies to persons who develop hearing deficits later in life.
- Language around mental health conditions is evolving with treatment advances and growing understanding about how these conditions unfold across the life span. "Serious and persistent mental illness" is accepted by some as encompassing a range of conditions. Certain individuals prefer phraseology evoking the concept of "recovery," depending on the stage of their conditions.

Finally, the common phrases "wheelchair bound" and "confined to a wheelchair" suggest inaction, loss of control, and dependency, which no longer apply to many wheelchair users. New wheelchair technologies allow persons to independently and easily perform daily activities and beyond, from competing as elite athletes to traveling the world. The phrase "wheelchair user" substitutes simple active language for outdated and stigmatizing metaphors.

Legal Requirements

Health-care settings, practitioners, and staff must comply with the law. However, as suggested by the "secret shopper" survey described above, clinicians and other personnel are often unaware of their legal obligations to provide equal access to persons with disabilities. The key federal statutes are:

- ADA Title II, which applies to entities run by state and local governments (e.g., public hospitals, community health centers)
- ADA Title III, which applies to private entities offering public accommodations, such as health care (e.g., private hospitals, physician practices)
- Section 504 of the Rehabilitation Act of 1973, which covers all recipients of federal dollars, such as payments from Medicare, Medicaid, and other federal programs

These laws require health-care delivery systems, facilities, and practitioners to provide full and equal access to persons with disabilities.

Regulations that initially went into effect 2 years after the ADA's passage (July 26, 1992) cover the accessibility of fixed structures that are newly built or renovated. The US Access Board, an independent federal agency, produces accessibility guidelines and standards under the ADA, Section 504, and other federal laws. The US Internal Revenue Service offers tax credits to eligible private health-care providers for certain costs of complying with accessibility requirements. ADA regulations, overseen by the US Department of Justice Civil Rights Division, delineate what is required to comply with ADA provisions, including ensuring not only physical access but also effective communication. ADA requirements represent a bare minimum, and often additional accommodations are needed to ensure full accessibility and comfort [23].

ADA physical accessibility regulations cover physical structures and items attached to those structures, such as grab bars and toilets. Accessibility standards for medical diagnostic equipment are not addressed. To fill this gap, Section 4203 of the 2010 Patient Protection and Affordable Care Act (ACA) amends Title V of the Rehabilitation Act to require the US Access Board, in consultation with the Food and Drug Administration, to issue technical standards for accessibility of medical diagnostic equipment, including examination tables, stretchers, diagnostic imaging equipment, mammography equipment, and weight scales. The statute explicitly aims for standards that will allow persons with disabilities to use equipment independently to the maximum extent possible. Thus, the law envisions design features that permit individuals with disabilities to safely transfer onto diagnostic equipment (e.g., exam tables that can be automatically raised and lowered) with minimal assistance from other persons. Although these standards were to have been produced by 2012, they are not yet available. After these standards are finalized, the US Department of Justice will determine how widely health-care providers must comply with these diagnostic equipment accessibility standards.

Training Clinicians

Eliminating the stigmatization of persons with disabilities within health-care settings will require explicit training of health-care professionals. The social model of disability and WHO's disability definition (Table 1.1) suggest critical considerations in training clinicians to care for persons with disabilities: teaching that disability and health must be viewed within the entire context of patients' lives and social and physical environments where they live [34]. This all-encompassing perspective is particularly critical for physicians to ensure they provide patient-centered care. Comprehensive care for many persons with disabilities requires integrated teams of diverse health-care professionals and interdisciplinary coordination. However, medical schools and postgraduate training programs rarely teach young physicians to work effectively within interprofessional teams, including nursing, various rehabilitation therapies, and other clinical disciplines.

Table 1.3 suggests core competencies for training health-care professionals to care for persons with disabilities [35]. These competencies include not only technical skills but also an understanding of how environmental and social factors contribute to disability, legal obligations, basic etiquette for interacting with persons with disabilities, and recognition of the value persons with disabilities place on their lives. The *World Report on Disability* specifically recommends that educators worldwide "integrate disability education into undergraduate and continuing education for all health care professionals" [16]. In calling for "people-centered services," the report emphasizes that this imperative connects directly to the human rights advocacy for persons with disabilities articulated within the United Nations Convention on the Rights of Persons with Disabilities [16].

As noted throughout this chapter, persons with disabilities have had a complicated history with health-care professionals, especially physicians. Even today, persons with disabilities often sense that many doctors "just don't get" important aspects of their lives and their expectations of and preferences for care [23]. Because

Table 1.3 Proposed core competencies for physicians caring for persons with disabilities

	Description
1	Framing disability within the context of human diversity across the life span and within social and cultural environments
2	Skills training for assessment of disability and functional consequences of health conditions, considering implications for treatment and management
3	Training in general principles concerning etiquette for interactions with persons with disabilities
4	Learning about roles of other health-care professionals forming integrated teams to care for persons with disabilities
5	Understanding legal requirements of the 1990 Americans with Disabilities Act for accommodating disability in health-care settings, along with principles of universal design
6	Competency in patient-centered care approaches, including understanding patients' perceptions of quality of life

Adapted from: Kirschner and Curry [35]

of that, having today's physicians – even when genuinely well-intentioned – assume complete control over designing disability training curricula for future doctors may miss critical issues in caring empathically and effectively for persons with disabilities [34]. "Nothing about us without us!" may therefore also apply to designing disability training programs for health-care professionals. Involving persons with disabilities in identifying key teaching points and even implementing curricula for future physicians (e.g., participating in teaching activities) may be the best strategy to ensure their competency to provide patient-centered care to persons with disabilities.

Imperative of Demographic Trends

As indicated at this chapter's outset, according to the Institute of Medicine, "disability affects today or will affect tomorrow the lives of most Americans" [2]. Inexorable demographic shifts, particularly the aging of "baby boomers," will cause the numbers of Americans living with disabilities to grow considerably in coming decades. More than their parents, the so-called "silent generation," aging "baby boomers" will likely want to continue participating fully in their communities and traveling the world. Sally Anne Jones, who is in her late 50s and uses a power wheelchair because of multiple sclerosis (MS), feels that public leaders have missed the obvious:

> The "boomers" are coming. Despite MS and other diseases, they're going to live longer. We're not going to warehouse them in nursing homes. These "boomers" simply won't do that. They're not going to go quietly into the night. [36]

"Boomers" with disabilities will speak up and demand accommodations.

In addition, many children of "baby boomers" have attended schools where students with disabilities were mainstreamed; they have interacted with peers with disabilities since early ages. This familiarity may breed more comfort and acceptance of individuals with disabilities. New assistive technologies are daily expanding the capabilities of individuals with disabilities to live independently and productively in their homes and communities. Dramatic changes in societal attitudes are unlikely to occur easily or immediately. But over the next several decades, one can only hope that the stigmatization and discrimination that have disadvantaged persons with disabilities for millennia will finally largely disappear.

References

1. Ustun TB, Chatterji S, Kostansjek N, Bickenbach J. WHO's ICF and functional status information in health records. Health Care Financ Rev. 2003;24(3):77–88.
2. Institute of Medicine, Committee on Disability in America Board on Health Sciences Policy. Field MJ, Jette AM, editors. The future of disability in America. Washington, DC: The National Academies Press; 2007.

3. Oliver M. Understanding disability: from theory to practice. New York: St. Martin's Press; 1996.
4. Iezzoni LI, Freedman VA. Turning the disability tide: the importance of definitions. JAMA. 2008;299(3):332–4.
5. Stone DA. The disabled state. Philadelphia: Temple University Press; 1984.
6. World Health Organization. International classification of functioning, disability, and health. Geneva: World Health Organization; 2001. p. 20.
7. Shapiro JP. No pity: people with disabilities forging a new civil rights movement. New York: Times Books; 1994.
8. Baynton DC. Disability and the justification of inequality in American history. In: Longmore PK, Umansky L, editors. The new disability history: American perspectives. New York: New York University; 2001. p. 33–57.
9. Jefferson T. Notes on the state of Virginia. Thomas Jefferson Writings. New York: The Library of America; 1984. p. 123–325.
10. Kirschner KL, Gill CJ, Panko Reis JP, Hammond C. Health issues for women with disabilites. In: DeLisa JA, Gans BM, Walsh NE, editors. Physical medicine and rehabilitation: principles and practice. Philadelphia: Lippincott-Raven Publishers; 2005. p. 1561–82.
11. National Council on Disability. Rocking the cradle: ensuring the rights of parents with disabilities and their children. Washington, DC: National Council on Disability; 2012.
12. Gallagher HG. FDR's splendid deception. Arlington: Vandamere Press; 1994.
13. Gallagher HG. Black bird fly away: disabled in an able-bodied world. Arlington: Vandamere Press; 1998.
14. Stigma GE. Notes on the management of spoiled identity. New York: Simon & Schuster, Inc.; 1963.
15. Young JM. Equality of opportunity: the making of the Americans with disabilities act. Washington, DC: National Council on Disability; 1997.
16. World Health Organization and World Bank. World report on disability. Geneva: WHO Press; 2011.
17. Iezzoni LI, Kurtz SG, Rao SR. Trends in U.S. adult chronic disability rates over time. Disabil Health J. 2014;7(4):402–12.
18. Kanny D, Liu Y, Brewer RD, Garvin W, Balluz L. Prevalence of doctor-diagnosed arthritis and arthritis-attributable activity limitation--United States, 2007–2009. MMWR Morb Mortal Wkly Rep. 2010;59:1–36.
19. Erickson L, Lee C, von Schrader S. 2012 disability status report. Ithaca: Cornell University Employment and Disability Institute; 2014.
20. Bureau of Labor Statistics, Department of Labor. Persons with a disability: labor force characteristics – 2013. Available at: http://www.bls.gov/news.release/pdf/disabl.pdf. USDL-11-0921.
21. Altman B, Bernstein A. Disability and health in the United States, 2001–2005. Hyattsville: National Center for Health Statistics; 2008.
22. Agency for Healthcare Research and Quality. 2013 National Healthcare Disparities Report. 2014; Available at: http://www.ahrq.gov/research/findings/nhqrdr/nhdr13/2013nhdr.pdf. Accessed 27 Oct 2014. AHRQ Publication No. 14-0006.
23. Iezzoni LI, O'Day BL. More than ramps. A guide to improving health care quality and access for people with disabilities. New York: Oxford University Press; 2006.
24. Harrington AL, Hirsch MA, Hammond FM, Norton HJ, Bockenek WL. Assessment of primary care services and perceived barriers to care in persons with disabilities. Am J Phys Med Rehabil. 2009;88(10):852–63.
25. Mudrick NR, Breslin ML, Liang M, Yee S. Physical accessibility in primary health care settings: results from California on-site reviews. Disabil Health J. 2012;5(3):159–67.
26. Lagu T, Hannon NS, Rothberg MB, Wells AS, Green KL, Windom MO, et al. Access to subspecialty care for patients with mobility impairment: a survey. Ann Intern Med. 2013;158(6):441–6.

27. Bachman SS, Vedrani M, Drainoni M, Tobias C, Maisels L. Provider perceptions of their capacity to offer accessible health care for people with disabilities. J Disabil Policy Stud. 2006;17(3):130–6.
28. Gerhart KA, Koziol-McLain J, Lowenstein SR, Whiteneck GG. Quality of life following spinal cord injury: knowledge and attitudes of emergency care providers. Ann Emerg Med. 1994;23(4):807–12.
29. Satchidanand N, Gunukula SK, Lam WY, McGuigan D, New I, Symons AB, et al. Attitudes of healthcare students and professionals toward patients with physical disability: a systematic review. Am J Phys Med Rehabil. 2012;91(6):533–45.
30. Wen LS. A simple case of chest pain: sensitizing doctors to patients with disabilities. Health Aff (Millwood). 2014;33(10):1868–71.
31. Charlton J. Nothing about us without us. disability oppression and empowerment. Berkeley: University of California Press; 2000.
32. U.S. Department of Health and Human Services. HealthyPeople.gov. 2020 topics & objectives. Disability and health. 2014; Available at: http://www.healthypeople.gov/2020/topicsobjectives2020/overview.aspx?topicid=9. Accessed 27 May 2014.
33. Mairs N. On being a cripple. In: Saxton MS, Howe F, editors. With wings. New York: The Feminist Press at The City University of New York; 1987. p. 118–27.
34. Iezzoni LI, Long-Bellil LM. Training physicians about caring for persons with disabilities: "Nothing about us without us!". Disabil Health J. 2012;5(3):136–9.
35. Kirschner KL, Curry RH. Educating health care professionals to care for patients with disabilities. JAMA. 2009;302(12):1334–5.
36. Iezzoni LI. When walking fails. Mobility problems for adults with chronic conditions. Berkeley: University of California Press; 2003.

Chapter 2
Stigma In Persons with Obesity

Mark J. Gorman, W. Scott Butsch, Noreen A. Reilly-Harrington,
Janey Pratt, and Stephanie Sogg

Introduction

Obesity is a highly stigmatized disease that is one of the most common health problems facing our nation today. The purpose of this chapter is to describe the current understanding of how perceptions of people with obesity and the associated weight-related stigma ultimately impact treatment (including weight loss surgery), the healthcare system, mental health/psychosocial functioning, and other social determinants of behavior (e.g., employment, education, interpersonal relationships). Finally, a look at current interventions to address weight stigma and future directions for the field will be summarized.

Currently, the prevalence of adults with overweight or obesity in the USA is 69 %, and 35 % of adults in the USA have obesity [1]. This represents more than a 20 % increase in obesity since 1991 [2]. Overweight and obesity have been linked to a wide variety of chronic health conditions, including hypertension, hyperlipidemia, diabetes, cancer, coronary artery disease, congestive heart failure, stroke, sleep apnea, nonalcoholic fatty liver disease, and osteoarthritis [3, 4]. In addition to

M.J. Gorman, PhD (✉) • N.A. Reilly-Harrington, PhD • S. Sogg, PhD
MGH Weight Center, Massachusetts General Hospital, Boston, MA, USA

Department of Psychiatry, Harvard Medical School, Boston, MA, USA
e-mail: mjgorman@mgh.harvard.edu

W.S. Butsch, MD, MSc
MGH Weight Center, Massachusetts General Hospital, Boston, MA, USA

Department of Medicine, Harvard Medical School, Boston, MA, USA

J. Pratt, MD
MGH Weight Center, Massachusetts General Hospital, Boston, MA, USA

Department of Surgery, Harvard Medical School, Boston, MA, USA

© Springer International Publishing Switzerland 2016   23
R. Parekh, Ed W. Childs (eds.), *Stigma and Prejudice: Touchstones in Understanding Diversity in Healthcare*, Current Clinical Psychiatry,
DOI 10.1007/978-3-319-27580-2_2

the significant health risks conferred by obesity, obesity and its associated comorbidities contribute to markedly reduced health-related quality of life and psychosocial functioning [5]. Among patients with severe obesity, higher current and lifetime rates of a number of different psychiatric disorders have been found, including mood disorders and anxiety disorders, such as PTSD, social phobia, and panic disorder [6–14].

Individuals with obesity encounter inequities in numerous domains, such as employment, education, healthcare, media, and interpersonal relationships [15]. As obesity rates continue to rise, the stigma associated with obesity also appears to be intensifying and expanding across cultures [16]. Within the USA, recent national estimates indicate that the prevalence of weight discrimination has increased by 66 % in the last decade, now comparable to racial discrimination [17].

Unfortunately, as Jeffrey Friedman, MD, notes, "People often reserve their harshest judgments for those conditions about which the least is known" (p. 563) [18]. An important contributor to weight bias is the lack of understanding of the biological basis of obesity and the complex multifactorial etiology of the disease [19]. For decades, obesity has been mislabeled as a behavioral problem, and individuals with obesity have been stereotyped as being lazy, unintelligent, and weak willed. Sadly, in the one area where prejudice would be least expected – healthcare – providers are not immune. These negative assumptions translate into pervasive stigmatization, leaving individuals with obesity the target of derogatory comments by healthcare professionals and, more concerningly, subject to unequal care [20].

Perceptions of People with Obesity

Research has shown that individuals with obesity are viewed by members of the general public as lazy, unmotivated, lacking in self-discipline, less competent, noncompliant, and sloppy [15]. In one study of 318 adults with overweight and obesity, respondents reported that close relationship partners were the most frequent source of their worst stigmatization and that the most common weight-based stereotypes described were attributions of laziness, overeating/binging, lack of intelligence, and lack of willpower/self-discipline [21].

Attribution models have been employed to illuminate the origins of obesity stigma, and it has been noted that stigmatization of specific conditions may arise because individuals characteristically search for causes for the condition, which affects their reactions and opinions about those with that condition. A widespread perception persists among the general public that individuals with obesity are personally to blame for being overweight, despite much empirical evidence suggesting that body weight is highly physiologically regulated and the result of a complex interaction of biological, behavioral, and environmental factors [22].

This perceived controllability of obesity is a fundamental component of weight-related stigma, demonstrated by many experimental studies. For example, by presenting vignettes describing a healthy-weight adolescent girl and an adolescent girl with obesity who was or was not described as having a glandular condition, De Jong et al. [23] found that when no medical cause for obesity was identified, respondents viewed the girl with obesity as less self-disciplined and less liked than the girl with healthy weight and the girl with obesity presumably due to the glandular disorder.

Sociocultural messages from the diet industry and the media may also reinforce the perception of personal responsibility for obesity, exacerbating weight-related stigma. Diet industry advertising emphasizes the idea that weight is easily modifiable with personal effort. Our cultural value of thinness in children and adults is exacerbated in movies and television, where individuals who are overweight are frequently ridiculed and portrayed as engaging in unhealthy eating behaviors, while thin characters are often assigned more desirable attributes and behaviors [15]. The view of obesity as being due to lifestyle choices versus a chronic disease with a complex combination of genetic, medical, environmental, and behavioral causes contributes to weight-related stigma and negative biases.

Effects of Weight Stigma

For the purposes of this chapter, the focus is primarily on healthcare; however, the role of social determinants of health is also very important. Therefore, other areas of concern that may ultimately impact health will also be highlighted. The documented effects of weight stigma are wide ranging, affecting numerous domains including employment, education, interpersonal relationships, and even healthcare [15, 24]. In addition, some have suggested that individuals with obesity may even experience bias during jury selection, denial of the right to adopt, or more difficulty obtaining housing [25].

Employment

Social inequalities resulting from weight discrimination are apparent in employment settings. Individuals with obesity are consistently denigrated in the workplace and are less likely to be hired, paid less, and receive fewer promotions compared to slimmer individuals, despite equal qualifications [26, 27]. Weight-based employment discrimination is 12 times more likely to be reported by adults who are overweight, 37 times more likely by adults with obesity, and 100 times more likely by adults with severe obesity than by nonoverweight individuals [28].

Education

Evidence shows that overweight students are subject to weight-related prejudice on the parts of their teachers. For instance, teachers have reported feeling that their overweight students are less tidy, more emotional, and less likely to succeed at work [29]. It has also been found that physical educators hold lower expectations across a wide range of domains (social, reasoning, physical, and cooperation skills) for children with obesity versus their healthier-weight peers [30]. This is concerning given that teacher expectations have been demonstrated to have a significant impact on academic attainment [31]. In one study, 92 % of adolescents reported having seen their classmates with overweight or obesity being teased at school [32]. Weight-based teasing and bullying may account for the finding that elementary students with obesity miss more school [33]. The long-term ramifications are considerable. Several studies have found that students who have obesity by 16 years of age have fewer years of education and are less likely to attend college [34, 35]. Sadly, it has also been shown that parents are less willing to financially support a child with obesity to attend college than they are for their children who are of a normal weight [24].

Weight-Related Stigma, Mental Health, and Psychosocial Functioning

Empirically, there is a lack of consistent evidence that obesity, in and of itself, is associated with higher rates of psychopathology [36], particularly among individuals with mild obesity [37]. However, research suggests that patients with severe obesity tend to exhibit more psychopathology than healthy-weight individuals or those with milder obesity [7, 38–43]. These findings are particularly true among those seeking medical weight loss treatment (i.e., pharmacological or surgical interventions), compared to those seeking behavioral weight loss treatment [37]. Few studies have examined the relationship between obesity and personality disorders, and findings from these studies are mixed and inconclusive [7, 9, 11].

The elevated prevalence of certain forms of psychopathology among individuals with obesity likely reflects bidirectional causal pathways. The adverse effects of obesity, including physical limitations, medical burden, and social stigma, likely contribute to or exacerbate mood and anxiety symptoms in many individuals [38, 39, 44, 45]. At the same time, the symptoms of, and pharmacological treatment for, various psychiatric disorders may also promote weight gain [38, 39, 41, 45]. While it is important to acknowledge the high psychosocial burden that obesity places on many individuals, and to recognize the elevated prevalence of psychological comorbidity among individuals with severe obesity, it is also important to note that there is a great deal of variation within this population in terms of psychosocial functioning. Individuals with obesity occupy all points along the continuum of mental health and emotional adjustment [36, 42, 46]. It should not be assumed on the basis of severe obesity alone that a patient is psychologically impaired.

A large body of empirical research demonstrates the deleterious impact that experiencing weight stigma has on mental health and psychosocial functioning. Experiencing weight-related discrimination has been found to be associated with a higher risk of psychiatric symptoms and disorders, with greater perceived discrimination being associated with a higher likelihood of having more than one psychiatric disorder [47, 48]. Perceived weight-related stigma or discrimination is associated with a higher risk for depression [47, 49, 50], anxiety [50], low self-esteem [47, 50, 51], and body image distress [47, 50]. Because these relationships are generally found to be independent of actual body mass index ([BMI] = weight (kg)/[height (m)]^2), it appears that it is the experience of stigma, rather than the degree of obesity itself, that is most deleterious to individuals' well-being [48, 52].

Interestingly, individuals with obesity tend to hold the same weight-related stereotypes and prejudices evident in the general population [47, 53–56]. A growing body of research suggests that people with obesity, independent of the degree of bias and discrimination they have actually experienced, often internalize the derogatory attitudes and pervasive stereotypes about weight in our society [21, 57, 58]. Research suggests that the psychosocial impact of weight-related stigma is considerably greater among individuals with internalized weight bias compared to those who have not internalized this bias [47, 49, 59]. Higher levels of depression [47, 60, 61] and anxiety [61], poor self-esteem [47, 52], social and behavioral problems [61], maladaptive cognitive and behavioral patterns related to eating and body image [47, 61–63], and an overall poor quality of life [61] have been associated with internalized weight bias. The impact of internalized weight bias extends beyond psychosocial domains to medical- and health-related domains as well; Hilbert et al. [64] found that internalized weight bias not only was associated with poorer overall health but a greater utilization of healthcare services.

Weight-Related Stigma and Weight Gain

Although popular belief might hold that experiencing weight-related stigma will help to motivate individuals with obesity to engage in healthy habits and efforts to lose weight, research strongly suggests that the opposite is actually the case [58, 65]. One study did find that individuals who reported a history of more stigmatizing experiences lost more weight and had better weight maintenance following a behavioral weight loss intervention [66]. However, evidence from a large population-based study suggests that experiencing weight-related stigma is not associated with weight loss; instead, it is strongly related to weight gain and an increased risk of developing obesity over the following several years [67]. Individuals who report such stigmatization consistently engage in behaviors that are likely to pose barriers to weight loss, or even promote weight gain. For instance, individuals with obesity have been found to report eating more, or specifically refusing to diet, as a way of coping with weight-related stigmatization [68]. This effect was also demonstrated in a laboratory setting, in which overweight women who watched a weight-stigmatizing video consumed more than three times as many calories as overweight women who had viewed a neutral video or average-weight women who had watched either video, during a snacking period immediately following the video presentation [65]. Weight stigma has also been implicated in attrition from weight loss treatment [15].

Weight-related stigmatization is also associated with maladaptive or disordered behaviors. For instance, internalized weight bias, independent of the degree to which one has personally been the target of such bias, has also been found to be associated with binge eating [58, 62], bulimic symptoms [59], emotional eating [63], and deliberate avoidance of physical activity and exercise [59]. Thus, far from being a motivating factor, weight stigma appears to promote behaviors that interfere with weight loss and may even lead to weight gain.

Weight-Related Stigma and Interpersonal Relationships

A growing body of research demonstrates that weight-related stigma has a significant impact on interpersonal interactions and relationships for people with obesity, beginning as early as childhood. Obesity-related bias has been well documented even among young children [69, 70]. Teenage boys and girls with obesity report significantly more overt and relational victimization (respectively) by their peers than same-age healthy-weight adolescents [71]. Young adults have also been found to hold a high degree of weight-based bias [70]. Unsurprisingly, the experience of weight-related stigma by one's peers not only has a deleterious impact on adolescents' self-confidence but also creates barriers to establishing or improving peer relationships, as it engenders feelings of isolation and anxiety around approaching new people and developing peer relationships [72]. It appears that the cumulative experience of weight-related stigma and bias may actually create social deficits that further compound these difficulties. In one study, college students talking by phone to women, though blind to those women's actual weights, rated the women with obesity lower in likability, social skills, and even attractiveness – judgments that were echoed in the ratings of observers of these conversations, who listened but did not participate themselves [73].

Weight bias also affects romantic relationships among people with obesity. Individuals with obesity tend to be viewed as less desirable as romantic partners, among both adolescents and adults [71, 74]. Overweight adolescent boys and girls both report being less likely to date than their average-weight peers [71], and among adults, people with obesity are ranked as less desirable as dating partners than individuals with drug addiction [74], sexually transmitted diseases [75], or severe physical disabilities [75]. In addition, large-scale, longitudinal research suggests that individuals with obesity have lower rates of marriage than healthy-weight peers [75, 76].

Poignantly, individuals of both genders who have obesity report that the most severely stigmatizing encounters they experience tend to occur at home and to involve close relationship partners, such as friends, parents, and spouses [21, 77]. Not surprisingly, there is a significantly higher degree of relationship strain and poorer family support among individuals with severe obesity [15].

Weight-Related Stigma in the Healthcare System

One of the central tenets of healthcare workers, regardless of profession, is to provide unrestricted care with compassion and respect for human dignity. However, instead of support and encouragement, patients with obesity are often treated with judgment and insensitivity by their healthcare providers. Physicians share the general population's strong anti-obesity bias [78], which, as reported by more than half of female patients in one study, is experienced on multiple occasions [68]. In one study, more than half of primary care physicians surveyed reported viewing individuals with obesity as "awkward, unattractive, ugly, and non-compliant with therapy" (p. 1174) [79]. Not surprisingly, the level of stigma may be greater toward those individuals with more severe obesity; nearly two-third of one sample of patients seeking bariatric surgery reported having experienced inappropriate comments from physicians [50].

Studies have shown that weight bias is widespread throughout the healthcare system, among nurses, dietitians, psychologists, and even those clinicians and researchers who specialize in obesity [20, 80, 81]. The structure of the healthcare system and the culture of healthcare professions, particularly in medical education and training, may provide some explanation for the pervasiveness of weight stigma in the clinical environment. For example, much of medical education is delivered by practicing physicians, and clinical experience may influence both the attitudes and clinical practice of physician trainees. Preclinical medical students are thus good examples of the effects of both implicit (unconscious) and explicit (conscious) weight bias. Surveys show more than 40 % of medical students have significant implicit weight bias [82], yet few are aware of their bias [83]. Unfortunately, the degree of weight stigma does not decrease with accumulating medical education or clinical experience. Therefore, it comes as no surprise when medical students report the use of derogatory humor by their peers, residents, and faculty physicians [84]. In addition, not only does the appearance of obesity alone bias medical students' impressions of the patient and the patients' ability to adhere to weight loss treatment recommendations [85] but also medical students report feeling uncomfortable when interviewing patients with obesity. As a result, these negative attitudes become barriers to discussing weight and thus may impede appropriate treatment of obesity [86].

Because of patients' experiences of discrimination and awareness of their highly stigmatized status, individuals who are overweight or those with obesity are more likely to delay or avoid routine medical care and, when they do seek care, often receive suboptimal care [87]. It is clear that the quality of healthcare delivery is not uniform for patients of different sizes. Several studies highlight potential mechanisms by which a healthcare provider's negative attitudes toward patients with obesity may affect the quality of clinical care [88–90]. Lack of trust or respect for the patient with obesity is one proposed explanation for why primary healthcare providers may provide suboptimal weight-related counseling or communicate less effectively. Hebl and Xu [91] found that poor allocation of time during a patient

Table 2.1 Types of weight bias in healthcare settings

Types of weight bias	Examples[a]
Language	Obese, morbid, fat, recidivism
Attitudes	"Obese patients" are lazy, lacking in self-discipline, and noncompliant
Behavior	Negative comments or facial gestures while weighing patients; weighing patients in a non-private setting
Built environment	
Office environment	Small waiting room chairs, small doorways/hallways
Medical equipment	Lack of appropriately sized patient gowns, examination tables, blood pressure cuffs, speculums, scales, stretchers, wheelchairs, and radiologic equipment

[a]Adapted from Rudd Center, http://www.yaleruddcenter.org/resources/bias_toolkit/module1.html

encounter was demonstrated in a study of primary care physicians. The authors found that physicians not only spent 29 % less time with patients with obesity compared to average weight patients but were more likely to consider the encounter a waste of time [91]. Furthermore, young physicians have been reported to over-attribute symptoms and other problems to obesity, ignoring important avenues for treatment. When presented with virtual patients with shortness of breath, for instance, medical students were more likely to prescribe a medication to manage symptoms in the normal-weight patient, while the patient with obesity was more likely to receive lifestyle counseling [85]. Providers fail to consider other, potentially effective treatment options for patients with severe obesity beyond lifestyle modification [92].

Numerous studies have shown that patients with obesity, and women with obesity in particular, are less likely to receive preventative care – for example, cervical, breast, and colorectal cancer screening – even though the incidence of these conditions is actually higher among individuals with obesity, making appropriate screening even more critical for this population [93–95]. Although the majority of research focuses on negative weight-related attitudes and language in healthcare settings, there are many other subtle and overt forms of bias, as highlighted in Table 2.1.

To reiterate, weight bias in the healthcare system is rooted, in large part, in the belief that obesity is a character flaw and that body weight is easily modifiable through volitional behavior alone. Despite substantial research highlighting a strong biological basis to weight regulation, many healthcare providers continue to believe that obesity is strictly a result of poor behaviors. Healthcare settings should be safe havens in which patients with obesity feel supported and receive appropriate treatment for their weight and other medical and mental health issues. Instead, many patients experience the same disrespect and prejudice in healthcare settings as in other environments they encounter. As a result of weight bias, the healthcare provider-patient relationship is damaged, treatment decisions are influenced, and quality of care is compromised.

Weight-Related Stigma and Weight Loss Surgery

In 1991, an NIH consensus conference reviewed all available treatments for severe obesity and concluded that patients with a BMI over 35 with major comorbidities or a BMI over 40 benefit most from weight loss surgery (WLS) [96]. However, due to the underlying bias and misperceptions among both healthcare providers and patients regarding the risks of weight loss surgery, the mechanisms by which it is effective, and the etiology of obesity, there is strong bias against surgery as a treatment option. Despite the NIH recommendations, both physicians and patients are reluctant to choose weight loss surgery, which continues to be viewed as a "last resort" or "drastic measure" for the treatment of severe obesity [79, 92, 97].

Physicians are less likely to refer severely obese patients for weight loss surgery when they have not been educated on the subject. A recent study of family physicians showed that in practices with a large volume of patients with severe obesity, providers recommended bariatric surgery less than 50 % of the time. This seemed to be related to a lack of information on the part of the physician, as the study also found that increased provider knowledge about weight loss surgery was associated with significantly more surgical referrals [98].

Another factor underlying suboptimal acceptance of bariatric surgery among both clinicians and patients is a fundamental misunderstanding of the mechanisms by which surgery works, which is directly related to the lack of understanding, noted above, of obesity as complex, multifactorial, and often genetic. Bariatric surgery is often viewed as working solely through limiting patients' caloric intake. There was a long-held belief that the mechanisms of weight loss surgery included restriction of intake and malabsorption of nutrients, thus acting like a tool to control patient behavior. New research provides evidence that weight loss surgery works through metabolic mechanisms due to changes in secretion patterns of gut hormones after surgery [99, 100], highlighting the influence of physiological mechanisms rather than patient behavior. Restriction of intake may play a role in the early months after surgery, but is not thought to be responsible for the majority of weight loss.

This simplistic and erroneous understanding of how weight loss surgery works continues to promote the notion that obesity is a failure of the patient's willpower. More recently, the American Medical Association has recognized obesity as a disease, supporting the body of evidence found within the field of obesity medicine. While it will take time for this view to be disseminated among the medical/surgical, nursing, nutrition, and psychological communities, one would hope that this may lead to better understanding of treatment options, including weight loss surgery. In addition, patients and the lay public could also benefit from additional education about the causes of obesity and the empirical evidence of bariatric surgery as the leading or "gold standard" intervention at this time.

Research on patients presenting for surgery provides some of the most compelling evidence for the pervasive existence of weight bias. At times, experiences of weight-related bias and prejudice become most clear as patients notice changes in how they are treated after losing weight with surgical intervention. Along with the significant weight loss that typically results from surgery, patients often report that they experience less weight-related bias and prejudice. Although most patients still remain in the overweight or obese category after surgery, many report that people treat them quite differently after the weight loss. Some patients note that they had felt "invisible" before surgery and that after they lose weight, people notice them more, or are more likely to talk to them in the hallway at work, open doors for them, or make positive comments about their appearance. A striking illustration of how much weight loss surgery patients value the weight loss they achieved, and how adversely they view returning to their former, higher weight is that in one study, postoperative patients reported on a survey that they would rather be deaf, dyslexic, diabetic, and have serious acne or even serious heart disease than return to their previous weight [101].

Interventions to Address Weight Stigma

A variety of interventions have been developed with the aim of combating weight stigma and its impact on the quality of life, psychosocial functioning, interpersonal interactions, and even healthcare of people with obesity. Based on the empirically supported premise that inaccurate weight bias results, in large part, from the inaccurate belief that weight is under the individual's full, volitional control [53, 56], a number of studies have focused on the impact of providing information about etiological contributors to obesity that are not controllable by the individual. In general, these interventions have yielded mixed results [102]. Studies have demonstrated that educational interventions about the etiology of obesity do increase the extent to which participants explicitly endorse beliefs that uncontrollable factors contribute to obesity [15, 56, 102–104]. However, with some exceptions [53, 104], this type of strategy has not been found to be effective in decreasing negative attitudes and stereotypes about obesity [15, 56, 102, 103].

Other interventions, aimed at evoking empathy for individuals with obesity, have demonstrated a positive effect among medical students [105]. However, two different empathy-evocation interventions studied more recently with participants drawn from the general population were unsuccessful in reducing either implicit or explicit weight bias [56].

One potentially promising strategy is the social consensus approach. This approach is based on the premise that stigmatizing attitudes are influenced by one's perceptions about what others believe [106]. A series of experiments manipulating perceived consensus about attitudes toward obesity demonstrated that providing feedback that others held favorable attitudes toward people with obesity changed both participants' beliefs about the causality of obesity and their negative attitudes about people with obesity, even though no information about causality was included in the intervention. In fact, this approach was more effective in changing negative attitudes toward people with obesity than either an intervention that provided education about the uncontrollable causes of obesity or one that provided education demonstrating that common obesity-related stereotypes are inaccurate [22].

A different type of intervention that holds some promise for reducing weight bias is based on a cognitive dissonance model. In one study, participants' attention was drawn to the fact that their own views about people with obesity were at odds with several of their own self-reported core values. Though this intervention did not reduce total bias scores, scores on several specific types of weight bias decreased following the intervention. The cognitive dissonance intervention employed in this study had a significantly greater impact on weight bias than did the social consensus-based intervention to which it was compared [106].

In the medical field, interventions to reduce weight stigma have primarily involved medical students. One innovative approach used a standardized patient encounter to influence students' attitudes and beliefs about obesity and their confidence in communication. Although there was an immediate and medium-term post-intervention improvement in empathy for patients and self-efficacy around providing obesity-related counseling, 1-year follow-up data showed a return of students' attitudes back to baseline [107]. Another study demonstrated that the use of theatrical readings, in place of a lecture, on obesity could diminish explicit obesity bias; however, it did not change levels of implicit bias or empathy [108]. Educational strategies emphasizing the complex etiology and physiological regulation of body weight have resulted in positive attitudes about patients with obesity among medical students [104]. Despite the overall mixed results in similar education interventions, strategies aimed at improving obesity medicine education in undergraduate medical and nursing curricula must be part of a larger effort to change the attitudes and actions of young physicians, nurses, and other healthcare providers.

Future Directions

Obesity has been observed to be, "one of the last acceptable forms of prejudice" (p. 1037) [109]. Not only is weight bias pervasive in our society, leading to inferior care of people with obesity, but it blocks needed progress in finding solutions to the epidemic of obesity. In a recent review, Phelan et al. [110] succinctly described several potential strategies to reduce weight bias in healthcare, from improving provider attitudes and altering the clinic environment to empowering patients to better cope with stigmatized encounters and better advocate for equality of care. However, it is clear that advances at multiple levels must take place to ensure sustainable progress.

At the federal level, the shared common belief that obesity is a character flaw and a behavior problem of weak-willed individuals has bled into policy. For years, US obesity prevention strategies, built on initiatives focusing on behavioral change, remain stagnant and have ranked below those of other countries [111]. A clear understanding of the biological basis of obesity and the multitude of contributing factors beyond personal control may foster greater initiative and growth.

Obesity has an enormous health cost to both the individual and to society. Because weight bias is seen as socially acceptable, there has been little effort to create legal protections from or consequences for weight-related discrimination. One of the most effective ways to change societal discrimination of individuals is through federal law; however, currently there are no federal laws that exist to protect individuals with obesity. Despite a high level of popular support for laws to extend the same protections to people with obesity as persons with physical disabilities, particularly in the employment setting, there has been little progress in developing such laws [26].

One state law that exists to prohibit weight discrimination is the Elliot-Larsen Civil Rights Act in Michigan. In 1977, a law was enacted to prohibit discrimination in ten categories, including weight, in areas relating to education, employment, housing, etc. Although there was initial criticism from the opposition that this law would open the floodgates of litigation on weight discrimination, there has been no evidence that this has happened. In 2013, a Labor and Workplace subcommittee in the State of Massachusetts passed a similar employment law, but it has not yet come to a full state congress vote.

To combat weight-related bias and discrimination in the healthcare system, educational strategies focused on obesity education must be implemented specifically in interprofessional training programs (e.g., kinesiology, nursing, psychology, physical therapy, and medicine). Special attention must be paid to improving the language and attitudes of healthcare students and increasing awareness of counterproductive explicit beliefs (see Table 2.1). In addition, the assessment of implicit attitudes (e.g., using the Implicit Association Test [IAT], specifically the Weight IAT [https://implicit.harvard.edu/implicit/takeatest.html]) can provide information to students of their internal beliefs at an early stage in their training, when time remains to shift these beliefs. In combination with an appropriate education on the multifaceted process of weight regulation, this may engender in students a more positive attitude about patients with obesity.

At the professional level, the formation of a new medical subspecialty, obesity medicine, has established a career pathway for physicians, nurses, dietitians, and psychologists to develop the necessary skills and attitudes to adequately care for patients with obesity. In 2012, the American Board of Obesity Medicine was formed and the first certification test in Obesity Medicine was administered. To date, there are over 1000 physicians who are board certified in obesity medicine. This new generation of advocates, who better understand the etiological complexities of obesity, will be more effective in addressing and managing obesity.

Furthermore, the clinic environment must also be an arena for change, creating a more welcoming and supportive patient experience and improving patient adherence. Several types of weight bias can be addressed in the clinic (see Table 2.1). Efforts to properly address the behavior of staff and providers (e.g., by creating a zero-tolerance policy for negative comments that stereotype or degrade patients based on their appearance) and to purchase medical equipment (chairs without arms, examination tables, gowns, scales, blood pressure cuffs, etc.) of the appropriate size for proper use in the care of patients with obesity are encouraged [110]. Lastly, using "person-first" language such as "patients with obesity" instead of "obese patients," which acknowledges the person before their disability or disease, chips away at the historical view of obesity as a behavioral problem and may have a profound effect on reducing weight stigma in the profession and community [112].

People with obesity experience stigma, prejudice, and discrimination in many facets of their everyday lives. Weight bias has significant and wide-reaching consequences for the social functioning, mental health, education, employment, and healthcare of people with obesity. A considerable body of research has demonstrated the ubiquity of weight-related stigma and bias; the task before us now is to develop effective ways to prevent and combat this discrimination and reduce the impact that this has on the well-being of individuals with obesity.

References

1. Flegal KM, Carroll MD, Kit BK, Ogden CL. Prevalence of obesity and trends in the distribution of body mass index among US adults, 1999-2010. JAMA. 2012;307(5):491–7.
2. Flegal KM, Carroll MD, Ogden CL, Johnson CL. Prevalence and trends in obesity among US adults, 1999-2000. JAMA. 2002;288(14):1723–7.
3. Hartz AJ, Barboriak PN, Wong A, Katayama KP, Rimm AA. The association of obesity with infertility and related menstrual abnormalities in women. Int J Obes. 1979;3(1):57–73.
4. National Institutes of Health. Clinical guidelines on the identification, evaluation, and treatment of overweight and obesity in adults--the evidence report. National Institutes of Health. Obes Res. 1998;6 Suppl 2:51S–209.
5. Anandacoomarasamy A, Caterson ID, Leibman S, Smith GS, Sambrook PN, Fransen M, et al. Influence of BMI on health-related quality of life: comparison between an obese adult cohort and age-matched population norms. Obesity. 2009;17(11):2114–8.
6. Greenberg I, Perna F, Kaplan M, Sullivan MA. Behavioral and psychological factors in the assessment and treatment of obesity surgery patients. Obes Res. 2005;13(2):244–9.
7. Kalarchian MA, Marcus MD, Levine MD, Courcoulas AP, Pilkonis PA, Ringham RM, et al. Psychiatric disorders among bariatric surgery candidates: relationship to obesity and functional health status. Am J Psychiatry. 2007;164(2):328–34.
8. Lester D, Iliceto P, Pompili M, Girardi P. Depression and suicidality in obese patients. Psychol Rep. 2011;108(2):367–8.
9. Mauri M, Rucci P, Calderone A, Santini F, Oppo A, Romano A, et al. Axis I and II disorders and quality of life in bariatric surgery candidates. J Clin Psychiatry. 2008;69(2):295–301.
10. Pawlow LA, O'Neil PM, White MA, Byrne TK. Findings and outcomes of psychological evaluations of gastric bypass applicants. Surg Obes Relat Dis. 2005;1(6):523–7; discussion 528–9.
11. Petry NM, Barry D, Pietrzak RH, Wagner JA. Overweight and obesity are associated with psychiatric disorders: results from the National Epidemiologic Survey on Alcohol and Related Conditions. Psychosom Med. 2008;70(3):288–97.
12. Rosik CH. Psychiatric symptoms among prospective bariatric surgery patients: rates of prevalence and their relation to social desirability, pursuit of surgery, and follow-up attendance. Obes Surg. 2005;15(5):677–83.
13. Wadden TA, Sarwer DB. Behavioral assessment of candidates for bariatric surgery: a patient-oriented approach. Obesity. 2006;14 Suppl 2:53S–62.
14. Wadden TA, Sarwer DB, Fabricatore AN, Jones L, Stack R, Williams NS. Psychosocial and behavioral status of patients undergoing bariatric surgery: what to expect before and after surgery. Med Clin North Am. 2007;91(3):451–69.

15. Puhl RM, Heuer CA. The stigma of obesity: a review and update. Obesity. 2009;17(5): 941–64.
16. Brewis AA. Stigma and the perpetuation of obesity. Soc Sci Med. 2014;118:152–8.
17. Andreyeva T, Puhl RM, Brownell KD. Changes in perceived weight discrimination among Americans, 1995-1996 through 2004-2006. Obesity. 2008;16:1129–34.
18. Friedman JM. Modern science versus the stigma of obesity. Nat Med. 2004;10(6):563–9.
19. Allison DB, Downey M, Atkinson RL, Billington CJ, Bray GA, Eckel RH, et al. Obesity as a disease: a white paper on evidence and arguments commissioned by the Council of the Obesity Society. Obesity (Silver Spring). 2008;16(6):1161–77.
20. Schwartz MB, Chambliss HO, Brownell KD, Blair SN, Billington C. Weight bias among health professionals specializing in obesity. Obes Res. 2003;11(9):1033–9.
21. Puhl RM, Moss-Racusin CA, Schwartz MB, Brownell KD. Weight stigmatization and bias reduction: perspectives of overweight and obese adults. Health Educ Res. 2008;23(2): 347–58.
22. Puhl RM, Brownell KD. Psychosocial origins of obesity stigma: toward changing a powerful and pervasive bias. Obes Rev. 2003;4(4):213.
23. de Jong J, van Ramshorst B, Gooszen H, Smout A, Tiel-Van Buul M. Weight loss after laparoscopic adjustable gastric banding is not caused by altered gastric emptying. Obes Surg. 2009;19(3):287–92.
24. Puhl R, Brownell KD. Bias, discrimination, and obesity. Obes Res. 2001;9(12):788–805.
25. Puhl R, Brownell KD. Stigma, discrimination, and obesity. In: Fairburn C, Brownell KD, editors. Eating disorders and obesity: a comprehensive handbook. 2nd ed. New York: The Guilford Press; 2002. p. 108–12.
26. Puhl RM, Heuer CA. Public opinion about laws to prohibit weight discrimination in the United States. Obesity. 2011;19(1):74–82.
27. Rudolph CW, Wells CL, Weller MD, Baltes BB. A meta-analysis of empirical studies of weight-based bias in the workplace. J Vocat Behav. 2009;74(1):1–10.
28. Roehling MV, Roehling PV, Pichler S. The relationship between body weight and perceived weight-related employment discrimination: the role of sex and race. J Vocat Behav. 2007;71(2):300–18.
29. Neumark-Sztainer D, Story M, Harris T. Beliefs and attitudes about obesity among teachers and school health care providers working with adolescents. J Nutr Educ Behav. 1999; 31(1):3–9.
30. O'Brien KS, Hunter JA, Banks M. Implicit anti-fat bias in physical educators: physical attributes, ideology and socialization. Int J Obes (Lond). 2007;31(2):308–14.
31. Hinnant JB, O'Brien M, Ghazarian SR. The longitudinal relations of teacher expectations to achievement in the early school years. J Educ Psychol. 2009;101(3):662–70.
32. Puhl RM, Luedicke J, Heuer C. Weight-based victimization toward overweight adolescents: observations and reactions of peers. J Sch Health. 2011;81(11):696–703.
33. Geier AB, Foster GD, Womble LG, McLaughlin J, Borradaile KE, Nachmani J, et al. The relationship between relative weight and school attendance among elementary schoolchildren. Obesity (Silver Spring). 2007;15(8):2157–61.
34. Fowler-Brown AG, Ngo LH, Phillips RS, Wee CC. Adolescent obesity and future college degree attainment. Obesity (Silver Spring). 2010;18(6):1235–41.
35. Sargent JD, Blanchflower DG. Obesity and stature in adolescence and earnings in young adulthood. Analysis of a British birth cohort. Arch Pediatr Adolesc Med. 1994;148(7):681–7.
36. Davin SA, Taylor NM. Comprehensive review of obesity and psychological considerations for treatment. Psychol Health Med. 2009;14(6):716–25.
37. Malik S, Mitchell JE, Engel S, Crosby R, Wonderlich S. Psychopathology in bariatric surgery candidates: a review of studies using structured diagnostic interviews. Compr Psychiatry. 2014;55(2):248–59.
38. Berkowitz RI, Fabricatore AN. Obesity, psychiatric status, and psychiatric medications. Psychiatr Clin North Am. 2005;28(1):39–54, vii–viii.

39. Berkowitz RI, Fabricatore AN. Obesity, psychiatric status, and psychiatric medications. Psychiatr Clin North Am. 2011;34(4):747–64.
40. Gariepy G, Nitka D, Schmitz N. The association between obesity and anxiety disorders in the population: a systematic review and meta-analysis. Int J Obes. 2010;34(3):407–19.
41. McElroy SL, Keck Jr PE. Obesity in bipolar disorder: an overview. Curr Psychiatry Rep. 2012;14(6):650–8.
42. Scott KM, Bruffaerts R, Simon GE, Alonso J, Angermeyer M, de Girolamo G, et al. Obesity and mental disorders in the general population: results from the world mental health surveys. Int J Obes (Lond). 2008;32(1):192–200.
43. Wadden TA, Butryn ML, Sarwer DB, Fabricatore AN, Crerand CE, Lipschutz PE, et al. Comparison of psychosocial status in treatment-seeking women with class III vs. class I-II obesity. Obesity. 2006;14 Suppl 2:90S–8.
44. Atlantis E, Baker M. Obesity effects on depression: systematic review of epidemiological studies. Int J Obes. 2008;32(6):881–91.
45. Simon GE, Von Korff M, Saunders K, Miglioretti DL, Crane PK, van Belle G, et al. Association between obesity and psychiatric disorders in the US adult population. Arch Gen Psychiatry. 2006;63(7):824–30.
46. Van Hout GC, Leibbrandt AJ, Jakimowicz JJ, Smulders JF, Schoon EJ, Van Spreeuwel JP, et al. Bariatric surgery and bariatric psychology: general overview and the Dutch approach. Obes Surg. 2003;13(6):926–31.
47. Friedman KE, Reichmann SK, Costanzo PR, Zelli A, Ashmore JA, Musante GJ. Weight stigmatization and ideological beliefs: relation to psychological functioning in obese adults. Obes Res. 2005;13(5):907–16.
48. Hatzenbuehler ML, Keyes KM, Hasin DS. Associations between perceived weight discrimination and the prevalence of psychiatric disorders in the general population. Obesity. 2009;17(11):2033–9.
49. Fettich KC, Chen EY. Coping with obesity stigma affects depressed mood in African-American and white candidates for bariatric surgery. Obesity. 2012;20(5):1118–21.
50. Friedman KE, Ashmore JA, Applegate KL. Recent experiences of weight-based stigmatization in a weight loss surgery population: psychological and behavioral correlates. Obesity. 2008;16(S2):S69–74.
51. Carr D, Friedman MA. Is obesity stigmatizing? Body weight, perceived discrimination, and psychological well-being in the United States. J Health Soc Behav. 2005;46(3):244–59.
52. Davison KK, Schmalz DL, Young LM, Birch LL. Overweight girls who internalize fat stereotypes report low psychosocial well-being. Obesity. 2008;16(S2):S30–8.
53. Crandall CS. Prejudice against fat people: ideology and self-interest. J Pers Soc Psychol. 1994;66(5):882–94.
54. Rudman L, Feinberg J, Fairchild K. Minority members' implicit attitudes: automatic ingroup bias as a function of group status. Soc Cogn. 2002;20(4):294–320.
55. Schwartz MB, Vartanian LR, Nosek BA, Brownell KD. The influence of one's own body weight on implicit and explicit anti-fat bias. Obesity. 2006;14(3):440–7.
56. Teachman BA, Gapinski KD, Brownell KD, Rawlins M, Jeyaram S. Demonstrations of implicit anti-fat bias: the impact of providing causal information and evoking empathy. Health Psychol. 2003;22(1):68–78.
57. Carels RA, Wott CB, Young KM, Gumble A, Koball A, Oehlhof MW. Implicit, explicit, and internalized weight bias and psychosocial maladjustment among treatment-seeking adults. Eat Behav. 2010;11(3):180–5.
58. Puhl RM, Moss-Racusin CA, Schwartz MB. Internalization of weight bias: implications for binge eating and emotional well-being. Obesity. 2007;15(1):19–23.
59. Vartanian LR, Novak SA. Internalized societal attitudes moderate the impact of weight stigma on avoidance of exercise. Obesity. 2011;19(4):757–62.
60. Durso LE, Latner JD. Understanding self-directed stigma: development of the weight bias internalization scale. Obesity. 2008;16(S2):S80–6.

61. Roberto CA, Sysko R, Bush J, Pearl R, Puhl RM, Schvey NA, et al. Clinical correlates of the weight bias internalization scale in a sample of obese adolescents seeking bariatric surgery. Obesity. 2012;20(3):533–9.
62. Durso LE, Latner JD, Hayashi K. Perceived discrimination is associated with binge eating in a community sample of non-overweight, overweight, and obese adults. Obes Facts. 2012;5(6):869–80.
63. Durso LE, Latner JD, White MA, Masheb RM, Blomquist KK, Morgan PT, et al. Internalized weight bias in obese patients with binge eating disorder: associations with eating disturbances and psychological functioning. Int J Eat Disord. 2012;45(3):423–7.
64. Hilbert A, Braehler E, Haeuser W, Zenger M. Weight bias internalization, core self-evaluation, and health in overweight and obese persons. Obesity. 2014;22(1):79–85.
65. Schvey NA, Puhl RM, Brownell KD. The impact of weight stigma on caloric consumption. Obesity (Silver Spring). 2012;19(10):1957–62.
66. Latner JD, Wilson GT, Jackson ML, Stunkard AJ. Greater history of weight-related stigmatizing experience is associated with greater weight loss in obesity treatment. J Health Psychol. 2009;14(2):190–9.
67. Jackson SE, Beeken RJ, Wardle J. Perceived weight discrimination and changes in weight, waist circumference, and weight status. Obesity. 2014;22(12):2485–8.
68. Puhl RM, Brownell KD. Confronting and coping with weight stigma: an investigation of overweight and obese adults. Obesity (Silver Spring). 2006;14(10):1802–15.
69. Latner JD, Stunkard AJ. Getting worse: the stigmatization of obese children. Obes Res. 2003;11(3):452–6.
70. Latner JD, Stunkard AJ, Wilson GT. Stigmatized students: age, sex, and ethnicity effects in the stigmatization of obesity. Obes Res. 2005;13(7):1226–31.
71. Pearce MJ, Boergers J, Prinstein MJ. Adolescent obesity, overt and relational peer victimization, and romantic relationships. Obes Res. 2002;10(5):386–93.
72. Griffiths LJ, Page AS. The impact of weight-related victimization on peer relationships: the female adolescent perspective. Obesity. 2008;16(S2):S39–45.
73. Miller CT, Rothblum ED, Barbour L, Brand PA, Felicio D. Social interactions of obese and nonobese women. J Pers. 1990;58(2):365–80.
74. Sitton S, Blanchard S. Men's preferences in romantic partners: obesity vs addiction. Psychol Rep. 1995;77(3 Pt 2):1185–6.
75. Chen EY, Brown M. Obesity stigma in sexual relationships. Obes Res. 2005;13(8):1393–7.
76. Fu H, Goldman N. Incorporating health into models of marriage choice: demographic and sociological perspectives. J Marriage Fam. 1996;58(3):740–58.
77. Falkner NH, French SA, Jeffery RW, Neumark-Sztainer D, Sherwood NE, Morton N. Mistreatment due to weight: prevalence and sources of perceived mistreatment in women and men. Obes Res. 1999;7(6):572–6.
78. Sabin JA, Marini M, Nosek BA. Implicit and explicit anti-fat bias among a large sample of medical doctors by BMI, race/ethnicity and gender. PLoS One. 2012;7(11):e48448.
79. Foster GD, Wadden TA, Makris AP, Davidson D, Sanderson RS, Allison DB, et al. Primary care physicians' attitudes about obesity and its treatment. Obes Res. 2003;11(10):1168–77.
80. Budd GM, Mariotti M, Graff D, Falkenstein K. Health care professionals' attitudes about obesity: an integrative review. Appl Nurs Res. 2011;24(3):127–37.
81. Teachman BA, Brownell KD. Implicit anti-fat bias among health professionals: is anyone immune? Int J Obes Relat Metab Disord. 2001;25(10):1525–31.
82. Phelan SM, Dovidio JF, Puhl RM, Burgess DJ, Nelson DB, Yeazel MW, et al. Implicit and explicit weight bias in a national sample of 4,732 medical students: the medical student CHANGES study. Obesity (Silver Spring). 2014;22(4):1201–8.
83. Miller Jr DP, Spangler JG, Vitolins MZ, Davis SW, Ip EH, Marion GS, et al. Are medical students aware of their anti-obesity bias? Acad Med. 2013;88(7):978–82.
84. Wear D, Aultman JM, Varley JD, Zarconi J. Making fun of patients: medical students' perceptions and use of derogatory and cynical humor in clinical settings. Acad Med. 2006;81(5):454–62.

85. Wigton RS, McGaghie WC. The effect of obesity on medical students' approach to patients with abdominal pain. J Gen Intern Med. 2001;16(4):262–5.
86. Pedersen PJ, Ketcham PL. Exploring the climate for overweight and obese students in a student health setting. J Am Coll Health. 2009;57(4):465–9.
87. Drury CA, Louis M. Exploring the association between body weight, stigma of obesity, and health care avoidance. J Am Acad Nurse Pract. 2002;14(12):554–61.
88. Huizinga MM, Cooper LA, Bleich SN, Clark JM, Beach MC. Physician respect for patients with obesity. J Gen Intern Med. 2009;24(11):1236–9.
89. Beach MC, Roter DL, Wang NY, Duggan PS, Cooper LA. Are physicians' attitudes of respect accurately perceived by patients and associated with more positive communication behaviors? Patient Educ Couns. 2006;62(3):347–54.
90. Bertakis KD, Azari R. The impact of obesity on primary care visits. Obes Res. 2005;13(9): 1615–23.
91. Hebl MR, Xu J. Weighing the care: physicians' reactions to the size of a patient. Int J Obes. 2001;25(8):1246–52.
92. Afonso BB, Rosenthal R, Li KM, Zapatier J, Szomstein S. Perceived barriers to bariatric surgery among morbidly obese patients. Surg Obes Relat Dis. 2010;6(1):16–21.
93. Harper DM, Else BM, Bartley MJ, Arey AM, Barnett AL, Rosemergey BE, et al. In a safety net population HPV4 vaccine adherence worsens as BMI increases. PLoS One. 2014;9(7), e103172.
94. Ostbye T, Taylor Jr DH, Yancy Jr WS, Krause KM. Associations between obesity and receipt of screening mammography, Papanicolaou tests, and influenza vaccination: results from the Health and Retirement Study (HRS) and the Asset and Health Dynamics Among the Oldest Old (AHEAD) Study. Am J Public Health. 2005;95(9):1623–30.
95. Wee CC, McCarthy EP, Davis RB, Phillips RS. Screening for cervical and breast cancer: is obesity an unrecognized barrier to preventive care? Ann Intern Med. 2000;132(9):697–704.
96. NIH Consensus Development Conference Panel. Gastrointestinal surgery for severe obesity. Consensus Development Conference Panel. Ann Intern Med. 1991;115(12):956–61.
97. Stanford FC, Kyle TK, Claridy MD, Nadglowski JF, Apovian CM. The influence of an individual's weight perception on the acceptance of bariatric surgery. Obesity. 2015;23(2): 277–81.
98. Ferrante JM, Piasecki AK, Ohman-Strickland PA, Crabtree BF. Family physicians' practices and attitudes regarding care of extremely obese patients. Obesity. 2009;17(9):1710–6.
99. Ionut V, Burch M, Youdim A, Bergman RN. Gastrointestinal hormones and bariatric surgery-induced weight loss. Obesity (Silver Spring). 2013;21(6):1093–103.
100. Lo Menzo E, Szomstein S, Rosenthal RJ. Changing trends in bariatric surgery. Scand J Surg. 2015;104(1):18–23.
101. Rand CS, Macgregor AM. Successful weight loss following obesity surgery and the perceived liability of morbid obesity. Int J Obes. 1991;15(9):577–9.
102. Lippa NC, Sanderson SC. Impact of information about obesity genomics on the stigmatization of overweight individuals: an experimental study. Obesity. 2012;20(12):2367–76.
103. Anesbury T, Tiggemann M. An attempt to reduce negative stereotyping of obesity in children by changing controllability beliefs. Health Educ Res. 2000;15(2):145–52.
104. O'Brien KS, Puhl RM, Latner JD, Mir AS, Hunter JA. Reducing anti-fat prejudice in preservice health students: a randomized trial. Obesity. 2010;18(11):2138–44.
105. Wiese HJ, Wilson JF, Jones RA, Neises M. Obesity stigma reduction in medical students. Int J Obes Relat Metab Disord. 1992;16(11):859–68.
106. Ciao AC, Latner JD. Reducing obesity stigma: the effectiveness of cognitive dissonance and social consensus interventions. Obesity. 2011;19(9):1768–74.
107. Kushner RF, Zeiss DM, Feinglass JM, Yelen M. An obesity educational intervention for medical students addressing weight bias and communication skills using standardized patients. BMC Med Educ. 2014;14:53.
108. Matharu K, Shapiro JF, Hammer RR, Kravitz RL, Wilson MD, Fitzgerald FT. Reducing obesity prejudice in medical education. Educ Health (Abingdon). 2014;27(3):231–7.

109. Stunkard AJ, Sorensen TI. Obesity and socioeconomic status--a complex relation. N Engl J Med. 1993;329(14):1036–7.
110. Phelan SM, Burgess DJ, Yeazel MW, Hellerstedt WL, Griffin JM, van Ryn M. Impact of weight bias and stigma on quality of care and outcomes for patients with obesity. Obes Rev. 2015;16(4):319–26.
111. Institute of Medicine. Evaluating obesity prevention efforts: a plan for measuring progress. In: Medicine Io, editor. Washington, DC: The National Academies Press; 2013.
112. Kyle TK, Puhl RM. Putting people first in obesity. Obesity. 2014;22(5):1211.

Chapter 3
Religious Minorities and Medicine: The Collision of Health Care and Faith

Shirin N. Ali

Introduction

Most of the research about prevention, diagnosis, and treatment disparities in minority patients in the medical literature focuses only on ethnic minority populations. This chapter will provide a description of religious minorities in the United States and the way in which their religious identification can impact the care that they receive in the medical system. For practitioners, researchers, and educators, particularly in major metropolitan areas, faith or religion-based values may present challenges to the way health care is typically delivered. Religious minority patients may have differences in terms of their dress, diet, or gender interactions, or the way in which they view reproduction and fertility, or may have a different view of end of life care. Their views could interfere with standard medical care.

In this chapter, I hope to provide an overview of religious minorities in the United States and discuss aspects of their faiths that can impact their interactions with the health-care system. While there is not much medical literature available, this chapter will review what literature is available on important topics such as reproductive/fertility issues, patient and medical team communication, end of life care, mental health care, and preventive medicine. While all of these areas may lead to potential conflict with medical personnel, there are also numerous examples within the literature of instances in which patients have received culturally competent care and interventions targeted to their specific needs.

When one considers working with any group of people, it is important to recognize the diversity within the group and to understand that each patient's approach to

S.N. Ali, MD
Department of Psychiatry, New York state Psychiatric institute,
New York, NY, USA
e-mail: sna2116@cumc.columbia.edu

© Springer International Publishing Switzerland 2016   41
R. Parekh, Ed W. Childs (eds.), *Stigma and Prejudice: Touchstones in Understanding Diversity in Healthcare*, Current Clinical Psychiatry,
DOI 10.1007/978-3-319-27580-2_3

his or her health will also be informed by socioeconomic, cultural, lingual, developmental, and psychological factors independent of, but perhaps related to, the person's religious and spiritual life. Through reading this chapter, the reader will hopefully gain more knowledge about different religious minority health beliefs and values and integrate this into his unique approach to his practice of medicine, medical education, or research. This chapter will include several blended cases based upon my work, cases of colleagues, and literature from different fields of medicine. These cases will help the reader to synthesize the different topics and themes discussed in the chapter and consider their application to realistic clinical scenarios. These cases will demonstrate the complexity and diversity of religious minority patients and hopefully provoke thought on how to work with these patients in a culturally sensitive manner. While some health-care professionals may feel that religion and spirituality do not necessarily have a place in discussions with patients, this chapter will illustrate that many health-care professionals are actually engaged in these discussions with patients and their families and will also illustrate the importance of incorporating the principles in their daily work.

Who Are Religious Minorities in the United States?

The Pew Research survey in 2008 involved results of interviews with 35,000 adults in the United States about their religious views [1]. Among Christians in the United States, minority groups include Mormons, who make up 1.7 % of the population surveyed, Jehovah's Witnesses who comprise 0.7 % of the population, and Eastern Orthodox Christians, who are 0.6 % of the population [1]. The Christian Orthodox population is divided between Greek and Russian Orthodox adherents. Jews comprise 1.7 % of the US population, and this chapter will mainly focus on adherents who identify as being Orthodox Jews, who are less than 0.3 % of the US population, and less so on conservative Jews who are 0.5 % of the population. People who identify as belonging to other religions are even less populous, including Buddhists who make up less than 0.7 % of the population. The percentage of Buddhists is divided between Theravada, Tibetan, and Zen Buddhists [1]. Muslims comprise 0.6 % of the population, which is divided between a majority of Sunnis and a minority of Shias and other smaller factions. Hindus and Seventh-Day Adventists are only 0.4 % of the population. Other minority religions include Unitarian Universalism, New Age, and Native American religions; a significant population of the United States identifies as unaffiliated, 16.1 % [1].

There are religious population-specific factors that may be distinctive and are useful to keep in mind when working with these populations. For example, Muslims and Mormons are among the more rapidly growing groups; they are the two religious minority groups with the largest families. Over 20 % of Mormons and 15 % of Muslims have more than three children currently living in their home [1]. The vast majority of Muslims and Hindus are immigrants, in contrast to most Buddhists. Three out of four Buddhists are converts to Buddhism [1]. While they may have specific religious or spiritual values that pertain to Buddhist beliefs, it is less likely that they will have stories of immigration that inform their experiences. Interestingly, only one-third of Buddhists identify themselves as Asian. With regard to socioeconomic factors that also impact health literacy and access to health care, Hindus and Buddhists have higher income levels among religious groups. With regard to educational background, half of Hindus, one-third of Jews, and one quarter of Buddhists have a graduate education, which is much higher than the general population in the United States in which 10 % of adults have a graduate education [1]. Interestingly, many Jehovah's Witnesses leave the religion; only 37 % of people who were raised Jehovah's Witness remain Jehovah's Witness. While a patient may identify as being raised as a Jehovah's Witness, it would be worth asking them about how much their religious background informs their current approach to their health and medical care. A review of all of these different religions and their major beliefs is beyond the scope of this chapter; summaries of their major principles and the way in which they relate to health care is summarized below (Table 3.1).

Is There Evidence of Stigma of Religious Minority Patients?

The components of stigma potentially faced by religious minority patients have not been rigorously studied in a way that compares outcomes between populations. In medicine, generally, there is now greater awareness of stigma and disparities in the health care of ethnic and racial minority patients, and there are efforts to address these differences in care examined in the Institute of Medicine Report from 2002 [2]. Many of the studies addressing religion and stigma address the stigma of having a specific disease, such as HIV/AIDS, within a faith-based community and describe interventions to increase access to care. The goal of these studies is not to understand the belief structure about the religion or values to decrease the stigma associated with the diagnosis, but rather to help patients use the resources and structures within their religious community. With regard to religious minority patients, much of the literature is limited to case studies, pilot studies, small controlled studies, or descriptive literature about clinical experiences in working with a specific population. Additionally, there are particular populations on whom there may appear to be a disproportionate amount of research, like the Orthodox Jewish population, which makes up a significant religious minority patient population in larger cities, such as New York City. This literature is reviewed in this chapter, and some of the studies in this chapter may be drawn from countries that have more studies on religious minority populations like the United Kingdom.

What Barriers to Treatment May Be Relevant for Religious Minority Patients?

Different aspects of stigma can occur within a particular group or community and can emerge in the interaction between the medical establishment and the patient from the target population. If one is diagnosed with an illness, such as bipolar

Table 3.1 Review of beliefs and health-related values of religious minorities [3, 5, 7, 10, 17, 22, 23, 29, 31–34]

Religion	Major tenets	Summary of views related to health care
Christian Science	A view of God, Jesus Christ, as the creator of a good universe and a benevolent deity who did not create evil Strong belief in prayer as a way to cope with life's difficulties of all kinds Strong emphasis on healing oneself and others through prayer and this being a central part of the religion	Emphasis on spiritual healing, mind, and power of prayer to heal illness Emphasis on prevention of medical conditions Indications of illness are mental, not physical; may be due to a spiritual problem or evil Emphasis on each person being free to make decisions about health care
Mormonism	Similar to other Christian denominations, but belief in an American Zion Belief in a "Celestial Family," an eternal family Emphasis on self-restraint and free agency Strong community, emphasis on mission in young adulthood for men Emphasis on baptism and marriage	Emphasis on marrying young and having a large family, particularly for women Prohibition of alcohol, tobacco, caffeine, drugs, gambling, premarital sex, masturbation Emphasis on modesty (use of sacred undergarments) and on relying on faith as a way to negotiate difficulties Observation of Sabbath on Sunday
Orthodox Judaism	Monotheistic religion Reliance on rabbi and religious authorities for decision-making Can have limited interaction with the secular world Specific gender roles—women may focus on family and children; men may focus on study Emphasis on rites of passage related to: circumcision (bris), bar/bat mitzvahs, holidays, rituals related to reproduction Priority on religious life and community life, more interdependent rather than individualistic life	Rituals around purification with regard to menses (*mikvah*) and abstaining from intercourse around menses (*niddah*), thought to signify impurity Separation of genders; modesty for both men and women Emphasis on marriage and having a large family Reliance on rabbinical authorities for guidance in everyday life and medical care When life begins and ends may be controversial and dependent on religious authorities Higher risk of birth defects May have arranged marriages
Hinduism	Polytheistic religion originating in India No great distinction between religion and culture Belief in karmic life cycle, that people are born and reborn again and their soul exists in another body Accountability for deeds of past life Modesty valued Communal, interdependent culture with an emphasis on filial piety	Belief in karmic cycle, may impact view of end of life care, organ donation or transplantation, and deity May believe that illnesses are a result of something done in a past life and interfering with this may interfere with the order of things Ayurvedic view of the individual: integration of mind, soul, and body within the context of family, culture, and nature; view of imbalance of humors May have values related to arranged marriage and stigma about how psychiatric illness may impact marital prospects Values of purity with respect to gender (male bias), auspiciousness

Table 3.1 (continued)

Religion	Major tenets	Summary of views related to health care
Buddhists	Many Asian immigrants and converts; for Asian immigrants there may be an overlap of religion and cultural beliefs People pursue enlightenment which is attainable There is a cycle of suffering and rebirths that everyone must endure Principle of not harming other creatures	Views on non-harm may impact diet (vegetarianism), views on end of life care or organ donation or transplantation Belief in cycle of rebirths and pursuing a peaceful death may impact health-care decisions Views may be quite individual driven; no central authority exists
Islam	Monotheistic religion, similar to Judaism and Christianity No centralized authority, though some Muslims may have particular religious authorities they respect Some Muslims may observe five daily prayers and annual 30-day fast (Ramadan) Can be intermingling of religious and cultural beliefs	Rituals around purification with regard to menses and other bodily fluids, thought to signify impurity Separation of genders; modesty for both men and women; some women may wear the *hijab* Prohibitions against alcohol, recreational drugs, premarital sex, eating pork products When life begins and ends may be controversial and dependent on religious authorities May have arranged marriages
Jehovah's Witnesses	Identify as Christians, but do not believe in the Holy Trinity They do not believe in the need for a religious authority Do not believe in an immortal soul Do not celebrate Christmas or Easter or birthdays Do not participate in war	General refusal to accept blood or blood products, though individual beliefs may be different Patients may look to family or church members for guidance about medical decisions No centralized religious authority
Sikhs	Majority of Sikhs are from Punjab region in India; most Sikhs are Punjabi Belief in karma and rebirth, similar to Hinduism Also family-oriented culture in which duty is prioritized Belief in community service and social responsibility Most people do not understand Sikhism—confusion about this religion post 9/11	May be at risk for particular illnesses like diabetes; may have higher likelihood of being uninsured Similar to Hinduism in that it is a patriarchal culture Similar to Hinduism in views of purity and integrated view of mind, body, soul, and social, family, and natural context

disorder, the patient may fear that others within their group will avoid him or his family or mistreat him or his family because of the diagnosis [3, 4]. Additionally, if there is a belief that a certain group of patients does not typically use a service, such as genetic counseling, the patient may be worried that medical professionals may avoid members of their particular group or treat members of the group differently than other patients [5]. Additionally, the health-care practitioners may also feel uncomfortable or ignorant when approaching members of this population in the clinical setting. Due to these tensions in the communication between health-care provider and patient, some patients may be less likely to pursue care they could benefit from. For example, a belief among health-care providers that an Amish patient may not be interested in technologically advanced treatments may lead to the medical team not offering a patient the latest reproductive technology due to a bias in thinking about the Amish as "conservative." Another example might be a gynecologist acting on an assumption about a Muslim woman not being open to discussing sexual health. This assumption could lead to the physician avoiding offering a female Muslim routine preventive care such as a pap smear or offering her contraception, due to assumptions about the patient having sexually conservative values. Additionally, cultural beliefs associated with religion or faith-based values may interfere with standard medical treatment for patients.

One of the most publicized cases in the past two decades that relates to religious and cultural values interfering with treatment is the story behind the nonfiction book *The Spirit Catches You and You Fall Down*, which is now often part of a medical school curriculum for this reason. This book details the story of a Hmong girl with a history of severe epilepsy. Because of her family's religious and cultural beliefs that epilepsy was a holy occurrence, her family did not wish to treat her with anti-epileptic medications, leading to a massive breakdown in the communication with her health-care team and negative outcomes in multiple ways for this patient and her family (see box below). While many subtle clashes may occur on a daily basis in medicine, this book illustrates a particularly extreme case with dire consequences for the patient and for her family [6].

Text Box 1

The Spirit Catches You and You Fall Down is a frequently read book in medical humanities courses in medical school. Anne Fadiman's 1997 nonfiction book describes the clash between medical culture and religious culture of a young Laotian Hmong girl with epilepsy in Merced, California. The child is diagnosed with epilepsy, and the medical team recommends standard medical treatment with antiepileptic medications after they repeatedly treat the patient when she presents to the hospital with a seizure. In the family's spiritual belief system, epilepsy is caused by a spiritual problem, and the family consults with a shaman to address this problem. The family does not adhere to instructions regarding the patient's prescribed antiepileptic medication, and the patient continues to have seizures, eventually leading to the frustration of the medical community and removal of the child from the family and her placement in the foster care system. This is a disturbing illustration of negative outcomes when the medical system and religious beliefs clash and communication between the patient and family completely down. Since the publication of the book, the Merced medical community has worked to train Hmong shamans about medical procedures and has become more knowledgeable about Hmong culture. Additionally health-care professionals have started to incorporate Hmong shamans into medical care and worked to facilitate trust between the Hmong community and medical community [6].

Potential Areas of Conflict Between Patients and Medical Teams

Various beliefs and traditions related to religious or spiritual views may prevent the creation of a good rapport between patients and medical teams or lead to difficulties in maintaining a therapeutic alliance. Common areas of conflict might include issues that interfere with standard medical treatment or procedures (Table 3.1). These issues are usually circumscribed to particular areas, involving gender interactions, conceptions of modesty, health care involving reproduction or death, and dietary issues.

For some individuals from particular religions, notably Islam, Hinduism, and Orthodox Judaism, a man or woman may be uncomfortable being physically examined with a cross-gender health-care provider. Or, he or she may be uncomfortable discussing sexuality or bodily functions, even if they are within the scope of what the health-care provider usually discusses with all patients [7–9]. A female Muslim patient may have discomfort with standard-issue medical gowns in the operating room or on a ward and request to be able to wear her own dress that she feels safeguards her modesty. Issues related to gender may also occur with male patients. A male Orthodox Jewish patient may express concern about sitting alone in a room with the door closed with a psychologist of the opposite gender, even in the confidential, individually tailored meeting, which might prove challenging for the practitioner who is used to having a door shut for confidentiality reasons.

Diets can prove to be difficult in more medically controlled settings, such as an inpatient unit. For example, an Orthodox Jewish family may be understood to observe kosher laws, but the hospital staff may not know about the difference between a patient observing standard kosher laws and observing kosher regulations for Passover. Or the patient may have more specific rules regarding the degree to which they are observant that the hospital staff may not be familiar with. Religious minority patients may require more time or space than is typical for family meetings. For example, when discussing options for a pregnant woman with an identified genetic defect in her fetus with a physician or a genetic counselor, the patient may request that multiple family members, including an elder family member, and a religious or cultural representative may also participate in the meeting. This may be unusual for a health-care professional, who may be used to a more individualistic approach in health-care decision-making. This may be true in South Asian Muslim or Hindu families, Orthodox Jewish families, and also in Mormon families.

The hospitalization of religious minority patients may lead to unanticipated areas of conflict in the hospital setting. Depending on the patient's wishes, medical team members may need to prepare to have discussions about the patient's treatment with multiple family members or community leaders as described above. They may need to extend visiting hours and visiting privileges to include a larger maximum number to account for religious community members and extended family, rather than just the immediate family. For example, a hospitalized Christian Scientist patient may believe that his primary mode of treatment may be prayer and may request that he have nightly prayer meetings in his room with his religious community members.

Medical teams on every inpatient service may find that they have to consult religious authorities while advising the patient about treatment and may need to delay treatment in order to obtain permission or consent with ethics boards. For example, for a nonemergency procedure, an Orthodox Jewish patient may not want a Jewish physician or staff member working on the Sabbath as that violates the patient's own personal religious beliefs.

Patients may also request particular accommodations to standard procedures. An Orthodox Jewish patient may request to have regular access to their tefillin and prayer shawl and may wish to have a private space for prayer and to be not interrupted during hours of regular prayer for vital signs or meals. Meals may need to be reheated, which can be an extra burden for staff. A Muslim patient may wish to have a prayer rug, which may not be considered hygienic, if it cannot be properly sterilized. A Buddhist patient may wish to have incense or particular icons. Accommodations can be particularly challenging in a psychiatric unit in which all patients are ambulatory and are required to participate in the communal treatment in which it can be difficult not to have the appearance of giving one patient "special" privileges.

In multiple studies reviewed, the use of cultural brokers to assist in communication between patients and health-care teams was emphasized. In general, patients felt most comfortable with cultural brokers who were matched in ethnicity, religion, and language and were women [7, 10]. There have been instances in which one of these brokers may be part of a decision-making team that includes the patient, his family, an ethics board, religious officials, and the medical team to help the medical care determine the right course of the intervention [11] (Table 3.2).

Table 3.2 Guidelines to consider in providing culturally competent care for religious minority patients

1. Ask about a patient's religious and spiritual beliefs as they relate to health care and the medical problem you are treating them for early on in the treatment. Try to anticipate future areas of discussion

2. Try to understand your patient's individual beliefs and how they may differ from the family and cultural beliefs to understand areas of conflict for them, particularly with regard to reproductive or end of life care issues

3. Try to have a holistic point of view. Are there easy accommodations that can be managed without compromising care in a significant way and build the treatment alliance?

4. Try to open up the informed consent/decision-making procedure. Ask if a patient may want to include religious leaders, family members, or a cultural broker in any aspect of the discussion

5. When using cultural/religious brokers, try to avoid using family members and attempt to use someone who matches with ethnicity and language. Women may be perceived as less threatening as cultural brokers in religions with values around modesty

6. Try to have some familiarity with particular dietary, modesty, reproductive, and end of life care issues for minority religions who are represented in your patient base

7. Present all options available for treatment in a sensitive and open manner. A patient of a religious minority background should have all of the options open to them, even if they choose not to avail themselves of them

Reproduction-Related Religious Minority Issues

Many religions have beliefs and rituals associated with sexuality and reproduction, which may involve rules around when sexual activity can occur, rules around cleansing and purification related to bodily fluids, and observances around fertility and birth (Table 3.1). These views may impact care around reproduction, fertility, and women's health in a variety of ways, some of which will be reviewed here from the vantage point of several different faiths: Judaism, the Baha'i faith, and Mormonism.

Genetic counseling may be more challenging with members of a particular faith, such as Orthodox Judaism, who may be more at risk for particular illnesses or birth defects due to high rates of intermarriage among their community [5]. In the Orthodox Jewish community, for women, establishing a large family and caring for children and the household are a primary responsibility. The concept of genetic counseling, with its emphasis on individual freedom to choose, may be in contradiction to precepts in the Torah about the sanctity of life and about seeking rabbinical guidance for decisions [5]. Some patients would prefer to not see a genetic counselor and avoid possibilities of birth defects by consulting an Orthodox resource for arranging marriage with a suitable match who may not have a history of particular illnesses in his or her family [5]. Orthodox Jewish patients may be even more wary of genetic counselors given stories of bad experiences that they have heard from other community members. A study in which Orthodox Jewish patients, health-care professionals, and genetic counselors serve the same Orthodox community found that there were barriers to access for genetic counseling that impacted the referral and communication process [5].

Health-care professionals were biased against referring Orthodox Jewish patients for genetic counseling based on the assumption that they would not want to see a genetic counselor [5]. Additionally, "horror stories" had circulated through the Orthodox community, including by religious officials, depicting genetic counselors as unfamiliar with Orthodox traditions and paternalistic [5]. When interviewed, genetic counselors felt ignorant about Orthodox cultural and religious traditions and were also worried about asking about a patient's religious observance and suggesting counseling interventions [5]. Patients felt that the process of counseling was not very useful to them and often wished to involve rabbis in the counseling and decision-making process [5]. This was difficult for the counselors to accept as involving another nonmedical person in a discussion was unfamiliar. A religious belief that the authors speculated interfered with the counseling process was the belief that Orthodox patients may believe that hidden miracles that could heal a child might not occur once a diagnosis has been made [5]. For all of the reasons above, the authors of this study recommended increasing the awareness of Orthodox beliefs in health-care communities that are likely to serve the Orthodox populations and the creation of alliances between health-care providers and cultural brokers within Orthodox communities, such as the having a meeting between community members and health-care professionals to discuss children's health [5].

Some other religions also emphasize the importance of motherhood and have rituals and beliefs around health-related aspects of motherhood, such as breastfeeding and labor and delivery. One article reviewed the importance of breastfeeding in the Baha'i faith, which is a religion that had its inception in Iran in the nineteenth century [12].

Text Box
The Baha'i faith: Worldwide, there are five million followers who adhere to this monotheistic faith that incorporates a belief in a series of messengers including Abraham, Christ, Zoroaster, Muhammad, Moses, and Bah'a'ullah and beliefs from all of these religions. There is a belief in equality between genders, a harmonious relationship between faith and science, the importance of service to the community, universal peace, and social justice [12].

There are core values of peace, security, and unity and a reverence for breastfeeding in Baha'i texts. In other religions, the importance of breastfeeding is also emphasized. Muslim women are encouraged to breastfeed their children for up to 2 years in Islamic texts and are exempt from fasting for Ramadan while breastfeeding. In Judaism and Hinduism, breastfeeding is prioritized over other domestic responsibilities for women [13].

A qualitative survey study examined the significance of childbirth for Orthodox Jewish women and Mormon women. In both religions, there is a strong emphasis on the creation of a new family, and women in both groups viewed giving birth as an empowering and spiritually important process [14]. Orthodox Jewish women may view creating a new family as their duty in following the biblical commandment to expand the population of followers. Latter-Day Saints believe that their families are eternal and that they will exist in afterlife [14]. Mormon women view children as essential for their spiritual progression.

Compared to the Mormon women in the study, Orthodox women, who may be more unfamiliar with secular resources due to their separation from secular communities, were much less aware of community child-birthing resources. Both populations viewed having experiential knowledge of childbirth as being helpful in their own preparations to give birth [14]. With regard to the labor and delivery process, 73 % of Orthodox husbands were present during labor and only 37 % were present during birth, due to the prohibition of seeing their wives immodestly exposed and touching their wives when they were having vaginal bleeding. Mormon husbands did not have the same prohibition on contact with their wives and were present for the birth.

It is important for health-care professionals to know that an Orthodox Jewish husband may adhere to nidda (avoidance of his wife during her impure period), which could begin from the start of labor or later, depending on their sect, which may reduce his ability to coach her through labor [14]. The Orthodox women in this study felt supported by their husbands praying for them and supporting them spiritually through the process of labor. Some Mormon women may ask for a blessing for their families and unborn children during labor. In both communities, female family members may provide support during the birthing process [14]. Results of a survey study like this one could be shared with doctors, nurses, midwives, and doulas in obstetrics and gynecology that treat the Orthodox and Mormon communities to increase religious cultural understanding. These results could be very helpful for medical professionals involved in creating birth plans with patients and involved in the delivery process [14].

Informed Consent

The health-care professional's job with regard to informed consent is to present the patient with the risks, benefits, and alternatives to any particular procedure, medication, or device. In this process, it is useful for the physician to be aware of how a patient's religious beliefs may impact their medical decision-making. For example, various religions have rules about what can be taken into the body and what is supposed to stay out of the body, whether it is alcohol, recreational or prescription drugs, blood products, or various animal products. While there may be guidelines, these views are not monolithic, and there is tremendous individual variation in how each patient may conduct his behavior. For example, a strict Seventh-Day Adventist, who is a vegetarian, might not ingest a bovine-derived product, but may give consent to use a bovine-based mesh for a hernia repair that is placed in the body [15]. Most medical students learn that Jehovah's Witnesses do not accept blood products. While this may be generally true, a medical practitioner or educator may not want to assume this without asking the patient. A recent study on consenting pregnant Jehovah's Witness women who were about to give birth revealed that there may be more variability to their belief about blood products than may have been previously thought.

The belief against accepting blood products stems from passages in the Old Testament that urge people to not "eat from the bread of life." The risk of accepting blood for observant Jehovah's Witnesses is potentially facing eternal damnation or excommunication from the church. There may be fear that someone urging them to take blood products may be influenced by evil [16]. Some medical professionals actually find that the informed consent process with Jehovah's Witnesses is less complicated because the lines of what they will and will not accept with regard to blood products are clearer than with other populations [16]. In this vein, medical professionals believe that clarity prevents unexpected conflicts in medical care or in discussions with Jehovah's Witnesses.

A recent chart review study demonstrated a thoughtful, flexible approach of New York State and also of a hospital in informed consent around transfusions for Jehovah's Witnesses. The state Health Care Proxy form specific to Jehovah's Witnesses that pregnant women must fill out before giving birth includes options about what blood products the woman would want to receive if she is in need of transfusion, as delivery is a time in which healthy young women are first confronted with the risk of hemorrhage. There is a 44-fold increase in risk of death if the woman opts not to accept transfusions [17]. In addition to the standard New York State Health Care Proxy form for Jehovah's Witnesses, the hospital in this study also included additional questions to women about whether they would wish to receive whole blood, cryoprecipitate, fresh frozen plasma, albumin, isolated factor preparations, or none at all. A pregnant Jehovah's Witness at this hospital undergoes counseling to understand all options besides getting blood products. This process may be particularly useful for Jehovah's Witness women who may not want to receive donor blood, but may be willing to accept a transfusion of their own blood products or other blood products [16].

This widened informed consent leaves room for her the patient to be able to make her own decision around blood products. In the study, 39.3% of Jehovah's Witness women consented to accept a variety of donated blood products, and 9.8 % said that they would accept packed red blood cells. This survey refutes the idea that a Jehovah's Witness would never accept blood products and may help medical teams provide a better informed consent process and may decrease the stigma of the patient making a decision that might go against more standard beliefs of her religion [16]. This example illustrates that informed consent includes discussing all of the treatment and nontreatment options with all patients, even if the team has an assumption about what a patient from a particular population may or may not do. Similarly, while a Hindu family may feel that life is sacred and believe in reincarnation, they still may decide to terminate a pregnancy if the child will not survive due to a chromosomal abnormality, for the reason of not preventing the child from reentering the cycle of reincarnation more quickly [7].

End of Life Care

End of life care involves difficult discussions between medical teams and patients about beliefs around life and death. These discussions are informed by a patient and family's religious and cultural beliefs about organ donation, attempts to prolong life, and rituals around death. Reviews on end of life care include studies of religious and spiritual beliefs as they relate to end of life care often without looking at the general beliefs of a religious minority group and/or individual. In this section, I will review the beliefs of different religions on end of life care.

Islamic views around the end of life derive from the Qur'an and Sunnah, the transcribed words and deeds of the Prophet Muhammad, and include the main principle of avoiding harm for the patient. Generally, Muslims believe in avoiding precipitating death, but Islam permits the withdrawal of life support as this is viewed as allowing death to proceed without human interference. Unlike in Catholicism or in Orthodox Judaism, there is no centralized Islamic religious authority for Muslims as a whole. Instead Muslims may rely on various scholars who may have different views on bioethical or religious questions [18]. The Islamic Medical Association of North America (IMANA) advises all Muslims to have an advance directive in which they describe what life-sustaining procedures they would like in the event that they are critically ill [18]. According to the IMANA, Muslims are allowed to die with comfort measures only, which can include nutrition, hydration, and pain medication. Nutritional and hydration support are generally not considered optional. However, at one Shia hospital in Iran, patients are allowed to deny themselves parenteral hydration and nutrition. In contrast, in Saudi Arabia, the Saudi Commission for Health Specialties advises against withholding intravenous fluids and nutrition from patients too ill to eat [18].

In Orthodox Judaism, two principles guide decision-making with respect to end of life care. As with organ donation, the principle that life is of "utmost value" applies and also that a person's dignity should be maintained during death, which is viewed as a natural process, similar to Islam [19]. Active areas of debate in end of life care include the balance between a patient's autonomy and paternalism, managing nutrition and pain for a patient, and issues around the value of life and maintaining quality of life. To provide culturally competent care, medical professionals can encourage families to contact their rabbi and involve them in the end of life care discussions with the family and physician as soon as possible. In this way, there will be communication between all parties and that the rabbi and physician can have a direct dialogue, which can prevent misunderstandings about the clinical situation and the religious beliefs on either side [19]. Committing or omitting treatments that may hasten a patient's death is to be avoided in Orthodox Judaism. Orthodox patients may have a more circumscribed view of autonomy with regard to medical decision-making in their faith compared to secular medical patients. Advance directives are also encouraged for Orthodox patients, and administration of these directives may also involve the rabbi as part of the decision-making process.

Most religious authorities are in agreement with maintaining patient comfort with regard to pain even if it makes a patient less cognitively responsive. It is recommended that physicians communicate to patients that using opiate medication for pain management does not hasten death. Generally, like in Islam, hydration and nutrition are to be maintained throughout the dying process by non-forceful means. Many Jewish religious authorities are in agreement that restraining a patient to prohibit him from pulling out a feeding tube may be infringing upon the dignity for that patient [19]. With regard to do not resuscitate (DNR) or do not incubate (DNI) orders, most Orthodox religious authorities are in favor of performing CPR and defibrillation and for consulting religious authorities about artificial ventilation. Most religious authorities are against extubation, which is seen as an act that hastens death. However, they may permit a patient's automatic internal defibrillator (AID) to be turned off as a patient nears death or permit other comfort measures to occur, such as stopping blood draws. Due to the lack of consensus about the definition of death in the Orthodox religion, whether it is brain death or lack of cardiopulmonary function, states with many Orthodox Jews, like New York and New Jersey, have required hospitals to make accommodations for patients with a definition of death as cardiopulmonary death [20].

There is limited data on the end of life care views of the Hindus in the United States. One recent survey of Indo-Caribbean Hindus located in Queens studied a population that was mostly from Guyana and had limited formal education. As with any small survey study, it is not clear that this group's beliefs are representative of other Hindus in the United States or the rest of the world. Participants who were religiously observant felt strongly about adhering to Hindu rituals around death and believed that karma was a cause of suffering and pain in life [21]. As a whole, this group had negative attitudes toward life-preserving procedures in terminal illness and felt positively toward advance directives. Most people surveyed could not define cardiopulmonary resuscitation (CPR) or describe it and expressed the belief that surviving CPR would lead to survival for the patient [21]. It is not clear whether their lack of familiarity with medical terminology was due to socioeconomic status, low health literacy, and cultural or religious factors. Most individuals surveyed were not in favor of CPR or mechanical ventilation and wanted to die comfortably [21]. The results of this study suggest that it is worthwhile for physicians to define medical terms in plain language during discussion of advance directives with all patients and particularly, terminally ill patients.

Buddhist principles regarding end of life care have similarities to views in Hinduism, particularly, a belief in karma and suffering in life. The concept of Ahimsa, non-harm of living creatures, is the value that most informs the Buddhist view on end of life care [22]. Buddhist patients may have difficulty considering an intervention that may increase their comfort in death but may potentially hasten death, such as the use of opiates similar to Orthodox Jewish patients. A Buddhist patient may also wish to speak to a religious authority and family members before making a decision on this matter [22]. Theravada Buddhists may be likely to follow principles literally, while Mahayana and Tibetan Buddhists may be more likely to emphasize compassion and leniency when considering a religious belief as it pertains to medicine [22]. Most Buddhist authorities are comfortable considering death as brain death, as was redefined from cardiopulmonary death by the Ad Hoc Committee of the Harvard Medical School to Examine the Definition of Brain Death in 1968 [22].

With regard to artificial feeding and hydration, similarly to Orthodox Judaism, withdrawing nutrition, like a feeding tube, may be viewed as an act that hastens death. However, if tube feeding causes other complications, such as aspiration pneumonia and infections, or causes other suffering, discontinuing tube feedings may be considered [22]. Preventing a person from reaching their next rebirth by prolonging their life through tube feeding or mechanical ventilation is supported by some Buddhists and Buddhist authorities who may favor returning a person to a more "natural" process of death [22]. In the article reviewed for this chapter, the authors emphasize that it is important for medical teams to explore how important it is that the patient have a peaceful death, an approach that is applied to many religious minority patients and may be an entry point for a discussion about religious views on the dying process. Palliative and hospice care are supported by most Buddhists and are not in contradiction to any beliefs, besides those described above [22].

Organ Donation

Organ donation is a complex issue, and no religion expressly prohibits organ transplantation from a donor, live or dead, or organ donation. Rates for organ donation among minority groups in the United States are low [23]. Clearly almost all religious texts were written long before there was consideration of organ donation technology, and thus discussions about organ donation often involve the extrapolation and application of ancient religious beliefs to a very modern health-care problem.

There is some controversy or difference in beliefs about what is permissible use of the body according to each religion and also what the definition of death is [24]. In 2011, the UK Chief Rabbi released a statement defining death as cardiopulmonary failure, rejecting the notion of brain death as death, which had been accepted by medical establishments since 1968 and by the Rabbinical Council of America in 2010 [20]. The position statement in 2011 led to statements from other rabbis in Israel and the United States supporting the idea of brain death as constituting death [24]. There is also debate among Islamic authorities concerning brain death and organ donation, as well as a plurality of views among Muslims. In Islam, desecration of the body of a living or dead individual is forbidden; however, as in Judaism, the altruism of saving a life is seen as a good deed. The goodness of organ donation may mitigate breaking the rule of bodily desecration, as Jewish law states that each person should be buried with all of his or her parts [19]. In 1996, the Muslim UK Council ruled that organ donation is allowed in Islam [20]. However, many Muslim countries have low rates of organ donation, for unclear reasons.

In a survey conducted among Detroit-area Muslims, it was found that higher Islamic religiosity did not correlate with negative attitudes toward organ donation [25]. Rather a "negative coping attitude," one in which a Muslim has an insecure relationship with God and a more negative attitude toward the world, correlated with negative views of organ donation [25]. Interestingly, there was also a cultural component to the views on organ donation among various Muslims. African-American and South Asian Muslims were less in favor of organ donation than Muslims of Arab origin. One hypothesis about this difference is that Arab religious authorities are more in favor of organ donation than South Asian religious authorities [25]. This demonstrates that while there may be some general attitudes toward organ donation in a religious group, there certainly is within-group difference worth exploring in the clinical encounter, particularly in a very culturally diverse religious group like Muslims.

While adherents of Sikhism and Hinduism may believe in the karmic cycle, and there is no prohibition against organ donation, there may be a variety of beliefs on the topic. Some Hindus may not believe in taking organs from a cadaver and may feel that a person should be cremated with all of their body parts [15]. However, every person may have their specific beliefs, and some observant Hindus may want to consult with their own guru before making a decision. Other Hindus may believe that one passes on his or her experiences, sin, and good works through organ donation and that the recipient accepts the donor's sins and impurities, as part of karma [26]. Karma plays a role also in Buddhist and Jain philosophies regarding organ donation. In Tibetan Buddhism, while there is no prohibition on organ donation, there is a belief that the soul may rest in the body after death for several days, and some Buddhists believe that disturbing the body in any way may disturb karmic rebirth [20]. However, other more liberal Buddhist authorities have noted that the act of organ donation may bring good karma to the donor and will outweigh the suffering they may incur as part of the process [22].

It is worth noting that transplantation from cadaveric donors may be resisted in the following populations: Native Americans, the Roma people, Confucians, and Shintoists [24]. One survey study of Chinese Americans, who have a low rate of organ donation, investigated potential influence of religious and spiritual beliefs on these low rates. This study showed that Chinese Americans are influenced by Confucian beliefs that equate an intact physical body with demonstrating respect for one's ancestors and for nature, based on views of "filial piety," in which the body is considered a gift from one's parents and ancestors. Buddhist and Daoist beliefs may also be contributing factors [23].

With organ donation, varying the protocol may allow an organ to be donated in a way that is consistent with a patient's religious and spiritual beliefs. Organ transplant clinicians should have a discussion with a patient about their specific spiritual and religious beliefs in this area. For example, if a Buddhist believes that the spirit leaves the body after a certain number of hours, it is possible that they may be willing to donate organs after that time period has passed, which would pass along the precious commodity of an organ [23].

Mental Illness

This section will focus on the challenges related to accessing mental health care in particular religious minority populations, Orthodox Jews, Muslims, and Mormons. Teaching points from this section can be applied to work with other religious minority populations. The common themes that will be explored for all of these groups will include religious values regarding mental health, stigma, and barriers to accessing mental health treatment.

Among Orthodox Jews, compared to the non-Orthodox Jewish population, the stigma of mental health diagnoses frequently arises in the course of treatment and presents a barrier to treatment. Stigma may manifest in various ways, including increased levels of secrecy about discussing or disclosing a diagnosis in a family or in the community, delays in seeking or adhering to mental health treatment, and significant concerns about marital prospects for the patient and his or her family members [4]. One survey study using case vignettes examined attitudes toward depression in Orthodox Jews compared to non-Orthodox Jews and found that there was higher secrecy and stigma associated with seeking treatment and more stigma around marriage and family discussion and acceptance of depression [4]. However, there was actually no significant social distancing, which implied that members of the Orthodox Jewish community would not avoid a member of the community who had a diagnosis of depression. There were no significant intergroup differences between Jews and Orthodox Jews about modality of treatment, despite the authors hypothesizing that the Orthodox population might prefer more behaviorally oriented treatment, rather than insight-oriented treatment [4]. There was a general preference for individual therapy over group therapy in both populations, and there was no clear preference for setting of treatment.

Another study examined the question of whether or not medical models of psychiatric illness increased or decreased stigmatization of mental illness among Orthodox Jews, using OCD as an example [3]. A common clinical technique of attempting to decrease stigma of psychiatric treatment and psychiatric illness is to liken psychiatric illnesses to chronic physical illnesses like diabetes. Physical illnesses are more accepted as "biological" in origin and may not be evident to others if well managed. Describing a psychiatric condition as equivalent to a medical condition ideally would make it more difficult to "blame" patients for their illness or attribute mental illness to a character weakness. Unexpectedly, this study found that for Orthodox Jewish families, the concept of mental illness having a biomedical cause might actually increase stigma particularly related to marital concerns and social distancing [3]. In this study, the stigma of psychiatric illness extended to the siblings of the psychiatrically ill individual and other family members [3]. These concerns about marriage eligibility due to the high rate of arranged marriages and the importance of maintaining social connections might be present with Muslim and Hindu patients.

These authors suggest specific approaches to discussion of treatment and diagnosis with family and community members of psychiatrically ill Orthodox patients. The authors recommend de-emphasizing genetic or biological factors and emphasizing behavioral factors, environmental factors, the stress-diathesis model of psychiatric illness, and relapse prevention. The emphasis on factors that are external to the person may help decrease stigma and increase access to and adherence to mental health treatment and help avoid shame and stigma for the patient and their family [3]. During an initial meeting with a patient and his or her family members, the clinician can gauge their attitudes toward medical models of mental illness and exert caution when discussing issues around diagnosis and treatment before being familiar with their religious and cultural context [3]. Though a patient may be in remission for his psychiatric illness, the fact that he or she may want to marry may lead to incredible stress for the patient and his family, whether or not he or she uses a matchmaker. Some patients and families may not disclose history of mental illness to a matchmaker or even to the patient's potential spouse or their family until much later, even after the marriage [27].

Another article examining the challenges of delivering mental health services to the ultra-Orthodox populations suggested that it would be most helpful for the therapist to try to explain the diagnosis from the patient's view of the world [27]. For example, a psychiatrist may need to explain the mechanisms of action of an antipsychotic as a spiritual barrier between a patient and demons and de-emphasize a biological explanation as described above [27], Additionally, while the goals of psychiatric rehabilitation often focus around work and independence, this may not be culturally appropriate for an ultra-Orthodox patient, who lives in a more communalistic and interdependent culture. Their culture emphasizes the study of the Torah as a full-time occupation particularly for men, rather than necessarily pursuing work outside of the yeshiva. These authors also recommend the use of a cultural broker within psychiatry. With patients who are treated with psychiatric medications, there may be many questions about the genetic risk of psychiatric illness, the effect of medications on breastfeeding, contraception, and the impact of medications on fertility, due to the emphasis of marriage in Orthodox culture [27]. It would not be surprising if this line of questioning were similar in Muslim, Hindu, or Mormon patients who also have religious cultures that emphasize the importance of marriage and/or having a large family.

Case Box
A 31-year-old female ultra-Orthodox Jewish patient, married, with three children, with a prior history of obsessive-compulsive disorder (OCD), is hospitalized for a manic episode. It is Passover, and the patient is barely eating any food because she is concerned about violating kosher laws and starts losing weight precipitously. Her family brings in food to the hospital as well as kosher grape juice, which is difficult for the hospital staff to accommodate with regulations about patients not having food in their rooms. Additionally, the patient requests to drink a nutritional supplement, which is not kosher, and the team feels confused about whether or not to allow the patient to do this. The patient needs the calories, but the team is worried about disrespecting the patient's wishes and also religious observances and offending the family. The team is worried that the patient can't necessarily consent to having nonkosher food because of her mental state. Throughout the treatment, the patient's parents do not want the team to use the term "bipolar disorder," particularly in front of the patient's husband and her in-laws and prefer the diagnosis of OCD.

Stigma may also prevent children with intellectual impairments from accessing adequate services. A study in the United Kingdom examined disparities in the care of Muslim children with cognitive impairments. In the United Kingdom, there was a notable lack of use of available services by Pakistani and Bangladeshi families with children with cognitive disabilities. Muslim children were more impaired than Hindu and Caucasian families with children with intellectual problems [28]. In this survey study, it appeared that Muslim mothers were not aware of services that were available for their children, though this did not appear to be due to religious factors [28]. The Islamic practices varied from family to family, with some families practicing Islam in a way that was more influenced by folk and cultural beliefs, which was confusing to health-care practitioners. Common Islamic beliefs included the belief that all humans are created equally and that cognitive impairment could be due to hereditary factors. Most Muslim families believed that they were expected to meet all of the child's needs without any expectation of help from their surrounding community [28]. It was not clear where this belief originated. While this study could not separate the complicated relationship between class, education, religion, and culture and how they impacted the access to care, the main recommendation was that individual care plans need to be developed for Muslim patients and that not speaking English and having lower educational factors may have led to disparities in care [28].

Mormons are another religious minority population that has difficulty accessing mental health care due to their belief system and also due to the relative dearth of Mormon mental health clinicians. The Mormon religion states that faith in Christ allows people to overcome their difficulties and heal themselves from pain, which leads to a Mormon patient feeling ashamed or spiritually weak in seeking psychiatric care [29]. Additionally, as there is not much familiarity with Mormon beliefs, Mormon patients may feel worried about being understood by non-Mormon practitioners [29]. In general, Mormons are encouraged to be hardworking, perfectionistic, and able to exert will power with regard to abstaining from premarital sex and alcohol and drugs. A Mormon who has homosexual feelings or is unhappy in a marriage may feel very pressured to remain in his or her situation and very uncomfortable seeking help for these problems [29]. Initially, if a Mormon has a mental health problem, he may be encouraged to consult with a priest first; as Mormonism favors men being leaders in the community, there may be a preference for seeing a male therapist by patients of both genders [29]. Due to the potential centrality of Mormon beliefs for a particular patient, it may be very helpful for a therapist to be Mormon. If the therapist is non-Mormon, he ought to familiarize himself with major principles within the culture and also try to understand how the patient relates to their culture [29].

For religious minority populations, accessing mental health care can be particularly challenging, due to stigma within their religious community, worry about the diagnosis and treatment impacting marital prospects, lack of culturally matching practitioners, religious beliefs that are in favor of spiritual treatment over psychiatric treatment, as well as cultural and socioeconomic factors.

Successful Interventions in Preventive Medicine with Religious Minority Patients

Underserved religious minority populations not targeted by traditional outreach programs may benefit from culturally sensitive interventions that incorporate religious and spiritual values. In this section I will review efforts designed to address health screening and prevention for three different religious minority communities.

In 2014, researchers from New York University conducted a pilot study to test a culturally informed lifestyle intervention program targeted to help prevent diabetes in the Indian Sikh community in New York City. South Asians are at high risk for diabetes, and Sikhs comprise a substantial portion of the South Asians in New York City. The experimental group participated in six community health worker lead group sessions on nutrition, diabetes prevention, exercise, and health care, while the control group participated in standard preventive care from their current providers and were followed for 6 months. The community health workers were bilingual in Punjabi and English and were Asian Indians. The educational materials were targeted toward the Sikh population [10]. For instance, the Sikh value of community service was used to underscore the importance of preventive medicine. A Sikh nutritionist adapted Punjabi recipes to make them healthier and provided them to participants. Culturally appropriate visual images and language were used in materials discussing exercise as part of spiritual practice [10]. The experimental groups demonstrated significant improvements in weight, diet, waist circumference, blood glucose, blood pressure, and total cholesterol [10]. Of note, the researchers did not create their materials and instead adapted materials available from the National Heart, Lung, and Blood Institute and the National Diabetes Education Program. This pilot study demonstrates that it is possible to design a culturally informed intervention by collaborating with local religious minority communities to help improve the health of a specific religious minority population.

Another article for health-care professionals details a clinical approach to discussing cervical cancer screening with Muslim women, who may hold religious beliefs that place importance on modesty in their clothing and interactions with male individuals who are unrelated to them, similar to Orthodox Jewish women. Muslim female patients articulate concerns about their modesty in health-care interactions and may have difficulty discussing reproductive and sexual health issues with a stranger, male or female [3]. Many Muslim women may not get gynecological care until after marriage unless there is an acute symptom or problem [3]. Female Muslim immigrants may not have had access to regular gynecological care before moving to the United States and are unlikely to be vaccinated for HPV. Additionally, there may be ignorance about the risks of HPV or reluctance to get regular gynecological care. The authors of this article, which was written for educational purposes for health-care professionals, recommend screening Muslim women while remaining sensitive to values of modesty throughout the initial discussion and procedures [3]. For example, a Muslim woman patient may respond better to a female clinician and may feel most comfortable if the practitioner states plainly that no men will enter the room during their discussion or physical exam. When recommending the HPV vaccine, using phrases such as "no one is immune" rather than "everyone is at risk" might be helpful in decreasing any shame or stigma associated with sexuality or HPV [3]. Like with other patients, only uncovering what needs to be examined may be helpful during a physical exam of a Muslim woman. The modifications to the standard annual gynecological exam procedure suggested by the authors of the article are subtle and easy to incorporate and are a great example of providing a culturally sensitive intervention to Muslim women.

Conducting focus groups of minority populations can be an effective way to learn more about tailoring screening and prevention to the specific needs of the population. Researchers from Wayne State University conducted focus groups among Orthodox Jewish women in cooperation with rabbis and community members to learn more about barriers to cancer screening in the Orthodox Jewish population. Ashkenazi Jewish women are at higher risk for carrying the BRCA genes, which increases their risk for breast, ovarian, and other types of cancer. Orthodox Jewish populations in particular may be at higher risk for cancer due to intermarriage, lower rates of screening, and poor health behaviors related to diet and exercise [30]. Themes emerged in the focus groups that impacted whether or not these women chose to be screened: the idea of preserving hidden miracles, fate, cost, having other priorities such as family, the absence of culturally relevant programming for screening, lack of information about screening, and fear [30].

Similar to the Muslim women described above, many Orthodox women adhere to the value of modesty in dress and behavior and might feel uncomfortable discussing gynecological topics in mixed-gender company. It may be for this reason family history of gynecological cancer or breast cancer may not be known by a patient. Additionally, as alluded to in the focus groups, Orthodox women may be busy with their family lives and may prioritize cooking, preparing for Sabbath, arranging religious observances, and taking care of their families over their own health. Some women expressed concern that pursuing screening would mean that there would be "nothing left to pray for" [30]. Some felt that whether or not one would be diagnosed with cancer was a matter of fate, not screening, and therefore screening had little utility [30]. Barriers similar to those faced by other minority populations include Orthodox women having relatively high rates of being uninsured or underinsured [30]. There is also a specific word in Yiddish "yenne machlah" that may be used instead of the word cancer, which can be considered scary to use. Taking together all of the insights into views of Orthodox women on cancer screening, the authors suggest that providing Orthodox women with culturally appropriate education would improve screening rates among Orthodox women [30]. Additionally, similar to the preventive intervention designed for the Sikh community in New York City, Orthodox women receiving endorsement about health screening from rabbis and community leaders would likely improve adherence to screening recommendations. Getting a mammogram or a pap smear could be framed as an important spiritual or family responsibility, just as eating healthily and exercising was framed as an important spiritual duty for Sikhs.

Case Box

A 21-year-old recently married Muslim woman newly immigrated from Somalia presents for a new patient visit at the gynecologist. She has never been to see a gynecologist before. She is wearing a *hijab* (scarf covering her hair and neck, leaving her face exposed) and jeans and a sweater. She is hesitant in discussing her sexual history with the physician and appears nervous about whether any male nurses or attendants will come into the room when she is getting a pelvic exam. She appears worried about the pelvic exam itself. The female physician meets with the patient for a consultation while the patient is fully clothed in a separate room before going to the exam room for the pelvic exam. During the pelvic exam, she makes an effort to keep the patient covered for as much of the exam as possible. During the initial consultation, the physician was surprised when the young woman asks about the HPV vaccine that she has heard about from other students at her college and asks whether or not it is recommended for her. The physician explains the purpose of the HPV vaccine and states that "no one is immune" to HPV. The physician sensitively explores contraceptive options and makes herself available for questions from this young woman in the future after she explains that she wishes to discuss them with her husband.

Culturally Competent Adapted Treatment Protocols

Some hospital centers that treat a significant number of religious minority patients have adapted treatment protocols to meet the needs of particular religious minority populations. In sharing their results, they provide a model of how other medical settings could provide culturally competent care to religious minority populations. Two particular areas of medicine where religious cultural issues come to bear frequently are around reproduction and fertility and end of life care.

As New York City has a particularly diverse patient population and a large number of Orthodox Jewish patients, one of the major academic medical centers has many Orthodox patients in its well-known Reproductive Endocrinology and Infertility program. For Orthodox women and men, there is a period of time called *niddah,* from the onset of menses through seven days after menses end during which intercourse is forbidden. After menses end, women visit the *mikvah* for ritual purification. Orthodox men are forbidden to masturbate during *niddah* as well [31]. One uncommon cause of infertility in Orthodox couples is a woman having a short cycle or missing the opportunity for intercourse if she is unable to go to the *mikvah.* Because having ritual purification is important to this patient population, the medical team at the hospital altered their in vitro fertilization (IVF) protocol to include one extra day of ovarian stimulation [31]. This one-day gap enabled Orthodox women to go to the *mikvah* before receiving their HCG trigger injection to prepare them for egg retrieval [31]. In comparing the outcomes of this modified protocol to the control protocol, the team demonstrated that there were no significant differences with regard to embryo implantation, pregnancy, and live birth between these women and controls, despite the perception of infertility treatment being quite rigid [31]. Muslim women also do a ritual purification after their menses, though they do not have to go to a specific location to perform their ritual cleansing. As many religions include rituals and beliefs around reproduction, sex, and sexuality, it is useful for infertility specialists to familiarize themselves with the specific beliefs around particular religious minority patient populations.

Another case report from a hospital in New York City describes a productive collaboration between a Hasidic female cancer patient, her family, an ethics board, religious authorities, and the medical team. In patients who are critically ill, ECMO (extracorporeal membranous oxygen) may be used for cardiopulmonary support. Physicians and medical teams may hesitate to start ECMO in a patient who is likely to stop life-sustaining treatment. In the case of the 40-year-old Hasidic Jewish woman, the medical team felt strongly that she could benefit from ECMO as a treatment "bridge" to chemotherapy, which they felt could potentially save her life [11]. However, the patient's religious tradition prohibited the cessation of life-sustaining treatment. Through the medical team's discussion with religious authorities and the ethics board, as well as the patient and her family, it was decided that ECMO could be considered a non-life-sustaining treatment for this patient [11]. The chemotherapy was then reframed as the life-sustaining treatment for this patient. This case illustrates that through reaching a consensus about the objectives behind each medical intervention, the patient did not have to violate her religious beliefs about stopping life-sustaining treatment, which ECMO is usually considered to be. This case is a good model of a productive discussion among members of the ethics board, the religious authorities, cultural brokers, the patient, and her family, which facilitated the patient being able to access lifesaving treatment [11].

Conclusions and Future Directions

Religion and spirituality are complex facets of an individual's identity and frequently inform his or her approach to health, the body, ethics, and rituals around reproduction and the end of life. Compared to other countries, many generations of people have come to our nation in pursuit of religious, cultural, and political freedom, which has led to the tremendous diversity in our country. The population of religious minorities in the United States continues to grow, and their health-care needs will continue to grow as well. This chapter has highlighted that there is a lack of data about these populations, their level of health knowledge, health care seeking, and barriers to access to health care. While there may be tremendous intergroup diversity of beliefs and approaches to health, there is also much diversity among each specific religious group, whose beliefs are multiply determined by class, ethnicity, education, language, and other personal factors. This complexity, as with any facet of identity, makes information gathering and research methods quite complicated, particularly qualitative research that may give health-care professionals a more nuanced approach to thinking about creative effective interventions. Larger scale survey studies may capture the breadth of views among a certain religious group, but a qualitative study may lead to a deeper understanding of the different views within the group.

This missing information makes the task of developing targeted interventions to decrease stigma and increase awareness of medical and psychiatric conditions quite difficult, though some good efforts to do so were reviewed in this chapter. A realistic appraisal of potential disparities in care in religious minority patients is an important future direction for researchers, and questions about religion and spirituality should be included in any assessment of aspects of identity. The Institute of Medicine report on health-care disparities in 2000 was quite significant in helping health-care professionals become aware of disparities among ethnic minority groups and to start to address them. The next assessment of progress since that report could also include information about the health-care needs and treatment of religious minority groups. This would help emphasize the importance for all researchers of assessing the prevalence and incidence of different diagnoses in religious minority groups and subgroups to help target effective interventions in the areas of treatment, screening, and prevention. Religion and spirituality are important factors to include in any large- or smaller scale study of health care in an ethnic minority population, and while they may add complexity to analyses of data, it would greatly enhance our understanding of these issues.

Another significant area of further exploration is the utilization of cultural brokers with religious minority patients, which is well studied in ethnic and lingual minority patients. While religious minority populations are quite different from one another, there are commonalities between groups. Certainly the approach to one group may be very useful to apply to another group. While the medical community has come a long way from *The Spirit Catches You and You Fall Down*, it is worthwhile to remember that that case occurred in the 1990s, which is very recent history. That case illustrates that when it comes to the health of religious minority populations, it is imperative that clinicians, researchers, and educators work to further characterize and meet their health-care needs and to prioritize religion and spirituality as crucial factors that impact a person's approach to his or her health and health care.

References

1. Pew U.S. Religious landscape survey. 2008. Available at http://religions.pewforum.org/reports.
2. Unequal treatment: confronting racial and ethnic disparities in health care. http://www.iom.edu/reports/2002/unequal-treatment-confronting-racial-and-ethnic-disparities-in-health-care.aspx. Accessed 20 Mar 2015.
3. Pirutinsky S, Rosen DD, Shapiro Safran R, Rosmarin DH. "Do medical models of mental illness relate to increased or decreased stigmatization of mental illness among orthodox Jews?". J Nerv Ment Dis. 2010;198(7):508–12.
4. Baruch DE, Kanter JW, Pirutinsky S, Murphy J, Rosmain DH. Depression stigma and treatment preferences among Orthodox and Non-Orthodox Jews. J Nerv Ment Dis. 2014;202(7):556–61.
5. Mittman IS, Bowie JV, Maman S. Exploring the discourse between genetic counselors and Orthodox Jewish community members related to reproductive genetic technology. Patient Educ Couns. 2007;65:230–6.

6. Laws T, Chilton JA. Ethics, cultural competence, and the changing face of America. Pastoral Psychol. 2013;62(2):175–88.
7. Coward H, Sidhu T. Bioethics for clinicians: 19. Hinduism and Sikhism. Can Med Assoc J. 2000;163(9):1167–70.
8. Guimond ME, Salman K. "Modesty matters: cultural sensitivity and cervical cancer prevention in Muslim women in the United States". Nurs Womens Health. 2013;17:212–7.
9. Padela AI, Gunter K, Killawi A, Heisler M. Religious values and healthcare accomodations: voices from the American Muslim community. J Gen Intern Med. 2011;27(6):708–15.
10. Islam NS, Zanowiak JM, Wyatt LC, Kavathe R, Singh H, Kwon S, Trinh-Shevrin C. Diabetes prevention in the New York city Sikh Asian Indian community: a pilot study. Int J Environ Res Public Health. 2014;11:5462–86.
11. Meltzer EC, Ivascu NS, Acres CA, Stark M, Furman RR, Fins JJ. Extracorporeal membrane oxygenation as a bridge to chemotherapy in an Orthodox Jewish patient. Oncologist. 2014; 19(9):985–9.
12. What Bahais Believe. http://www.bahai.org/beliefs/. Accessed 20 March 2015.
13. Setrakian HV, Rosenman MB, Szucs KA. "Breastfeeding and the Bahá'í Faith". Breastfeed Med. 2011;6(4):221–5.
14. Callister LC, Semenic S, Foster JC. Cultural and spiritual meanings of childbirth. Orthodox Jewish and Mormon women. J Holist Nurs. 1999;17(3):280–95.
15. Jenkins ED, Yip M, Melman L, Frisella MM, Matthews BD. Informed consent: cultural and religious issues associated with the use of allogeneic and xenogeneic mesh products. J Am Coll Surg. 2010;210(4):402–10.
16. Curlin FA, Roach CJ, Gorawara-Bhat R, Lantos JL, Chin MH. When patients choose faith over medicine: physician perspectives on religiously related conflict in the medical encounter. Arch Intern Med. 2005;165:88–91.
17. Gyamfi C, Berkowitz RL. Responses by pregnant Jehovah's Witnesses on health care proxies. Obstet Gynecol. 2004;104(3):541–4.
18. Alsolamy S. Islamic views on artificial hydration and nutrition in terminally ill patients. Bioethics. 2014;28(2):96–9.
19. Loike J, Gillick M, Mayer S, Prager K, Simon JR, Steinberg A, Tendler MD, Willig M, Fischbach RL. The critical role of religion: caring for the dying patient from an Orthodox Jewish perspective. J Palliat Med. 2010;13(10):1267–71.
20. Editorial Staff. "Religion, organ transplantation and the definition of death". Lancet. 2011;377:271.
21. Rao AS, Desphande OM, Jamoonda C, Reid CM. Elderly Indo-Caribbean Hindus and of end of life care: a community-based exploratory study. J Am Geriatr Soc. 2008;56:1129–33.
22. McCormick AJ. Buddhist ethics and end-of-life care decisions. J Soc Work End Life Palliat Care. 2013;9(2):209–25.
23. Lam WA, McCullough LB. Influence of religious and spiritual values on the willingness of Chinese-Americans to donate organs for transplantation. Clin Transplant. 2000;14:449–56.
24. Bruzzone P. Religious aspects of organ transplantation. Transplant Proc. 2008;40:1064–7.
25. Padela AI, Zaganjor H. Relationships between Islamic religiosity and attitude toward decreased organ donation among American Muslims: a pilot study. Transplantation. 2014;97(12): 1292–9.
26. Hutchcinson JF, Sharp R. Karma, reincarnation, and medicine: Hindu perspectives on biomedical research. Genomic Med. 2008;2:107–11.
27. Greenberg D, Witztum E. Challenges and conflicts in the delivery of mental health services to ultra-orthodox Jews. Asian J Psychiatr. 2013;6(1):71–3.
28. Kaur-Bola K, Randhawa G. Role of Islamic religious and cultural beliefs regarding intellectual impairment and service use: a South Asian parental perspective. Community Med. 2012;9(3): 241–51.
29. Lyon SJ. Psychotherapy and the Mormon Faith. J Relig Health. 2013;52:622–30.

30. Tkatch R, Hudson J, Katz A, Berry-Bobovski L, Vichich J, Eggly S, Penner LA, Albrecht TL. Barriers to cancer screening among Orthodox Jewish women. J Community Health. 2014;39:1200–8.
31. Reichman DE, Brauer AA, Goldschlag D, Schattman G, Rosenwaks D. In vitro fertilization for Orthodox Jewish couples: antagonist cycle modifications allowing for mikveh attendance before oocyte retrieval. Fertil Steril. 2013;99(5):1408–12.
32. Dunner GA. "When the symptoms appear." Christ Sci Sentinel. 1973;75:36. Available at http://sentinel.christianscience.com/shared/view/2827i9v48wy?s=cs.
33. "What is Christian Science?". Available at http://christianscience.com/what-is-christian-science#basic-teachings. Accessed 20 Mar 2015.
34. "Frequently asked questions about Jehovah's Witnesses." http://www.jw.org/en/jehovahs-witnesses/faq/. Accessed 20 Mar 2015.

Chapter 4
The Poor and Economically Vulnerable in Public and Safety Net Healthcare Institutions: Outcomes and Attitudes

Lior Givon

> **Case**
> A young adult male with history of depression was brought from a private university to a local public hospital emergency department endorsing suicidal ideation, with intent and plan to harm himself. The psychiatric emergency team as well as his outpatient providers agreed that he needed to be hospitalized emergently on a locked inpatient psychiatric unit for safety, mood stability, evaluation of treatment options, and support. While the patient was waiting for a bed to open at the institution's psychiatric unit, the patient's parents arrived and insisted they are taking him out of the emergency department to a private psychiatric facility, saying, "Our son will not be admitted to a hospital with poor and homeless people."

Introduction

This chapter is a product of years of interactions with patients and their families and conversations with physicians from different medical disciplines, colleagues, and investigators who are interested in healthcare inequalities and economic vulnerabilities. While much has been published on the relationship between racial, ethnic, and gender disparities and healthcare outcomes, there is a paucity of research on the

L. Givon, PhD, MD
Department of Psychiatry, Cambridge Health Alliance, Cambridge, MA, USA

Harvard Medical School, Boston, MA, USA
e-mail: lgivon@challiance.org

© Springer International Publishing Switzerland 2016   67
R. Parekh, Ed W. Childs (eds.), *Stigma and Prejudice: Touchstones in Understanding Diversity in Healthcare*, Current Clinical Psychiatry,
DOI 10.1007/978-3-319-27580-2_4

quality of medical care in institutions that provide care for a disproportionate number of the economically disenfranchised. This chapter reviews the relationship between poverty, health outcomes, attitudes, and perceptions held by healthcare providers, patients, and the public toward the poor. Specifically, it focuses on healthcare delivery systems that treat and service economically vulnerable groups that are supported by state and government health insurance, are uninsured or underinsured.

Healthcare is more than direct medical attention provided to patients. It involves access to preventive and continuity of care, health insurance, medications, health education, advocacy, and community resources. State and federal financial support, public policy and sponsorship, as well as societal attitudes toward the poor and poverty determine the availability and allocation of these services. While the United States ranks among the five highest nations on the Human Developmental Index (a summary measure of achievements of potential human development) [1], its statistics on poverty are striking: In 2013, the national poverty rate was 14.5 %, with 45.3 million people living below the poverty line. In that same year, the poverty rate for children under age 18 years old was almost 20 %. Despite a decline in the national poverty rate, the 2013 regional poverty rates were unchanged from the previous year [2]. Poverty is associated with racial and gender disparities. In 2012, 18.9 million non-Hispanic whites, 13.6 million Hispanics, and 10.9 million African Americans were living in poverty, with 8.4 million non-Hispanic whites, 5.4 million Hispanics, and 5.1 million African Americans living in deep poverty [3]. In 2010, 23 % of Native American families earned income below the poverty line, with the highest poverty rates recorded in South Dakota (43–47 %) [4]. In 2012, over five million more women than men were living below the poverty line and two million more women than men were living in deep poverty. Almost 30 % of households headed by a single woman were living below the poverty line, nearly five times the poverty rate for families headed by two parents and twice the poverty rates of households headed by a single male [3].

There are few conversations and little training in medical schools and postgraduate programs on the relationship between economic insecurities and health outcomes and even fewer discussions on stigma, attitudes, and perceptions held by healthcare professionals toward the poor. As a consequence, healthcare providers do not think routinely of economic predicaments having direct implications on their patients' physical and mental well-being.

The sociologist Erving Goffman [5] conceptualized social stigma in discrete layers of societal perceptions that include physically visible characteristics, unique behaviors, and group affiliations. Most often, the poor do not exhibit these attributes, making it difficult to identify and provide them the specialized medical attention and social services they frequently require. Unlike racial and ethnic features or unique physical characteristics such as physical disabilities, the poor are indistinguishable from other patients. They are "visibly invisible" in hospitals and clinics, awaiting their turn in line to the pharmacy, on a gurney in the emergency department (ED), or in the reception room at their primary care clinics. A silent and often shamed population that carries lifelong economic challenges, health vulnerabilities, legal and immigration liabilities, unemployment, chronic substance use, and a stagnate future.

The Effects of Poverty on Health

Poverty is a complex and fluid construct that first and foremost is defined by income disparities and inconsistent and unreliable access to basic needs such as food, shelter, and clothing [6]. In its broader conceptualization, poverty in the United States is about economic uncertainties. It restricts access to societal resources such as healthcare and health insurance, suitable housing, sanitation, healthy nutrition, educational opportunities, stable employment, and access to local and global information sources. As a result, poverty reduces life expectancy, quality of life, and future prospects for socioeconomic upward mobility [7].

Poverty has lifelong and permanent consequences on the health and welfare of the economically vulnerable. In addition to inadequate access to acute and preventive care, income disparities are related to worse health outcomes and are correlated with increased morbidity and mortality. Three decades of data demonstrated that those with income below 200 % of the poverty level were at increased cumulative odds ratio risk for diabetes (1.74), arthritis (1.35), back pain (1.29), hypertension (1.21), chest pain (1.13), and heart disease (1.05), as well as increased risk of death (1.29–1.70). Additionally, poverty was associated with increased risk for depression (3.24) and decreased cognitive functioning (4.60) [8]. Geographical areas with higher rates of low-income households were associated with worse medical outcomes, such as elevated rate of amputations and vision loss as a result of diabetes mellitus [9, 10]. A 4-year observational study found that while physical health [hypertension, non-insulin-dependent diabetes mellitus, acute myocardial infarction (AMI), and congestive heart failure (CHF)] declined at a similar rate in both poverty and non-poverty groups, mental health improved significantly for the non-poverty group but did not improve for the poverty group [11].

The effects of poverty on health start in childhood and last a lifetime. Children who grew up in poverty were more likely to develop and die earlier from cardiovascular disease and diabetes mellitus when adults. The health effects of childhood poverty have lifelong enduring consequences on health outcomes and overshadow poverty alleviation and economic improvement during the adult years [12]. Childhood poverty is associated with increased stress, resulting in a chronically dysregulated stress response. The longer the time spent in poverty during childhood, the less efficient is the hypothalamic-pituitary-adrenal axis response to acute stressors [13].

The effects of economic vulnerability on health are well established. Poverty is associated with cumulative risk for acute and chronic diseases, shorter life span, higher mortality, and physiological changes that permanently affect the psychological and cognitive well-being of the poor population. In turn, these health consequences prevent those raised in poverty from achieving economic independence and upward social mobility, creating a cycle of perpetually physical, psychological, and social vulnerabilities.

Healthcare Institutions That Care for the US Poor Population

A large part of the healthcare provided to the economically vulnerable population in the United States takes place in public and health safety net (HSN) hospitals. Public hospitals are owned or maintained by government funding; receive financial support from local, state, and federal agencies; and accept state and federal health insurance in the form of Medicaid and Medicare, in addition to commercial insurance. Mostly in urban areas, public hospitals provide a disproportionate high percentage of uncompensated care and are often considered "safety nets" for uninsured patients who have otherwise little access to medical care. Historically, public hospitals have been the main venue for medical care delivery to the ethnically, racially, and economically disadvantaged [14]. They emerged from charity institutions (almshouses) in large crowded urban areas from the late 1700s through the early 1900s, to control and prevent the spread of infectious diseases [15]. The number of US public hospitals has been declining [16, 17] and they are being replaced by HSN institutions whose mission is to reduce healthcare disparities [18]. As a result, the majority of the research on healthcare outcomes provided to the economically vulnerable population in the United States is carried out in HSN hospitals.

Designated HSN hospitals provide a "disproportionate amount of care to vulnerable populations" [19] and are legally committed "to caring for populations without stable access to care, specifically public hospitals or private hospitals with Medicaid caseload greater than one standard deviation above their respective state's mean private hospital Medicaid caseload" (pg 240) [20]. Safety net hospitals emerged in the 1980s in response to the needs of geographically depressed communities and vary in their financial structure. In one neighborhood, a local public hospital might serve as the HSN facility, while in another locality, a community and/or privately owned hospital carries this designation [21]. Some HSN institutions are nonprofit, while others are for-profit, a designation associated with the institution's tax status. A nonprofit designation indicates that the organization does not pay local, state, or federal income tax because it is considered a charity. For-profit or investor-owned health organizations are quicker to respond to changes in profitability of medical services than public and nonprofit health organizations [22]. A community hospital designation is a loosely used term that describes local, general, nonfederal hospitals, mostly for short-term patient care that is either nonprofit or for-profit. These financially diverse health institutions may be academically affiliated with a medical school and have postgraduate training programs.

A survey by the American Hospital Association showed that as of 2013, there were a total of 5,686 registered hospitals in the United States, of which 4,974 were community hospitals, 2,904 nonprofit hospitals, 1,060 for-profit hospitals, 1,010 state and local government community hospitals, and 409 nonfederal psychiatric hospitals [23].

Health Outcomes in Public and HSN Hospitals Serving the Economically Vulnerable Population

In 2012, Pauline Chen M.D. published an article in the New York Times [24] contrasting a patient's perception of the poor care he thought he would receive at his local HSN hospital with recently published health outcome data on the medical care provided to patients in HSN hospitals. She writes, "When I asked him why (he did not seek the urgent medical care he needed), he looked disgusted. Have you ever been in that hospital? he snorted rolling his eyes. The halls were dingy, he continued… the waiting rooms were veritable dens of human misery, filled with patients and their families in endless holding patterns. Who knows what kind of care I would have gotten in one of those hospitals, he said with a shudder."

In the past decade, health policy specialists and government agencies echoed similar concerns as Dr. Chen's patient did regarding the medical care provided to the poor in hospitals that treat a disproportionate number of the economically disadvantaged. The Center for Medicare and Medicaid Services (CMS) and other groups investigated national benchmarks and performance outcomes in HSN, public, and nonprofit healthcare institutions. These studies focused on some of the most prevalent, chronic, and costly diseases that are associated with high mortality and morbidity among the US population. Heart disease was a major target because homelessness and low socioeconomic status (SES) are associated with increased burden of cardiovascular disease risk factors as well as morbidity and mortality [25].

Examination of performance changes in hospitals with low (5 %) and high (40 %) percentage of Medicaid beneficiaries for 2004–2006 demonstrated that institutions with low percentage of Medicaid beneficiaries had higher performance gains in AMI, CHF, and pneumonia treatment. The study authors concluded that "safety-net hospitals were less likely to be identified as top performers" (pg. 2184) [26]. The study was criticized for defining HSN hospitals "solely on the percentage of patients insured by Medicaid" and trivializing "the effects community hospitals have on the US health care system" (pg. 1651) [27].

In 2010, CMS published aggregate performance reports comparing over 1200 HSN and non-HSN hospitals on outcome measures such as readmission rates for AMI, CHF, and pneumonia, as well as mortality rates for these illnesses, as indicators of the hospitals' quality of care. Data for 2006–2008 [28, 29] demonstrated that HSN hospitals (24.5 %), serving a larger proportion of low-income patients, performed modestly worse on risk-standardized readmission rates (RSRR), but "there was a substantial overlap in RSRR in all income quartiles" (pg. 17). While 30-day risk-standardized mortality rates (RSMR) were slightly higher for the HSN hospitals, there was also "a substantial overlap in RSMR between these two types of hospitals" (pg. 18).

In 2011, CMS analyzed RSRR for AMI, CHF, and pneumonia for 2007–2009 [30], comparing HSN to non-HSN hospitals, teaching and nonteaching hospitals, as well as urban versus rural hospitals. The initial assumption was that "certain types of hospitals are generally expected to have better performance, including those with greater financial and clinical resources" (p. 31). Similar to the previous publication, results indicated that there was "a substantial overlap in distribution of hospital RSRR among HSN and non-HSN hospitals for all three medical conditions and minimal differences in performance" (pg. 35). Interestingly, RSRR for pneumonia admissions was higher for teaching hospitals (0.4 %) compared to non-teaching hospitals, with no difference for AMI and CHF. Furthermore, RSRR for AMI and CHF was similar across US hospitals regardless of geographical location [urban vs. rural], with a slightly higher RSRR for pneumonia in urban hospitals. In summary, it was concluded that "safety-net hospitals have a similar range of performance as non-safety net hospitals…despite caring for a large number of vulnerable patients" (p. 35).

In response to worries that "some stakeholders are concerned that hospitals caring for large numbers of poor or minority patients may not perform well on the outcome measures" (pg. 12), CMS published in 2012 RSMR for AMI comparing hospitals with different proportions of Medicaid beneficiaries [31]. Despite differences in resources, hospitals with the highest proportion of Medicaid beneficiaries ($\geq$30 %) demonstrated similar benchmark quality performance to those with fewer Medicaid beneficiaries ($\leq$8 %). For RSRR measures, hospitals with higher Medicaid beneficiaries did slightly worse for AMI, CHF, and pneumonia.

In 2013, CMS expanded its report to risk-standardized complication rates (RSCR) associated with hip/knee arthroplasty [32]. Outcome data showed that hospitals serving fewer Medicaid patients had identical results to hospitals serving high percentage of Medicaid beneficiaries as were results from RSRR for hip/knee arthroplasty. Expanding health outcome performance measures, CMS published in 2014 results comparing mortality complication associated with CABG and stroke among hospitals serving a high proportion of Medicaid or African American patients. The investigators concluded that "Among hospitals with the lowest proportion of Medicaid patients, the median stroke RSMR was 0.3 % points lower than among hospitals with the highest proportion"(pg. 56) [33].

Colorectal cancer (CRC) care is of special importance to those concerned with healthcare disparities. It is the third most commonly diagnosed cancer and the third leading cause of mortality in both men and women in the United States [34]. Low SES patients account for a disproportionate high number of CRC patients in the United States. Analysis of over half a million records showed that "overall incidence of CRC was significantly higher among people who had low educational level or lived in low-SES neighborhoods" (pg. 3640) and was associated with an unhealthy diet, smoking, and obesity [35]. For these reasons, there is a special interest in CRC outcomes and care available to the poor population in HSN hospitals. Data from the Virginia Cancer Registry of 5488 uninsured and Medicaid-insured patients who underwent CRC resection between 1999 and 2000 showed that HSN hospitals reduced emergency surgeries, suggesting that CRC care in HSN hospitals was "timely and appropriate" for the uninsured and Medicaid patients compared to non-HSN facilities [36].

Because of disproportionate CRC mortality rates among poor patients, investigators asked whether patients utilizing HSN institutions experience delay in CRC diagnosis and care. A retrospective chart review of CRC patients for 2008–2012 demonstrated that one in two patients had advanced illness at the time of presentation to an HSN facility and a third of the CRC surgeries were performed on an urgent or emergent basis. Race, age, and gender did not predict treatment delays [37]. The study authors concluded that it is not the actual care patients received in HSN hospitals that contributed to the high burden of advanced illness but barriers such as lack of access to health insurance and preventive care that directly affected health outcomes.

Nursing care is paramount to the quality of care patients receive in clinics and hospitals. Nurse staffing ratio was compared in HSN and non-HSN hospitals while controlling for patients' acuity and technology. Of the 54 hospitals studied, 46 were designated HSN facilities and included urban and rural hospitals. A higher mortality from CHF was reported in HSN hospitals and those with a higher proportion of Medicare beneficiaries. Surprisingly, higher nurse staffing ratio in HSN hospitals was associated with increased mortality from CHF, while higher nurse staffing ratio in non-HSN hospitals was associated with lower CHF mortality, lower rate of iatrogenic infections, and lower length of stay. The explanation offered was that worse outcomes in HSN hospitals were not associated directly with the care but with patients' characteristics. The study authors concluded that "patients in health safety-net hospitals are more likely to be from lower socioeconomic groups, have poorer general health and have more co-morbid conditions. Therefore, they are more likely to have negative outcomes regardless of nurse staffing" (pg. 412) [38].

The number of emergency departments (EDs) in HSN hospitals has increased by about 50 % from 2000 to 2007 and since, EDs have been monitored for the care provided to disadvantaged and vulnerable populations. In a study looking at 396 hospital EDs, patients presenting to HSN ED facilities were younger, mostly of minority ethnicity, and with higher proportion of Medicaid or no health insurance. Those in HSN EDs had a shorter median ED length of stay by 7 %, and the length of stay for critical care admissions was also shorter by 5 %. Psychiatric admissions from HSN EDs were 22 % higher compared to non-HSN EDs, and the median length of stay for psychiatric patients was 13 % shorter [39]. The study authors concluded that length of stay measures for admissions, discharge, and transfer did not differ between HSN and non-HSN EDs.

Mental illness introduces additional economic hardship to already economically burdened individuals [40]. Since the 1960s, there has been a reduction in the number of beds in public psychiatric hospitals with 42 out of the 50 states having less than half of the minimum number of beds need to accommodate the mentally ill [41]. Historically, for-profit psychiatric facilities had a greater bed capacity and focused on inpatient services, with major reimbursements from private health insurance and out-of-pocket revenues to maximize profits [42]. In the past decade, services for mental and behavioral health have been mostly financed by public resources, mainly Medicaid [43, 44].

Review of ethnicity and SES disparities among the mentally ill demonstrates that minority groups are more likely to use emergency services in high-poverty areas and often present to hospitals as a last resort [45]. By the nature of psychiatric illnesses, many of the chronically and seriously mentally ill (SMI) do not have insight or acceptance of their illness, do not comply with treatment, and present in acute states to EDs and hospitals [46]. Often, they are unable to advocate for themselves due to cognitive impairments associated with psychosis, mania, or severe depression, are homeless and victims of violence in the community, and have a high comorbid substance use profile [47]. As expected, those with SMI are more likely to be admitted to public psychiatric hospitals [48, 49].

Little has been published in the mental health literature comparing health outcome measures in different hospital systems. A qualitative review of the literature compared for-profit to nonprofit psychiatric inpatient facilities for cost, quality of care, and performance assessment, between the years 1980–2002. Results showed that "the major – and unexpected – finding of this synthesis of studies was the performance superiority of the nonprofit psychiatric inpatient care providers compared with the for-profit providers" (pg. 185) [50].

The sample of studies reviewed demonstrates that medical and psychiatric care provided to the economically vulnerable treated in public, HSN, and nonprofit hospitals is comparable to non-HSN and for-profit facilities. Health safety net hospitals are as efficient in providing prompt and judicious care to those with state and federal health insurance or uninsured. When inconsistencies in care exist among the different types of healthcare facilities, it is attributed to the high acuity or advanced disease the poor and vulnerable patients present with. Many of those utilizing HSN facilities are sicker and need more intense medical care and rescue measures. Many investigators recognize that while the care of the poor is appropriate, layers of disparities still exist, that include barriers of access to preventive care, lack of education about the importance of continuity of care, and compliance with aftercare.

Perceptions and Attitudes Toward the Economically Vulnerable Population Among Healthcare Providers

In addition to medical attention, healthcare is about empathy, relationships, and collaborations among healthcare providers, patients, families, community advocates, and social organizations. Healthcare providers are expected to acquire cultural competence, knowledge, awareness, and communication skills that will encourage trust and promote long-lasting rapport with their diverse and vulnerable patients. What do healthcare professionals practicing in hospitals that serve the economically vulnerable know about the needs and lives of their patients and how do they perceive and relate to their patients? Unfortunately, there is little research on this topic. Much of the available studies focus on attributions and perceptions of the poor regardless of the system they are treated at and mostly by healthcare trainees.

Historically, the nursing profession has had a strong commitment and advocacy for the economically disadvantaged. Nurses' empathy and compassion for the poor improve health outcomes, enrich interactions with patients, and motivate the profession to create strategies to reduce healthcare disparities. Nurses practicing in a community hospital serving rural and urban areas demonstrated increased stigmatizing statements on the "Attitudes about Poverty and Poor Populations (APPPS)" scale. The more experienced and educated the nurse was, the more positive were the attitudes toward the poor, the fewer stigmatizing beliefs were expressed about poverty, and the more structural explanations were given [51]. Nursing student who underwent a "poverty simulation" training demonstrated improvement in post-training testing on the APPPS scale [52]. Nursing students in three Canadian universities were evaluated on their knowledge and beliefs about the relationship between poverty and healthcare and their personal and educational exposure to poverty. A greater exposure to poor patients and positive attitudes toward the poor predicted structural explanations of poverty. The study authors suggested that improving attitudes and structural explanations through education and exposure to those living in poverty would facilitate a better understanding of the relationship between health consequences and economic distress and would raise advocacy efforts [53].

Social workers have been an integral part of the healthcare system. They serve as part of interdisciplinary medical and mental health teams in hospitals and clinics and function as case managers, providing community resources, short-term therapy, and support. There are no studies looking at social workers' attitudes toward poverty in hospital settings [54], but social workers' general attitudes toward poverty and social advocacy have been studied. Comparing attitudes of social workers residing in New York in the mid-60s to those in the mid-80s revealed that the later group endorsed greater structural and societal explanations about poverty but was less committed to social activism as part of the profession's mission [55]. A more recent study assessed feelings about poverty, attributions, stereotypes, and sociopolitical ideologies among social worker students in a Midwestern college. Attitudes toward the poor were significantly more negative than those toward the middle class, blamed the poor for their poverty, and varied with the respondents' SES and demographic backgrounds [56]. Lastly, while graduate social worker students rejected both the personal attribute explanation of poverty and the aversive attitudes toward the poor, they underestimated the hardship poverty inflicts on individuals [57].

Physicians, medical students, and other healthcare professionals provide direct care to patients. Improving attitudes toward the economically vulnerable is of major importance because teaching hospitals and academically affiliated health institutions treat a disproportionate number of the poor and uninsured [58]. All physicians are bound by the Hippocratic Oath to care for patients regardless of economic status, "whatever may be the rank of those who it may be my duty to cure, whether mistress or servant, bond or free." Healthcare professionals that included medical students, physician assistants, social workers, and nurse practitioners participated in a federally funded clinical practicum program that aimed at reducing health disparities and increasing access to primary care. Comparing attitudes before and after participation in the program showed no change in cultural competence, with participants remaining in the "culturally aware" stage, not yet considered "culturally proficient or competent," even though participants found their experience with the underserved to be rewarding and humbling [59].

The only publication assessing perceptions and behaviors in an HSN hospital observed healthcare professionals' attitudes toward substance users in an ED setting [60]. After 2 years of direct observations, the study authors reflected that the majority of caregivers deliberately chose to provide compassionate care "to stigma-vulnerable substance-using patients" (pg. 1339) and that interacting with this population was challenging due to exposure to aggression, violence, and lack of reliable medical information. The study authors wrote: "The results suggest that the day-to-day care provision of substance-involved patients was both meaningful and challenging to providers…We observed a competent and experienced staff that was skilled at handling difficult cases and meeting the complex needs of substance-involved patients…our results do not provide definite conclusions about whether providers stigmatized substance-involved patients in this setting…" (pg. 1345).

Unfortunately, there are no studies on the public's attitudes and perceptions of the care provided in public and HSN hospitals to vulnerable patients. A blogger [61] described his mother-in-law complaining about the shortage of pillows in a public hospital. He wrote, "The next day I took in a pillow…She (the mother-in-law) was in a mental health unit. I was grateful for the support she got in (the) hospital but was puzzled to hear of shortage of pillows." Ironically, this account summarized the available evidence about healthcare in public and HSN facilities. While medical and mental health care in hospitals serving a disproportionate number of the poor are comparable to for-profit institutions, often the facilities in public institutions are old, crowded, and run-down, echoing the patient who refused to seek care at his local HSN hospital because of the "dingy" ED [24].

The little research available on stigma and attitudes held toward the poor in public and HSN hospital settings is telling. This population is a heterogeneous group that is not easily recognized and identified by distinct physical or behavioral characteristics. As a demographic group, the economically vulnerable are of different ethnic, racial, and national affiliations and varied in educational levels. What the poor population in the United States shares are health vulnerabilities. Caregivers have to familiarize themselves with their economically vulnerable patients, recognize their special needs, and understand their unique lifelong health burdens and struggles in order to promote better health outcomes.

Summary

Healthcare and Poverty: Expanding the Discussion

Healthcare finances, societal disparities, and misguided attitudes and perceptions affect health outcomes of the economically vulnerable. This chapter focused on a literature review of medical outcomes in hospitals providing care for a disproportionate number of the economically vulnerable and attitudes toward the poor among healthcare professionals. The detailed review demonstrated that in the past decade, medical care provided to the poor population in public and HSN hospitals has proven comparable to for-profit and other healthcare delivery systems. Patients served in HSN hospitals receive quality medical treatment for some of the most common and costly illnesses that carry high mortality and morbidity when measured by readmission, complication, and mortality rates [25–29]. Most often, the poor lack access to preventive and continuous medical care and present to hospitals with advanced illness, higher acuity, and greater morbidity that result in unfavorable health outcomes.

Negative attitudes toward vulnerable patients propagate inequitable healthcare provisions and affect relationships between patient and providers, lowering trust and satisfaction [62, 63]. Unfortunately, there is a paucity of research on attitudes toward the poor in HSN facilities, and the research that is available is either descriptive or not associated with direct patient care. Regardless, those engaged in direct patient care in HSN hospitals are committed to working with vulnerable populations. Rigorous studies are needed in order to promote better understanding of the stigma associated with attitudes toward the poor in healthcare institutions. This will provide healthcare professionals and healthcare delivery systems with the much needed tools necessary to screen and improve the health and quality of life of the economically vulnerable.

Poverty has lifelong physical and psychological harmful effects on children and adults. The effects of poverty on health outcomes, morbidity, and mortality are well established [8–13] and linked to multiple physical and psychological risk factors for children and adults. Infants and toddlers living in poverty die at a higher rate from infectious diseases and have increased rates of asthma [64], cognitive deficits [65], higher rate of hospitalization, and lower rates of vaccination [66]. Children living in poverty are exposed to increased rates of parental depression, maltreatment, and alcohol and substance use and witness community violence [64]. Adults living in poverty are at increased risk for morbidity and mortality from cardiovascular disease, diabetes, and cancer (lung, oral, CRC, cervical) and have higher rates of asthma, dental and oral disease, and mental illness [8–11, 66, 67].

These are the patients that use public and HSN hospitals for their medical care. With poor quality of life and chronic illnesses, they also experience decreased life expectancy, malnutrition, unemployment, homelessness, delinquency, and illiteracy. Sandy Buchman M.D. writes: "I recently completed a death certificate for Marie. She was 42 years old. I listed the cause of death as *cancer of the cervix, metastatic*. But I think I erred in completing the certificate. I really believe Marie died of her poverty" (pg. 709) [68]. Recognizing the relationship between poverty and health outcomes prompted Canadian hospitals and government agencies to develop poverty screening tools and make it a routine part of primary care practice [66, 69].

Healthcare and Poverty: The Roots of Stigma and Attitudes

Research on health outcomes in public and HSN hospitals that treat a disproportionate number of the poor was initiated by academic centers and government agencies that were concerned and made assumptions about disparities and inequalities in the healthcare provided in these facilities. The studies generated by CMS were in response to concerns from "stakeholders" about the perceived inferior medical care provided to the poor in HSN hospitals [31], and when healthcare outcomes proved comparable among HSN and non-safety net facilities, the investigators referred to the results as "unexpected." Organizations and individuals alike have similarly perceived and articulated their biases and preconceived notions regarding the medical care provided to the poor in public and HSN hospitals.

The roots of the misconceptions about the medical care the poor receive in public facilities originated with economic shifts and the emergence of public health institutions in the United States. This historical explanation is associated with the image of public hospitals in the "collective societal mind." The years between the mid-eighteenth century to the early nineteenth century are characterized by a transition from an agrarian to an industrialized economy in the United States. This resulted in population shifts of mass immigration from foreign countries and relocation from rural US communities to overcrowded cities with no adequate or nonexistent sanitation systems. As a result, large urban communities were exposed to repeated outbreaks of cholera, dysentery, TB, typhoid fever, influenza, yellow fever, and malaria. Public hospitals such as Bellevue Hospital in New York City and Charity Hospital in New Orleans were built in response to increased needs to care and shelter "the chronically ill, deprived, and disabled" residing in large urban areas [15, 70]. These epidemics were associated with high mortality rates due to ineffective treatments and strategies to contain them [71]. By the early 1900s, the incidence of many of these epidemics declined owing to efforts by public health institutions that improved sanitation and hygiene [72]. Health departments were established and progress in disease prevention and control, improvements in municipal infrastructure (sewage and waste disposal, water treatment, food safety), and public education about hygiene were endorsed and sponsored.

Society's "collective memory" associates and links public hospitals with care provided exclusively to the poor, homeless, and "infected," who were isolated and segregated from the rest of humanity in order to prevent the spread of TB, dysentery, and the "disease poverty" [73]. The historic images in the "public's mind" are of patients carrying communicable and fatal diseases, lying in long rows of beds, lined in large, poorly lit halls, separated from one another by a flimsy curtain, awaiting their death. This is why the highly educated parents quoted in the beginning of the chapter refused to hospitalize their son in a public facility. They displayed an irrational and unfounded belief that their son will be "infected" with diseases exclusively associated with poverty and homelessness, that his care will be substandard and of poor quality, and that, by association, he will be contaminated and "branded" by the "disease of poverty." The public's attitudes, concerns, and beliefs are similar to those expressed by health policy organizations and government agencies.

The second reason for the prevailing misconceptions about the care the poor population receives in HSN and public institutions relates to shifts in healthcare economics in the United States. In the past 35 years, the United States has witness a trend that has contributed to further healthcare disparities, namely, the "commodi-fication" and "consumerization" of healthcare [74], resulting from deregulation and privatization of health services and emphasizing cost-effectiveness. As a result, health services became a "commodity" and patients are viewed as "consumers." In this healthcare model, the responsibility for health insurance shifted from state and federal agencies to individuals who believe they are entitled to a fare return on their "health investment": Private health insurance and higher premiums, deductibles, and co-pays should provide health consumers with "better" and faster care and ame-nities such as private rooms. The resultant perception is that the "haves" should be treated in exclusive healthcare facilities where the care is "superior" and partitioned from those who spend less, have state and federal health insurance, or are uninsured. This trend is an extension and continuance of the historical segregation and isola-tion of the "have not" from the rest of society.

In reality, US health economic trends are complicated, unstable, and in constant flux and change, mainly because the concept of healthcare "value" is elusive. Different health delivery systems assign different monetary values to identical pro-cedures, equipment, and labor. Furthermore, healthcare is more than a fiscal exchange for rendered services. It is about providing long-term care to individuals and communities, health education, and advocacy and expanding opportunities and improving quality of life [75]. All hospitals, including public, HSN, and for-profit institutions are tightly regulated by state and federal agencies, have internal assess-ment mechanisms, and are subjected to consumer surveys and public scrutiny. In 2008, five CEOs and medical directors discussed the efforts their institutions embarked on in order to improve medical care, as well as their vision for the future of public and HSN hospitals. They all acknowledged the commitment to improve care and medical outcomes, the efforts to expand "good customer service" and accommodate the needs of the diverse and disenfranchised population they serve, as well as praising the "high-caliber staff" [76].

In economically progressive countries such as the United States, access and high-quality healthcare are basic societal rights, not privileges. With the decline in the number of public hospitals, and the emergence of HSN facilities, a large propor-tion of the vulnerable and economically disadvantaged patients are being treated side by side patients from higher SES. In fact, HSN hospitals are becoming "soci-etal equalizers" and a "laboratory" for healthcare equality. As the affordable care act is taking effect, it is creating a unique opportunity in the history of healthcare in the United States for collaborative and multidisciplinary initiatives to bring an end to healthcare disparities that afflict the economically vulnerable. Federal and state agencies, hospitals, medical schools, and public health departments should start conversations and develop rigorous research programs to evaluate care, perceptions, and attitudes held by healthcare providers, patients, and the public in facilities pro-viding care for the poor and vulnerable. Medical schools and postgraduate programs should make the study of poverty a priority and an integral part of their curricula to promote better screening tools and services, as well as empathy and compassion for the poor population.

References

1. United Nations Development Programme. The real wealth of nations: pathways to human development. Human development report, 20th anniversary edition. New York: United Nations Development Programme; 2010.
2. Social, economic, and housing statistics division: poverty. Poverty data sources. U.S. Census Bureau; 2014. https://www.census.gov/hhes/www/poverty/about/overview/index.html.
3. Poverty in the United States: a snapshot. National Center for Law and Economic Justice. New York. 2015. http://www.nclej.org/poverty-in-the-us.php.
4. 2013 American Indian population and labor force report. U.S. Department of the Interior, Office of the Secretary. Office of the Assistant Secretary – Indian Affairs. Simon & Schuster, New York, NY; 2014.
5. Goffman E. Stigma: notes on the management of spoiled identity. Upper Saddle River: Prentice-Hall; 1963.
6. Social transformations and intellectual dialogue: poverty. United Nations educational, scientific and cultural organization. http://www.unesco.org/new/en/social-and-human-sciences/themes/international-migration/glossary/poverty/.
7. Carlock H. A different type of poverty: journalist Sasha Abramsky looks at what it means to be poor in America. U.S. News and World Report, Washington, DC; 2013.
8. Lynch JW, Kaplan GA, Shema SJ. Cumulative impact of sustained economic hardship on physical, cognitive, psychological and social functioning. N Engl J Med. 1997;337(26): 1889–95.
9. Stevens CD, Schriger DL, Raffetto B, Davis AC, Zingmond D, Roby DH. Geographic clustering of diabetic lower-extremity amputations in low-income regions of California. Health Aff. 2014;33(8):1383–90.
10. Ko F, Vitale S, Chou CF, Cotch MF, Saaddine J, Friedman DS. Prevalence of nonrefractive visual impairment in US adults and associated risk factors, 1999–2002 and 2005–2008. JAMA. 2012;308(22):2361–8.
11. Ware JE, Bayliss MS, Rogers WH, Kosinski M, Tarlov AR. Differences in 4-year health outcomes for elderly and poor, chronically ill patients treated in HMO and fee-for-service systems: results from the medical outcomes study. JAMA. 1996;276(13):1039–47.
12. Raphael D. Poverty in childhood and adverse health outcomes in adulthood. Maturitas. 2011;69(1):22–6.
13. Evans GW, Kim P. Childhood poverty and health: cumulative risk exposure and stress dysregulation. Psychol Sci. 2007;18(11):953–7.
14. Public hospitals focus on reducing health care disparities: research brief. National Association of Public Hospitals and Health Systems. Washington, DC; 2008.
15. Matos R. Hospitals in United States: historical overview. Academia; 2015. https://www.academiapublishing.org/index.htm.
16. Public hospitals decline swiftly. The Washington Times; 2005.
17. Waitzkin H. Commentary-the history and contradictions of the health care safety net. Health Serv Res. 2005;40(3):941–52.
18. What is a safety net hospital? National Association of Public Hospitals and Health Systems. Washington, DC; 2004.
19. Wynn B, Coughlin T, Bondarenko S, Bruen B. Analysis of the joint distribution of disproportionate share hospital payments: what is a safety net hospital? Assistant Secretary of Planning and Evaluation. Washington, DC: U.S. Department of Health and Human Services, under contract with the Urban Institute; 2002.
20. Ross JS, Cha SS, Epstein AJ, Wang Y, Bradley EH, Herrin J, Lichtman JH, Normand S-LT, Masoudi FA, Krumholz HM. Quality of care for acute myocardial infarction at urban safety-net hospitals. Health Aff. 2007;26(1):238–48.
21. Hadley J, Cunningham P. Availability of safety net providers and access to care of uninsured persons. Health Serv Res. 2004;39(5):1527–46.

22. What is the difference between nonprofit hospitals and for-profit hospitals. The Medicare newsgroup. 2011–2012. www.medicarenewsgroup.com.
23. American Hospital Association Resource Center. Fast facts on US hospitals. Chicago: American Hospital Association Resource Center; 2015.
24. Chen PW. The fraying hospital safety net. The New York Times, New York, NY; 2012.
25. Jones CA, Perera A, Chow M, Ho I, Nguyen J, Davachi S. Cardiovascular disease risk among the poor and homeless – what we know so far. Curr Cardiol Rev. 2009;5(1):69–77.
26. Werner RM, Goldman LE, Dudley RA. Comparison of change in quality of care between safety-net and non–safety-net hospitals. JAMA. 2008;299(18):2180–7.
27. O'Connell GM. Comparisons of safety-net and non-safety net hospitals, letters to the editor. JAMA. 2008;300(14):1650–2.
28. Medicare Hospital Quality Chartbook: performance report on outcome measures for acute myocardial infarction, heart failure and pneumonia. Center for Medicare and Medicaid services, Yale Health System Corporation, Center for Outcomes Research and Evaluation, Baltimore, MD; 2010.
29. Ross JS, Bernheim SM, Lin Z, Drye EE, Chen J, Normand S-LT, Krumholz HM. Based on key measures, care quality for Medicare enrollees at safety-net and non-safety net hospitals was almost equal. Health Aff. 2012;8:1739–48.
30. Medicare Hospital Quality Chartbook: performance report on readmission measures for acute myocardial infarction, heart failure and pneumonia. Center for Medicare and Medicaid services, Yale Health System Corporation, Center for Outcomes Research and Evaluation, Baltimore, MD; 2011.
31. Medicare Hospital Quality Chartbook: performance report on outcome measures for acute myocardial infarction, heart failure and pneumonia mortality and readmission. Center for Medicare and Medicaid services, Yale Health System Corporation, Center for Outcomes Research and Evaluation, Baltimore, MD; 2012.
32. Medicare Hospital Quality Chartbook: performance report on outcome measures for acute myocardial infarction, heart failure, pneumonia, hip/knee arthroplasty. Center for Medicare and Medicaid services, Yale Health System Corporation, Center for Outcomes Research and Evaluation, Baltimore, MD; 2013.
33. Medicare Hospital Quality Chartbook: performance report on outcome measures for acute myocardial infarction, heart failure, pneumonia, COPD, ischemic stroke hip and/or knee arthroplasty and isolated CABG surgery. Center for Medicare and Medicaid services, Yale Health System Corporation, Center for Outcomes Research and Evaluation, Baltimore, MD; 2014.
34. Colorectal Cancer. Facts & figures 2014–2016. Atlanta: American Cancer Society; 2014.
35. Doubeni CA, Laiyemo AO, Major JM, Schootman M, Lian M, Park Y, Graubard BI, Hollenbeck AR, Sinha R. Socioeconomic status and the risk of colorectal cancer: an analysis of over one-half million adults in the NIH-AARP Diet and Health Study. Cancer. 2012;118(14):3636–44.
36. Bradley CJ, Dahman B, Sabik LM. Differences in emergency colorectal surgery in Medicaid and uninsured patients by hospital safety net status. Am J Manag Care. 2015;21(2):e161–70.
37. Millas SG, Alawadi ZM, Wray CJ, Silberfein EJ, Escamilla RJ, Karanjawala BE, Ko TC, Kao LS. Treatment delays of colon cancer in a safety-net hospital system. J Surg Res. 2015 [Epub ahead of print].
38. Blegen MA, Goode CJ, Spetz J, Vaughn T, Park SH. Nurse staffing effects on patient outcomes: safety-net and non-safety-net hospitals. Med Care. 2011;49(4):406–14.
39. Fee C, Burstin H, Maselli JH, Hsia RY. Association of emergency department length of stay with safety-net status. JAMA. 2012;307(5):476–82.
40. Hudson GC. Socioeconomic status and mental illness: tests of the social causation and selection hypotheses. Am J Orthopsychiatry. 2005;75(1):3–18.
41. Torrey EF, Entsminger K, Geller J, Stanley J, Jaffe DJ. The shortage of public hospital beds for mentally ill persons. Arlington: The Treatment Advocacy Center, Arlington, VA; 2008.

42. Culhane DP, Hadley TR. The discriminating characteristics of for-profit versus not-for-profit freestanding psychiatric inpatient facilities. Health Serv Res. 1992;27(2):177–94.
43. Garfield R. Mental health financing in the United States: a primer. Washington: The Kaiser Commission on Medicaid and the Uninsured, Washington, DC; 2011.
44. Pellegrini LC, Rodriguez-Monguio R. Medicaid provisions and the US mental health industry composition. J Ment Health. 2014;23(6):312–6.
45. Chow J, Jaffe K, Snowden L. Racial/ethnic disparities in the use of mental health services in poverty areas. Am J Public Health. 2003;93(5):792–7.
46. Moczygemba LR, Osborn RD, Lapane KL. Adherence to behavioral therapy and psychiatry visits in a safety-net setting in Virginia, USA. Health Soc Care Community. 2014;22(5):469–78.
47. Mental illness and homelessness. National coalition for the homeless. Washington, DC; 2009. http://www.nationalhomeless.org.
48. Olfson M, Mechanic D. Mental disorders in public, private nonprofit, and proprietary general hospitals. Am J Psychiatr. 1996;153(12):1613–9.
49. Shen JJ, Cochran CR, Moseley CB. From the emergency department to the general hospital: hospital ownership and market factors in the admission of the seriously mentally ill. J Healthc Manag. 2008;53(4):268–79.
50. Rosenau PV, Linder SH. A comparison of the performance of for-profit and nonprofit U.S. psychiatric inpatient care providers since 1980. Psychiatr Serv. 2003;54(2):183–7.
51. Wittenauer J, Ludwick R, Baughman K, Fishbein R. Surveying the hidden attitudes of hospital nurses' towards poverty. J Clin Nurs. 2015;24(15–16):184–91.
52. Patterson N, Hulton LJ. Enhancing nursing students' understanding of poverty through simulation. Public Health Nurs. 2012;29(2):143–51.
53. Reutter LI, Sword W, Meagher-Stewart D, Rideout E. Nursing students' beliefs about poverty and health. J Adv Nurs. 2004;48(3):299–309.
54. Social workers at work. Center for workforce studies. Washington, DC: National Association of Social Workers; 2008.
55. Reeser LC, Epstein I. Social workers' attitudes toward poverty and social action: 1968–1984. Soc Serv Rev. 1987;61(4):610–22.
56. Cozzarelli C, Wilkinson AV, Tagler MJ. Attitudes toward the poor and attributions for poverty. J Soc Issues. 2001;57(2):207–27.
57. Spenciner-Rosenthal B. Graduate social work students' beliefs about poverty and attitudes toward the poor. J Teach Soc Work. 1993;7(1):107–21.
58. Wear D, Kuczewski MG. Perspective: medical students' perceptions of the poor: what impact can medical education have? Acad Med. 2008;83(7):639–45.
59. Smith-Campbell B. A health professional students' cultural competence and attitudes toward the poor: the influence of a clinical practicum supported by the National Health Service Corps. J Allied Health. 2005;34(1):56–62.
60. Henderson S, Stacey CL, Dohan D. Social stigma and the dilemmas of providing care to substance users in a safety-net emergency department. J Health Care Poor Underserved. 2008;19(4):1336–49.
61. Shortage of pillows in public hospitals. Chloeplace. 2015. http://www.essentialbaby.com.au/forums/index.php?/topic/1147154-shortage-of-pillows-in-public-hospitals/.
62. Samra R, Griffiths A, Cox T, Conroy S, Gordon A, Gladman JR. Medical students' and doctors' attitudes toward older patients and their care in hospital setting: a conceptualization. Age Ageing. 2015;44(5):776–83.
63. LaVeist TA. Attitudes about racism, medical mistrust, and satisfaction with care among African Americans and white cardiac patients. Med Care Res Rev. 2000;57(4):146–61.
64. Krutsinger A, Tarr N. Poverty fact sheet: implications for infants and toddlers. Washington, DC: Zero To Three. National Center for Infants, Toddlers and Families; 2011.

65. Farah MJ, Shera DM, Savage JA, Betancourt L, Giannetta JM, Brodsky NL, Malmud EK, Hurt H. Childhood poverty: specific associations with neurocognitive development. Brain Res. 2006;1110:166–74.
66. Block G. Poverty: a clinical tool for primary care in Ontario. Toronto: Ontario College of Family Physicians. University of Toronto; 2013.
67. Steele CB, Rim SH, Joseph DA, King JB, Seeff, LC. Colorectal Cancer Incidence and Screening—United States. 2008;2010;53–60. In Health disparities and inequalities report United States. Morb Mortal Wkly Rep. 2013;62(3). Center for disease Control and Prevention, Atlanta.
68. Buchman S. Screening for poverty in family practice. Can Fam Physician. 2012;58(6):709.
69. Brcic V, Eberdt C, Kaczorowski J. Development of a tool to identify poverty in a family practice setting: a pilot study. Int J Family Med. 2011;2011:1–7.
70. History of Public Hospitals in the United States. America's Essential Hospitals. Washington, DC. [http://essentialhospitals.org/about-americas-essential-hospitals/history-of-public-hospitals-in-the-united-states/].
71. The worst disease outbreaks in history: from the smallpox epidemics in the 17th century to whooping cough outbreak of last year. Healthline editorial team, Healthline Network; 2013. http://www.healthline.com/health/worst-disease-outbreaks-history#Overview1.
72. Achievements in public health, 1900–1999: control of infectious diseases. Morb Mortal Wkly Rep. 1999;48(29):621–9. Center for Disease Control and Prevention, Atlanta.
73. Lieberman T. This doctor treats poverty like a disease. Center for Advancing Health; 2013. http://www.cfah.org/blog/2013/this-doctor-treats-poverty-like-a-disease.
74. Henderson S, Petersen A, editors. Consuming health: the commodification of health care. London: Routledge; 2002.
75. Poor health: poverty and scarce resources in U.S. cities. Pittsburgh Post-Gazette. 14 June 2014. http://newsinteractive.post-gazette.com/longform/stories/poorhealth/1/.
76. Janisse T, Wong WF. Innovation in our nation's public hospitals: interview with five CEOs and medical directors. Perm J. 2008;12(1):66–74.

Chapter 5
Stigma and Prejudice Against Individuals Experiencing Homelessness

Denise De Las Nueces

Introduction

For many Americans, homelessness is a specter of "otherness," one that haunts the lives of others but does not, and never could, affect their own. But the reality is that homelessness is a problem far larger than what many believe and can affect any of us at any time. National data prove that homeless individuals, often regarded by general society as not worthy of even a passing glance, are anything but invisible. Over two million people experience homelessness each year in the United States [1]. In a single night in January 2014, nationwide point-in-time estimates compiled by the US Department of Housing and Urban Development (HUD) revealed that 578,424 people across the United States were homeless, most staying in emergency shelters or transitional facilities across the country. Of these individuals, roughly a quarter of them were homeless children aged less than 18, and more than two-thirds of them were 25 years or older; 37 % of these individuals were members of homeless families, and 11 % of them were homeless veterans. The burden of homelessness is greatest in the State of California, at 20 % of the share of the national homeless population, with California, New York, Florida, Texas, and Massachusetts collectively accounting for more than half of the homeless population in the United States [2].

Those these numbers are not insignificant, homeless individuals every day struggle with experiences that make them feel marginalized, less than, and frankly

D. De Las Nueces, MD, MPH
Boston Health Care for the Homeless Program, 780 Albany Street,
Boston, MA 02118, USA

Department of Medicine, Boston University Medical Center,
Boston University School of Medicine, Boston, MA, USA
e-mail: ddelasnueces@bhchp.org

© Springer International Publishing Switzerland 2016   85
R. Parekh, Ed W. Childs (eds.), *Stigma and Prejudice: Touchstones in Understanding Diversity in Healthcare*, Current Clinical Psychiatry,
DOI 10.1007/978-3-319-27580-2_5

discriminated against. Individuals experiencing homelessness are subject to stigma that not only colors their day-to-day lives but also renders them exquisitely vulnerable to violence and can even affect the quality of health care they receive. This stigma can lead to perceptions of a second-class citizenship that can, implicitly and explicitly, render the very individuals experiencing homelessness seemingly powerless in their attempts to free themselves from their current circumstances. Stigma and prejudice against the homeless population can take the form of overt manifestations, as with anti-homeless violence, or insidious ones, as with measures that criminalize activities associated with homelessness.

This chapter will review the scope of anti-homeless stigma in society today, first by defining homelessness and then by examining the roots of anti-homeless sentiments through a review of the history of homelessness in the United States. The current manifestations of anti-homeless stigma as reflected in today's local legislation, violence against the homeless population, and health care disparities will also be examined. Lastly, recommendations on how to compassionately care for and attend to the health care needs of the homeless population will be reviewed, as well as future directions that can be taken to help eliminate anti-homeless stigma in health care settings.

Homelessness Defined

Before understanding the nature of and extent of stigma against the homeless population, one must first understand how homelessness is defined today and how homelessness has evolved over the course of American history. According to the McKinney-Vento Homeless Assistance Act of 1999, which provides federal funding for homeless shelters across the nation, the term *homeless* refers to an individual or family that (a) lacks a regular, adequate residence, (b) has a primary residence that is a private or public place not ordinarily used for sleeping accommodations, (c) resides in a supervised shelter, or (d) is at risk of imminently losing housing [3].

Homelessness is far from a homogenous, one-size-fits-all condition. Rather, it can take many forms, ranging from a transient to a more permanent lack of housing. *Chronic homelessness* refers to individuals who have been continuously homeless for one or more years or who have experienced at least four episodes of homelessness in the last 3 years. For individuals who are chronically homeless, shelter living is not a temporary emergency state, but rather a long-term condition. These individuals often struggle with concurrent long-term disability, debilitating chronic medical conditions (such as diabetes mellitus, chronic obstructive pulmonary disease, and congestive heart failure), mental health issues, or substance use disorders, all of which pose increased challenges to breaking the cycle of chronic homelessness. Individuals experiencing *transitional homelessness* are those who enter the shelter system for a limited period of time, often after a catastrophic event (such as a job loss, home foreclosure, or natural disaster), before transitioning back into stable permanent housing.

Lastly, *episodic homelessness* refers to those individuals who toggle back and forth between housing and homelessness, often due to concurrent challenges (such as mental health issues, substance use disorders, and/or disabilities) that impede their ability to maintain stable employment and permanent housing [4].

History of Homelessness in the United States

A true understanding of the state of stigma, prejudice, and discrimination against individuals and families experiencing homelessness today requires a look at the history of homelessness in the United States and how our unique history has set the foundation for and continues to shape anti-homeless sentiments today. Nineteenth-century poet Emma Lazarus' words, erected on the Statue of Liberty in New York's Ellis Island, boldly proclaim:

> Give me your tired, your poor,
> Your huddled masses yearning to breathe free,
> The wretched refuse of your teeming shore.
> Send these, the homeless, tempest-tost to me,
> I lift my lamp beside the golden door!

These words convey a sense of hope and the promise of a better life in the United States for society's downtrodden, homeless masses. But history reveals that for many, this promise was often a mere illusion, a false hope for those entering a nation that has historically viewed homeless individuals as victims of their own design who succumbed to the vice of idleness.

The history of homelessness in America, and anti-homeless sentiments, can be traced as far back as colonial times. During the seventeenth and early eighteenth centuries, most homelessness, referred to at the time as *vagrancy*, was rooted in the effects of warfare, which uprooted families from their settlements and forced them into coastal towns where they were often unwanted. The prevailing Puritan theology at the time, which upheld the spiritual value of work and productivity, led many to view vagrants quite negatively, as the moral dregs of society and the personification of sin and unworthiness. Vagrants and beggars were seen as a plague on civil society who should, in the words of a prominent Calvinist theologian at the time, be "taken as enemies of this ordinance of God." In 1679, Massachusetts passed an act requiring vagrants and beggars who held an "idle and riotous life" to be forced into labor as servants. Practices such as these underscored the belief that if vagrants would not willingly engage in productive labor, it was society's moral imperative to force them to do so. The Puritans distinguished between the "worthy" poor, those vagrants unable to work due to illness or age, and the "unworthy" wandering poor, whose unfortunate circumstances were viewed solely as manifestations of the sin of idleness and who had no place in civilized society. Towns established workhouses, where "rogues, vagabonds, common beggars, and other lewd and disorderly persons" were subject to corporeal punishment if they refused to engage in labor [5].

In the eighteenth century, the colonial population of vagrants and beggars increased periodically, mostly as a result of economic downturns in local and world markets. New York City, which had previously been witness to little poverty, experienced an influx of larger numbers of beggars and vagrants in the 1720s and 1730s. Its response was the construction, in 1734, of the first public building to incarcerate beggars, named the "Poor House, Work House, and House of Correction." That the city's first response to vagrancy was to criminalize homelessness in this way again reflects the era's prevailing philosophy that unemployed, idle vagrants were seen as a pestilence to society requiring not benevolence, but rather correction via the enforcement of labor [5].

The immigration of poor Europeans to the states during the nineteenth century, the very masses that Lazarus' words welcome on the Statue of Liberty, also spurred an increase in homelessness. These masses were greeted with as much scorn as their native-born counterparts. Public officials in Philadelphia and Boston often turned immigrants, many from Ireland, away, ordering to leave the towns at once. Public welfare was limited to use only by legal city residents in many Northern urban centers. Indentured servants and runaway slaves also contributed o the homeless population in Northern states. Though vagrants were present in the antebellum South, homelessness was not as significant a problem in the South as in the North at the time [5].

The nineteenth century marked the onset of the industrial revolution, and with it a rapidly growing divide between rich and poor that was especially notable in urban centers experiencing swift population growth. By the mid-nineteenth century, European immigrants comprised a large portion of the homeless population in urban settings. The rise in homelessness led authorities in many cities to turn to law enforcement to deal with the "scourge of vagrancy." Police stations began to offer overnight emergency lodging for homeless individuals, and anti-vagrancy laws were passed to enforce harsh penalties for begging outdoors. In light of the growing prevalence of homelessness, private charitable organizations were established to help combat poverty and homelessness. These organizations often espoused conflicting ideologies and approaches to almsgiving. In Philadelphia, the Western Soup Society was founded in 1837, in a year of economic depression. A first of its kind, this soup kitchen's mission was to provide soup daily to the poor, without regard to the "worthiness" or "unworthiness" of beneficiaries. Many critics at the time accused the organization of feeding into the idleness of the poor and disincentivizing individual industry and self-reliance. Other charitable organizations of the time were established based on a philosophy of "unsentimental, scientific" almsgiving aimed at serving only the "worthy" poor who were willing to engage in labor. One such organization, the New York Society for the Prevention of Pauperism, founded in 1817, once campaigned to outlaw all outdoor poor relief in favor of workhouses for the able-bodied poor. This ideology of scientific almsgiving also affected local governments' responses to homelessness. Outdoor relief efforts such as the distribution of food and clothing were outlawed for several years in the early- to mid-nineteenth century in Philadelphia and Chicago. Only in the mid-1800s did this moralistic view of poverty start to lose traction, as prominent literary authors (such as Charles Dickens and Victor Hugo) shed a sympathetic light on the plights of the poor, and economic downturns underscored that poverty was a consequence of unfortunate circumstances to which anyone was vulnerable [5].

The post-Civil War period defined a major turning point in the national conceptualization of homelessness. This time period marked the birth of the terms *tramp* and *bum*, both words with roots in the military, in reference to homeless vagrants. During the final years of the Civil War, soldiers would frequently go *tramping* about homes encountered along major roads, foraging the properties for food. After the war, many of these veterans, suffering from war-incurred physical disabilities and psychological trauma that complicated their reintegration into civilian life, continued to engage in such foraging, much to the dismay of landowners. This behavior laid the foundation for the national characterization of vagrants as aimless criminals and threatening figures. The terms tramp and bum, the latter of which is derived from the derogatory word bummer in reference to an idle person, thereafter emerged to describe homeless vagabonds in the post-bellum period [5].

The rise of the railroad and western expansion subsequently allowed these vagrants, who had previously been confined mostly to urban settings in the Eastern seaboard, to travel to rural territories in the Midwest and West Coast, where they were encountered with fear by settlers who had no prior experience with these downtrodden masses. Vagrants would often hitch rides in railroads, whose crew viewed them as a menace to fare-paying customers. By the end of the nineteenth century, the life of a vagrant 'tramp' was synonymous with one of laziness and criminality, a notion that was propagated in the literature and media of the time. Perhaps most illustrative of this are the words published in a Pennsylvania newspaper in the 1870s, where vagrant 'tramps' were described as leeches that sucked the lifeblood of society. New Jersey passed the nation's first "anti-tramp" law in 1876, allowing authorities to arrest vagrants and force them into brief sentences of labor in workhouses. Police station lodging in urban centers slowly grew out of favor, and wayfarer lodges, which provided meals and overnight emergency shelter to homeless individuals in exchange for labor, were established in several major cities [5].

Important demographic changes and shifts in the national attitudes on homelessness occurred in the twentieth century. Unlike their Reconstruction Era counterparts, turn of the century 'tramps' were no longer vilified, largely due to the aging out of Civil War veterans from the vagrant population and romanticization of the 'tramp' in literature and the arts, as with Charlie Chaplin's portrayals in several moving pictures. In addition, the early twentieth century saw a rise in the number of charitable organizations aimed at providing aid to homeless individuals and families, though many organizations still upheld the moralistic ideology that aid should only be given to impoverished individuals who were willing to work in exchange for support.

The Great Depression heralded an increase in the homeless population nationwide, as well as a notable increase in the population of homeless women, who alongside their families had fallen into homelessness during the Depression, and homeless African Americans, who were often the first to suffer from layoffs during the economic downturn. Urban settlements where homeless individuals fashioned shelters of tin, cardboard, and paper, called *shantytowns*, sprung up in several urban areas around the country. Homeless individuals were often not treated with the same hostility that had been historically witnessed in past economic downturns, likely reflecting a national awareness of the vulnerability of all individuals to unpredictable turns of fortune and circumstance. Formerly white collar workers such as store managers and sale clerks found themselves sharing breadlines and soup kitchens with the chronically homeless. During this era of national hardship, the term *tramp* was slowly replaced by the more neutral term *transient*, which unlike its predecessor bore no hint of judgment [5].

Whereas the provision of emergency shelter and aid had previously been exclusively the purview of municipal governments and private organizations, President Franklin D. Roosevelt's New Deal heralded the establishment in 1933 of the Federal Transient Service (FTS), the first federal agency in national history dedicated to providing relief services for homeless individuals. Under the FTS, several federally run shelters, called *transient centers*, arose around the country. These centers eschewed the traditional moralistic philosophy that had been upheld by many private and municipal charity organizations of the past. Though chores were expected of individuals who lodged at the centers, work was not a mandatory requirement to receiving aid. Furthermore, the transient centers innovatively focused not only on the provision of food and lodging but also on the delivery of health care, dental care, educational activities, and employment training opportunities. The transient centers were so successful that the number of transients in shantytowns and on the road decreased substantially while they were in operation. Unfortunately, the success of the FTS, though promising, was short lived. By 1935, the FTS had been dissolved as the Roosevelt administration shifted its attention to broader-scale federal projects such as social security [5].

Unsurprisingly, the number of shantytowns and the homeless population rose soon after the closure of the federal transient centers. As the nation moved from the Depression Era to World War II and increasing industrialization, the homeless population underwent yet another demographic shift to an older, more male-predominant and less mobile population. Chronic settlement in *skid rows*, segregated settlements of low-income temporary lodging in cities and towns, became more commonplace. African Americans, migrant Mexican and Mexican-American workers, and Puerto Ricans grew to comprise a larger portion of the homeless population in the Northeast and West Coast in the 1940–1960s. Stereotypes of homeless individuals as "idle 'bums'" reemerged. State and municipal governments attempted to crack down on the "nuisance" of homelessness by criminalizing activities related to homelessness. The threshold for arrest of homeless individuals, often for minor offenses such as public intoxication and disorderly conduct, grew lower, and police roundups of homeless individuals in skid rows became increasingly more common. By the 1970s, urban renewal efforts led to the eradication of skid rows in several cities around the country [5].

Over the ensuing 30 years, the homeless population again experienced a demographic transformation, shaped by the economic and political climate of the times. Increased safety net benefits for the elderly and a lack of parallel supports for the young rendered the homeless population younger, on average, than its skid row counterpart decades earlier. The economic recession of the 1980s disproportionately affected racial minorities, rendering the national homeless population more diverse than it had ever been by the mid-1990s (41 % Black and 11 % Hispanic). Police roundups and criminalization of activities related to homelessness continued [5].

Despite considerable advances in technology, health care, economics, and the sciences, a solution to homelessness remains elusive in the twenty-first century. Today, the causes of homelessness remain varied, complex, and multifactorial, but a few themes stand out as modern iterations of the same leitmotifs that have persisted throughout the history of American homelessness. Vulnerability to economic downturns is one such theme. The subprime mortgage crisis of 2007 heralded another era of economic recession, shrinking the middle class and catapulting many individuals and families into homelessness due to unforeseen home foreclosures. As domestic and international markets suffered, the national unemployment rate peaked at 9.9 % in 2009 [6]. Affordable housing remains elusive to many. The National Low Income Housing Coalition reports that in 2014, the two-bedroom housing wage (the hourly full-time wage a household must earn in order to afford a unit while spending no more than 30 % of total income on housing costs) was estimated at $18.92, more than 2.5 times the federal minimum wage and 52 % higher than it was in 2000 [7]. Racial and ethnic minorities continue to comprise up to 50 % of the nation's homeless population, with veterans representing up to a third of the homeless male population [8]. Families continue to be deeply affected, with approximately 2.5 million children (representing 1 child in every 30) experiencing homelessness in the United States in 2013 [9].

Discrimination Against the Homeless Population Today

The modern age has not heralded a solution to the problem of homelessness, and therefore it should come as no surprise that today's homeless population continues to struggle under the weight of oppressive discrimination and stigma. Foremost among this discrimination is the continued insidiousness, as in centuries past, of legislation aimed at criminalizing activities related to homelessness. A report by the National Coalition for the Homeless and the National Law Center on Homelessness and Poverty highlights that many cities have enacted ordinances placing severe restrictions on sleeping/camping, eating, sitting, and panhandling in public. Of 235 American cities surveyed for the report, 33 % had anti-camping laws restricting camping in certain public places, 17 % had city-wide restrictions on camping, and 47 % prohibited panhandling in certain public places, with 23 % instituting city-wide restrictions on panhandling. In one American city, the police department's focus on crime in the city's skid row resulted in disproportionate citations and arrests of homeless individuals, as highlighted by the arrest of the same 24 people a total of 201 times over an 11-month period in 2007. Homeless individuals in this city were also subject to selective enforcement of laws against certain activities—such as loitering or jaywalking—that would normally not have resulted in citations in other parts of the city [10].

Other American cities have even gone as far as prohibiting food sharing in public parks. The city of Orlando, Florida, passed a law in 2006 restricting groups from sharing food with more than 25 people more than twice a year in certain public parks. Legislators voiced safety and sanitation issues as the motivation behind the ordinance, but in essence the law created restrictions on public charity groups that provided regular weekly meal services to homeless individuals. In Lake Worth, Florida, legislation has been passed prohibiting the sharing of food, by a large group, with people experiencing homelessness in a public park. The city of Raleigh, North Carolina, does not completely eliminate the opportunity to distribute meals in public parks, but does require the purchase of a permit which costs up to $800 a day before such food distribution efforts can be legally executed [11]. One can argue that these ordinances are modern-day manifestations of the same ideology that led Philadelphia and Chicago to briefly abolish all outdoor relief efforts in the mid-1800s.

Anti-homeless practices today also take the form of city sweeps of public homeless encampments. In August 2014, the city of New Orleans, Louisiana, citing a public health hazard, cleared out a tent city encampment of over 140 people under a city expressway, an act reminiscent of the destruction of shantytowns by officials in the post-FTS era. A month later, in September 2014, the New Orleans City Council voted to ban tents and large items of furniture from public spaces in New Orleans [12].

Anti-homeless Violence

Anti-homeless discrimination today often takes much more brutal and overt forms than discriminatory legislation. A survey by the National Coalition for the Homeless (NCH) reports that from 1999 to 2013, a total of 1,437 acts of violence against homeless individuals by housed perpetrators were reported. Of those attacks, 347 proved fatal. In 2013, the NCH reported a total of 109 attacks, 18 of which were fatal. A review of these attacks by the NCH reveals that while 90 % of the victims in 2013 were middle-aged men, with an average age of 44 years, the housed perpetrators were most often young men (48 % of perpetrators in 2013 were under the age of 20). Case descriptions of these attacks reveal the heinousness of these crimes: from the murder of a 71-year-old homeless veteran, who was stabbed over 70 times by a 21-year-old man in Doylestown, Pennsylvania; the fatal assault of a 54-year-old homeless man by three teenagers in New Port Richey, Florida; the case of a disabled homeless veteran in Los Angeles, California, who had gasoline poured on him and was set on fire while sleeping in his wheelchair at a local library; to the assault of a mentally ill 52-year-old homeless man by police officers in Columbia, South Carolina, after his arrest for sleeping on the University of South Carolina campus [13].

Homeless individuals are also at risk of sexual assault, forced prostitution, human trafficking, and media exploitation, as the 2013 NCH report highlights. The report describes a case in which two homeless women were raped and assaulted by young men in Portland, Oregon in 2013. That same year, in Dania Beach, Florida, a 27-year-old man lured a homeless woman into forced prostitution by offering her shelter. In this age of multimedia, attacks on homeless individuals are often posted on public websites, where they can be viewed by many and can inspire copycat assaults. The NCH report cites a series of videos posted online over the past decade called "Bum Fights," where homeless individuals are lured to engage in fights or dangerous stunts in exchange for compensation of some form (such as food, drink, or cash). The NCH reports that these "Bum Fights" have incurred more than seven million views on YouTube, underscoring the popularity of these exploitative videos [13].

Health Care Disparities

Research reveals that anti-homeless stigma and discrimination reflected by the general population, municipal governments, and law enforcement unfortunately often spills into the health care system, marring homeless individuals' experiences in obtaining medical care. A 2008 qualitative analysis of 15 homeless adults who sought care at a free clinic in an inner city of Connecticut revealed how such stigma can pose barriers to homeless individuals' efforts to seek care. Patients' own words paint a picture of their experiences with stigmatization, disrespect, and devaluation on the basis of their homelessness, with one participant reporting: "They don't treat you like you're a human being. On the ward I was on, the workers treat you like you're stupid" [14]. A 2014 qualitative study surveying 20 homeless patients with diagnoses of active alcohol use disorder who frequented a safety net hospital in New York City further touches on the stigma that homeless patients, and in particular those struggling with addiction, can face when seeking care, with one participant reporting: "A part of me feels like I've abused the services, but I feel like after a while they kind of look at you—'Oh you again'—and they stick you in a corner and let you sleep it off, and then once they see that you can get up and walk around, they let you go home" [15]. Wen and colleagues identified similar concerns about anti-homeless stigma in the Canadian medical system after conducting a qualitative analysis of interviews of 17 homeless male and female clients of shelters in Toronto, Canada. Major themes that emerged in those interviews included experiences of health care encounters that were perceived by homeless individuals as rushed, rude, and disrespectful. One patient in the study notes that "...on two occasions I had reason to believe that because I'm in a shelter, it's like secondary treatment, not as how we envisage it should be when you go to accident and emergency [an emergency department]." Another stated "I get to the point where I don't really, I don't know, trust or like physicians. More and more I see it as almost they would sooner deal with rich people, people with good insurance, and everything else." And yet another patient reported "I'm not going to get treated like that, I'm not going through that again. I'd rather sit here and f---n'die on a bench than go over there" [16].

Reading these testimonies underscores how the stigma and discrimination that homeless individuals experience can affect their utilization of health care services. In a study of 558 homeless adults in Boston who died between 1988 and 1993, Hwang and colleagues noted that about one-quarter of the cohort had no evidence of direct contact with safety net health care institutions in the year prior to death [17]. Anti-homeless stigma and discrimination in the health care system may help explain why, in this cohort, homeless individuals seemed to underuse health care services even when death was most imminent. A recent study by Baggett and colleagues evaluated the responses of 966 homeless individuals who participated in the national 2003 Health Care for the Homeless Survey. The study revealed that 73 % of respondents reported at least one unmet health care need (as defined as medical or surgical care, prescription medications, mental health or counseling, eyeglasses, or dental care) in the past year, with 49 % of respondents reporting two or more unmet needs in that period of time [18]. The most common reasons cited by respondents for these unmet needs were inability to afford care and lack of insurance coverage, though one wonders whether the alienating and unwelcoming effects of anti-homeless stigma and discrimination in the health care delivery system also played an implicit role.

Anti-homeless stigma experienced by homeless individuals often manifests, as with other marginalized populations, in significant health care disparities. Research studies on mortality and health outcomes among homeless individuals have consistently revealed a relationship between homelessness and premature mortality. A recent review of the literature on premature mortality in homeless populations reveals that homeless persons are three to four times more likely to die than aged-matched controls in the general population, with the average age at time of death, in review of national and international research at the time, falling between 42 and 52 years for homeless individuals [19].

Research focusing on the homeless populations of individual American cities further underscores the alarming trend of premature mortality that characterizes this disadvantaged population. In Philadelphia, Hibbs and colleagues discovered that the age-adjusted mortality rates of a cohort of 6308 homeless individuals aged 17–74 years in Philadelphia between 1985 and 1988 were 3.5 times that of the city's general population [20]. Barrow and colleagues analyzed National Death Index data to study the mortality rate of 1260 homeless male and female clients of New York City shelters in 1987. Results revealed that age-adjusted mortality rates for these individuals were four times that of the general US population [21]. In Boston, Hwang et al. evaluated a cohort of 17, 292 adult individuals who were patients of the Boston Health Care for the Homeless Program from 1988 to 1993. The analysis revealed that among the predominantly male (68 %) cohort, the average age at time of death was 47 years. The leading cause of death among individuals aged 18–24 years and women aged 25–44 years was homicide. HIV/AIDS emerged as the leading cause of death among all individuals aged 25–44 years, while heart disease and cancer were identified as the leading causes of death among all individuals in the cohort aged 45–64 years [22].

This analysis was repeated and updated in 2013 by Baggett and colleagues, who evaluated the mortality rates of 28,033 adults who were patients at the Boston Health Care for the Homeless Program from 2003 to 2008. Though the study revealed no significant differences in adjusted mortality rates among this adult cohort as compared to the 1988–1993 cohort, several important distinctions did emerge. First, the mean age at time of death, though still low compared to the general population, increased from 47 years in the 1988–1993 cohort to 51 years in the 2003–2008 cohort. Importantly, the leading cause of death in the entire cohort was now drug overdose, reflecting the effects of the substance use disorder epidemic in Massachusetts [23]. A follow-up study by Baggett et al. on this same cohort revealed that 51.9 % of all deaths in the 2003–2008 cohort were attributable to substance use disorder (involving tobacco, alcohol, and/or illicit drugs) [24].

A Primer on Compassionate Care of the Homeless Population: Recommendations from Consumers and Staff Members at Boston Health Care for the Homeless Program

The author would like to use Boston Health Care for the Homeless Program (BHCHP) and the collective experience of some of its consumers and staff members to highlight a pragmatic approach to the compassionate care of homeless individuals for students, clinicians, and practitioners of all disciplines. The following pearls represent the collective expertise of consumers on BHCHP's active and talented Consumer Advisory Board, which consists of seven homeless or formerly homeless men and women who meet monthly to develop the program's advocacy agenda and provide feedback that helps shape clinical services at BHCHP. This approach has, in our programmatic experience, exemplified a patient-centered, compassionate, stigma-free model that has served as a foundation for the welcoming environment that characterizes the services provided at BHCHP.

Meet Patients Where They Are and Follow Their, Not One's Own, Agenda

Individuals experiencing homelessness by definition are struggling, on a day-to-day basis, to meet the basic human needs of finding food and shelter. This means that when they seek medical care, they may not be ready or able to address the care team's agenda for completion of tests and management of chronic diseases. The competing priorities inherent to a life of homelessness may render finding a warm bed, a meal, a roof over their heads, and a place to rest their weary feet the most important items on their agenda for an emergency room visit. A patient with advanced lung disease may not yet be ready to cut down on her excessive cigarette smoking, despite being at risk for worsened lung disease and lung cancer, if the comfort provided by those cigarettes helps allay the wearisome anxiety that accompanies a history of past trauma.

It is therefore of utmost importance for practitioners to meet homeless individuals where they are. Use every clinical encounter to learn what a homeless patient's agenda and goals may be for himself or herself. See every clinical encounter as an opportunity to learn more about the patient as a person and to develop a relationship that is grounded in trust. Listening to their stories, worries, and concerns is in and of itself truly powerful and moving and is a gift that is often not afforded to homeless individuals in the busy arena of health care. Once a foundation of trust and nonjudgment has been laid, clinicians will experience greater success in working with patients to help them achieve the patients' health care self-management goals.

Recognize the Power of Touch

The power of touch is often taken for granted by those of us who have never experienced homelessness. But having others avoid a simple handshake is not an uncommon experience for homeless individuals who may not have consistent access to showering and toileting facilities. This experience, in particular when persistent, can help further their sense of marginalization and alienation. Clinical encounters that begin with eye contact, a handshake, and a respectful salutation including the patient's last name ("Good morning, Mr. Jones") can make all the difference between starting a clinical encounter on a patient-centered and compassionate foot and initiating a clinical encounter that will be experienced by a homeless individual as degrading, rushed, and disrespectful.

The story of BHCHP's founding beautifully exemplifies the importance of touch. In his collection of stories and essays entitled *Stories from the Shadows: Reflections of a Street Doctor*, BHCHP's founder and current President, Dr. James O'Connell, chronicles his first experiences with the Nurse's Clinic at Boston's Pine Street Inn Shelter in 1985 [25]. There, Dr. O'Connell, who had just completed a rigorous internal medicine residency program at an intensive tertiary care medical center in Boston, discovered, under the tutelage of a dynamic nurse named Barbara McInnis, that all patient visits began with a footsoak and foot care. The symbolism of that footsoak—which upended the patient-clinician dynamic that homeless patients were so used to, putting clinicians at the feet of their patients as a representation of humility and service—helped set the tone for BHCHP upon its founding. Today, BHCHP's success as a homeless health care program can largely be attributed to its philosophy of trust building, humility, service, and compassion for the struggles faced by the homeless population.

Demonstrate Non-judgment

The most important part of a successful clinical interaction with individuals experiencing homelessness is grounding the interaction in nonjudgment. The homeless population already confronts the stigma of judgment based on their lack of housing, their appearance, etc. on a daily basis as noted above. We must strive to therefore foster clinical encounters that are rooted in nonjudgment. For instance, if a clinical encounter requires the collection of sensitive information from the patient, such as whether the patient engages in active substance use or whether a patient engages in sex work in order to earn an income, one recommendation is to preface the question by reassuring the patient that the question is a sensitive one, but one whose answer will help the clinical team provide better care. Similarly, the preface can include reassurance that the patient's response is confidential and will only be shared with those individuals who are involved in the patient's care and that the response will in no way affect how that patient is treated by the care team.

In addition, being mindful of past trauma that a homeless patient may have experienced and how that trauma may affect his or her response to the care team's recommendations is crucial in fostering an encounter rooted in trust and nonjudgment. A prime example is that of a homeless woman at risk of cervical cancer who is several years overdue for a Pap smear. During an initial clinical encounter with a new provider, she may adamantly decline a Pap smear, despite the health care provider's counseling on the importance of this screening test and her risk of cervical cancer. While one way to view this homeless patient's response as a clinician is to become frustrated and label the patient "noncompliant," a more compassionate and nonjudgmental approach is to gently inquire into why she is declining the exam. Over time, if a relationship of trust is built, the patient may reveal a history of sexual trauma, and she may even allow a trusted provider to proceed with the screening exam at a later clinical encounter.

Future Directions

The history of anti-homeless stigma in the United States, current manifestations of anti-homeless stigma and prejudice in the local government and law enforcement arenas, and poor health outcomes affecting homeless individuals all paint a dire picture of the unjust marginalization of and discrimination against the neediest among us. Concerted efforts are needed in order to ensure that anti-homeless sentiments is proactively addressed with the goal of eliminating anti-homeless stigma in the future.

Government and Law Enforcement

Continued advocacy is needed on the city, state, and national levels to urge policy makers to bring an end to legislation that criminalizes activities related to homelessness. Arrests of homeless individuals for minor offenses can contribute to a vicious cycle of homelessness. Once arrested, homeless individuals incur a criminal record that thereafter jeopardizes their chances of obtaining housing and employment, rendering them at risk of chronic homelessness during which they may, at times out of necessity, engage in the same activities for which they can again be arrested under anti-panhandling, anti-vagrancy, and anti-camping laws. In addition, concerted efforts to provide competency and sensitivity training on homelessness for law enforcement officials are sorely needed. Police officers, being on the front lines, are often the first to encounter homeless individuals in times of emergency and in times of need. It behooves us to provide law enforcement officials the training they need to not only manage their interactions with homeless individuals respectfully but also to view each encounter with a homeless individual not as an opportunity to catch a perpetrator, but rather as a chance to guide an individual in need toward homeless-based services in as compassionate a manner as possible.

Health Professional Competency Training and Tailored Primary Care Programs

In order to address the presence of anti-homeless stigma in the health care system, we must incorporate sensitivity and homeless competency training into the curriculum of mid-level practitioner graduate programs, nursing and medical assistant training programs, medical schools, and social work graduate programs. For maximal effectiveness in eliminating anti-homeless stigma among health care providers, these trainings must encompass an understanding of the history of homelessness, the many factors that contribute to homelessness today, and the marked disparities in health outcomes for the homeless population compared to the general population. The most powerful element that must not be overlooked in these trainings is the human one—exposure to individuals experiencing homelessness throughout training and the privilege of listening to and learning from their stories. Importantly, these sensitivity trainings must also be extended to all ancillary staff (such as nursing aides, licensed practical nurses, front desk staff, benefits staff, security and facilities staff, and phlebotomists) who may spend a considerable amount of time interacting with homeless individuals in health care settings. As interactions with many of these individuals may precede a homeless patient's interactions with health care providers, it is of utmost importance that health care organizations also engage ancillary staff in training on how to sensitively, compassionately, and respectfully serve homeless individuals.

Lastly, health care organizations that predominantly serve homeless patients should consider tailoring their services to the unique needs of the homeless population. Data suggest that homeless individuals' experiences seeking care at tailored primary care sites were superior to the experiences of homeless individuals seeking care in primary care settings where services were not tailored to their specific needs [26]. Tailored care of the homeless population should include outreach and engagement aimed at decreasing barriers to accessing health care services, as with clinics based at emergency shelter sites. In addition, the care should be multi-faceted, focusing not only on medical conditions commonly affecting homeless individuals (such as through the provision of dental and foot care) but also on intensive case management services that facilitate connection to needed benefits, food pantry services, and housing resources. Multi-disciplinary care that encompasses case management needs and behavioral health services and that encourages consistent and standardized communication between disciplines on individual patients' care teams is recommended in order to fully address the complex needs that characterize the homeless population [27]. A tailored primary care setting and a public health framework of care delivery (which focuses not only on provision of health care but also on population management, disease prevention, and addressing social determinants of health) form the foundation of superior, quality health care for homeless individuals [28].

As an example of primary care models tailored to the needs of the homeless population, at Boston Health Care for the Homeless Program tailoring of services is evident in the structuring of clinic hours to match the evening shelter schedule during which patients seek emergency shelter beds provision of clinical services specific to women's health at women's shelters, and collaboration with local hospital partners to eliminate barriers and wait times for important health care screening tests, such as through arrangement of same-day mammography for eligible patients. Such tailoring to meet the needs of the homeless population is also exemplified by the program's medical respite facility, named the Barbara McInnis House, which provides short-term, round-the-clock medical and recuperative care for homeless individuals who are too sick to stay in shelters but do not require acute inpatient care.

Research

Though city-specific premature mortality data have been instrumental in efforts to understand the health care challenges facing the homeless population, research analyzing the health care needs and outcomes of the national homeless population would help shed further light on the health care challenges unique to this population. In addition, such research could help further advance advocacy agendas by providing much needed evidence on the detrimental consequences of homelessness for state and national policy makers. More research on homeless individuals' experiences and interactions with the health care delivery system can also help further highlight the importance of competency training for all health care professionals on issues unique to the experience of homelessness.

Conclusion

There remains considerable hope that the future will bring what the past has not: an end to anti-homeless stigma and discrimination. The clinical recommendations and future directions noted above are just a few ways in which we can continue to work on improving, as a society, the day-to-day quality of life of homeless individuals by eliminating the preconceived stigma that colors how we—as lawmakers, law enforcement officers, neighbors, and health care providers—project implicit messages of homeless individuals' inherent worth. But though our progress has been slow in this regard and has been characterized by fits and starts, the very existence of the social service providers, homeless health care clinicians, national homeless advocacy agencies, and researchers devoted to homelessness today is a testament to how far we have come in working toward better understanding, characterizing, supporting, and accompanying this uniquely resilient population. In the immortal words of Franklin D. Roosevelt, "The test of our progress is not whether we add more to the abundance of those who have much; it is whether we provide enough for those who have too little." May we continue to strive to overcome this ultimate test of progress.

References

1. Burt M, Aron L, Lee E, Valente J. How many homeless people are there? Helping America's homeless: emergency shelter or affordable housing? Washington DC: Urban Institute; 2001. p. 23–54.
2. Henry M, Cortes A, Shivji A, Buck K. The 2014 annual homeless assessment report to congress. Office of Community Planning and Development. Washington DC: U.S. Department of Housing and Urban Development; 2014.
3. The McKinney-Vento Homeless Assistance Act. General definition of homeless individual. 42 U.S. Code § 11302; 2009.
4. Kuhn R, Culhane D. Applying cluster analysis to test a typology of homelessness by pattern of shelter utilization: results from the analysis of administrative data. Am J Community Psychol. 1998;26(2):207–32.
5. Kusmer K. Down & out, on the road. Oxford: Oxford University Press; 2002.
6. Bls.gov. Overview of BLS statistics on unemployment. [Internet]. 2015 [Cited 8 Feb 2015]. Available from: http://www.bls.gov/bls/unemployment.htm.
7. Arnold A, Crowley S, Bravve E, Brundage S, Biddlecombe C. Out of reach 2014. [Internet]. National Low Income Housing Coalition. 2014.
8. National Coalition for the Homeless. Who is homeless? Fact Sheet. [Internet]. 2009. Available from: http://www.nationalhomeless.org.
9. The National Center on Family Homelessness at the American Institutes for Research. America's youngest outcasts: a report card on child homelessness. Waltham; 2014.
10. The National Law Center on Homelessness and Poverty and the National Coalition for the Homeless. Homes not handcuffs: the criminalization of homelessness in U.S. Cities. 2009.
11. National Coalition for the Homeless. Share no more: the criminalization of efforts to feed people in need. Washington, D.C: National Coalition for the Homeless; 2014.
12. Webster R. Homeless given 3 days to leave encampment under Pontchartrain expressway. The Times-Picayune. [Internet]. 2014 [Cited 8 Feb 2015]. Available from: http://www.nola.com/politics/index.ssf/2014/08/homeless_given_3_days_to_leave.html.
13. National Coalition for the Homeless. Vulnerable to hate: a survey of hate crimes & violence committed against homeless people in 2013. Washington, D.C: National Coalition for the Homeless; 2014.
14. Martin D. Experiences of homeless people in the health care delivery system: a Descriptive Phenomenological Study. Public Health Nurs. 2008;25(5):420–30.

15. McCormack R, Hoffman L, Norman M, Goldfrank L, Norman E. Voices of homeless alcoholics who frequent Bellevue hospital: a qualitative study. Ann Emerg Med. 2015;65(2): 178–186.e6.
16. Wen C, Hudak P, Hwang S. Homeless people's perceptions of welcomeness and unwelcomeness in healthcare encounters. J Gen Intern Med. 2007;22(7):1011–7.
17. Hwang S, O'Connell J, Lebow J, Bierer M, Orav E, Brennan T. Health care utilization among homeless adults prior to death. J Health Care Poor Underserved. 2001;12(1):50–8.
18. Baggett T, O'Connell J, Singer D, Rigotti N. The unmet health care needs of homeless adults: a National Study. Am J Public Health. 2010;100(7):1326–33.
19. O'Connell J. Premature mortality in homeless populations: a review of the literature. Nashville: National Health Care for the Homeless Council, Inc.; 2005.
20. Hibbs J, Benner L, Klugman L, Spencer R, Macchia I, Mellinger A, et al. Mortality in a cohort of homeless adults in Philadelphia. New England J Med. 1994;331(5):304–9.
21. Barrow S, Herman D, Córdova P, Struening E. Mortality among homeless shelter residents in New York City. Am J Public Health. 1999;89(4):529–34.
22. Hwang S, Lebow J, Bierer M, O'Connell J, Orav E, Brennan T. Risk factors for death in homeless adults in Boston. Arch Intern Med. 1998;158(13):1454–60.
23. Baggett T, Hwang S, O'Connell J, Porneala B, Stringfellow E, Orav E, et al. Mortality among homeless adults in Boston: shifts in causes of death over a 15-year period. JAMA Int Med. 2013;173(3):189–95.
24. Baggett T, Chang Y, Singer D, Porneala B, Gaeta J, O'Connell J, et al. Tobacco-, alcohol-, and drug-attributable deaths and their contribution to mortality disparities in a cohort of homeless adults in Boston. Am J Public Health. 2015;105(6):1189–97.
25. O'Connell JJ. Stories from the shadows: reflections of a street doctor. Boston: BHCHP Press; 2015.
26. Kertesz S, Holt C, Steward J, Jones R, Roth D, Stringfellow E, et al. Comparing homeless persons' care experiences in tailored versus nontailored primary care programs. Am J Public Health. 2013;103(S2):S331–9.
27. King Jr T, Wheele M, Wheeler M. Medical management of vulnerable and underserved patients: principles, practice, and populations. New York: McGraw-Hill Medical Publishing Division; 2007.
28. O'Connell J, Oppenheimer S, Judge C, Taube R, Blanchfield B, Swain S, et al. The Boston health care for the homeless program: a public health framework. Am J Public Health. 2010;100(8):1400–8.

Chapter 6
VIP Patients: An Unexpectedly Vulnerable Population

Jonathan Avery, Daniel Knoepflmacher, Neel Mehta, and Julie Penzner

A well-known, former CEO, Mr. Miller, is admitted for a gastric bleed and hyponatremia to the "amenities" floor of a major quaternary academic hospital. He comes to the hospital with his own home health aide, a personal nurse, his adult daughter (who is his health-care proxy) and his girlfriend. Mr. Miller's daughter demands that his nurse and home health aide be directly involved in his care, despite the advice of the floor nursing staff, who argue that this is not the standard of care and will complicate his treatment. Both the physicians and nursing staff are reluctant to go to the room because they are anxious about being questioned and criticized for their work. An agreement is made to let the private nurse and home health aide collect vital signs and blood tests with a staff nurse present in the room.

One night, the daughter refuses vital signs, the sequential compression devices (SCDs), and evening blood tests, stating her father "has had enough of this." The physician speaks with Mr. Miller's daughter, and a compromise is reached where the evening blood test will be obtained by the home health aide and, in an

J. Avery, MD (✉) • D. Knoepflmacher, MD • J. Penzner, MD
Department of Psychiatry, Weill Cornell Medical College, New York, NY, USA
e-mail: Joa9070@med.cornell.edu

N. Mehta, MD
Department of Pain Medicine, Weill Cornell Medical College, New York, NY, USA

© Springer International Publishing Switzerland 2016
R. Parekh, Ed W. Childs (eds.), *Stigma and Prejudice: Touchstones in Understanding Diversity in Healthcare*, Current Clinical Psychiatry, DOI 10.1007/978-3-319-27580-2_6

effort to maximize the patient's comfort overnight, the vital signs and SCDs will be removed until the next morning. The next morning the nursing staff reports that morning vital signs show Mr. Miller to be hypoxic and tachycardic. Upon returning to the room, he is found to be hemodynamically unstable. The patient is transferred to the intensive care unit where it is discovered that he has a deep vein thrombosis and a life-threatening pulmonary embolism. The lack of the SCDs and monitoring overnight is thought to have led to this poor outcome.

Stature, power, money, and connections do not render an individual immune to mental or physical health problems. Therefore, very important people (VIPs) are bound to become patients too. Although it is often assumed that such individuals receive superior care as patients, a growing body of literature reveals that VIP patients are an unexpectedly vulnerable population [1–9]. While there is a need for more research on this topic, VIP individuals have been shown to receive subpar medical care and are often stigmatized in health care by providers, other patients, and the general public [1–9].

In this chapter, the authors provide an overview of the complex relationship between VIPs and the health-care system and discuss the effects of this relationship. The authors begin by describing the VIP population. They then discuss the attitudes of health-care professionals (HCPs) toward VIPs and the impact of these attitudes on the VIP patient's health care. VIP patient and family expectations of health care are also discussed. Additionally, the authors outline the impact of the care of the VIP patients on the health-care system. The chapter concludes with a discussion on ways to improve the treatment of VIPs and future directions for this underappreciated topic.

Who Are VIPs?

It is thought that Winston Churchill was the first to use the term *VIP* to refer to important and high-ranking government and military personnel [1, 10]. Over the years, *VIP* has come to also refer to celebrities, the wealthy, famous authors, artists, and other well-known or influential individuals [1, 7, 10, 11]. In the hospital setting, VIPs may also include HCPs, hospital administrators, and other hospital staff, as well as donors or other individuals associated with the hospital [5, 9, 12–14]. Family members of VIPs are at times considered VIPs in the health-care setting as well [11]. Given the large potential number of individuals who may be considered a VIP by HCPs, the authors of this chapter consider a VIP patient a patient in whom the health-care system has a special interest and has deemed important.

The literature provides many examples of how VIPs are treated as patients [7, 15–17]. One noteworthy case discusses the care of an internationally well-known celebrity who was admitted to a psychiatric inpatient unit for manic symptoms in a major academic hospital [7]. The patient was brought to the hospital at midnight with special accommodations. She was hostile and demanding upon arrival, asking for her room to be changed and for the treatment orders of her outpatient psychiatrist to be followed without deviation. Her presence in the milieu was extremely disruptive on the unit, where other patients and visitors asked for autographs, which she provided willingly. The news of her admission spread throughout the hospital, with staff from different divisions seeking ways to obtain autographs and other members of the house staff asking the resident who was treating her for details about her hospitalization. The patient was discharged against medical advice within 72 h at her request [7]. At the beginning of the chapter, the authors also provided the blended case of Mr. Miller to demonstrate how VIP status can result in substandard care and, in this case, an adverse outcome.

Maintaining Privacy and Safety of VIPs

The care of VIP patients is often different from the care of other patients due to concerns about patient privacy and safety. All patients have a right to privacy and safety; both may be compromised by other patients, staff, and the media in the health-care setting [1]. This often necessitates that the VIP patient be kept apart from other patients. It appears that most HCPs are in agreement with this practice. When emergency department medical directors were surveyed about expediting care – not providing different care – for VIP patients in the emergency room, for example, all but one endorsed the practice [9]. However, the separateness is accompanied by inherent vulnerability. For example, when VIP patients are treated in isolated areas of the hospital, it may make it harder for these patients to receive routine access to hospital resources and personnel.

There is also the temptation to spectate in the care of VIP patients. Although electronic health records have decreased the potential for in-chart observation that is not related to clinical care, hospital staff may loiter, chat in nursing stations, inquire, and otherwise ogle what is meant to be a private event. This is worrisome from the standpoints of both patient privacy and patient safety, as it increases distractedness and can shift focus away from health care and toward restrictions designed to condone privacy. Threats and realities of press involvement are critical, as they interfere with provider concentration and with patient privacy itself [1].

The Attitudes of Health-Care Professionals Toward VIPs

HCPs often have a host of reactions – both positive and negative – to VIP patients and the care that they receive. While more research is needed to further elucidate these attitudes, existing literature reveals the complex feelings that VIPs can generate in providers. VIPs can be regarded with awe and respect but also with disdain [1]. Envy, admiration, distractedness, anxiety, judgment, and the assumption by HCPs that they already "know" something about the VIP patient based on public reputation can create countertransferential hurdles with negative effects. Feelings can even change over the course of an interaction with a patient, resulting in a "VIP syndrome": "(1) the VIP succeeds in gaining certain priorities through the application of external pressures upon the hospital; (2) the hospital staff, fearful and angry, withdraws from the patient and isolates him on the ward; (3) a vicious circle of increased patient pressure and further staff withdrawal is created; (4) therapeutic failure inevitably follows with suicide and AMA discharge particularly to be feared" [4].

Given the complexity of the health-care system, it is not uncommon for different members of the treatment team to have different attitudes toward the VIP patient. The young physician may feel pride in being able to work with the VIP patient. The veteran nurse may be wary of the demands of the VIP patient and the large amount of resources consumed by just one individual. The administrator may see the treatment of the VIP patient in terms of the potential monetary and reputation benefit for the institution. In turn, the VIP patient himself has a host of his/her own feelings, some that predate health-care encounters and others that arise as a reaction to them. This transaction of the attitudes of HCPs and patient attitudes sets up high likelihood for misunderstanding, poor communication, and time-consuming distraction from the health-care issues at hand.

The Impact of the Attitudes of Health-Care Professionals on VIP Patient's Health Care

Given the need for more research, it is difficult to assess the full impact of the attitudes of HCPs on VIP health care. Case reports often focus on adverse outcomes. There is a paucity of literature on cases where attitudes toward VIP patients were neutral or resulted in positive outcomes for the patient.

As far back as the 1950s, however, there were studies and reports on worse care received by VIP patients. In one such study, physicians often delayed diagnosing or treating patients who were also a physician, secondary to overidentifying with the patient [5]. It has also been described how attitudes of hospital administration and personality traits possessed by the VIP patient led to worse care of VIP psychiatric patients [4].

The negative outcomes for VIPs are often thought to be due to a loss of objectivity by the HCP [1]. The role of the distracted HCP cannot be underemphasized. These conditions can lead to a departure from standard medical practice. The case of Mr. Miller also showed how the departure from standard medical practice can quickly lead to an adverse outcome.

VIP Patient and Family Expectations of Health Care

VIP individuals are accustomed to special treatment in many areas of their lives and often have quick access to whatever they may want or desire [4]. This is antithetical to the structure of organized health care, which relies on standard, evidence-based approaches and may lead to vulnerabilities for patients and providers [1]. When exceptions are made, it is difficult to predict outcome, as was demonstrated in the case of Mr. Miller. The authors recommend that VIP patients not be exempt from standards of practice, for example, from preadmission medical screens, in-depth initial assessments, and questions about substance use and sexual practices to other routine practices that may impact their care [8]. Although the temptation to "respect" VIP privacy by avoiding some more intrusive and possibly less relevant areas is real, the pitfall of failing to conduct a complete history, physical examination, and review of systems is more dangerous [8].

VIP patients and families may also desire quick results [4]. As with all patients and patients' families, it is important to take time to discuss pros and cons of procedures, research protocols, medications, and medical results in detail, emphasizing that there may not be a "quick fix" or that doing something may be worse than nothing at all. For example, back pain may lead to many opinions and interpretations of otherwise normal findings on an MRI. The VIP patient may push for a quick fix instead of physical therapy or patience and reassessment, resulting in multilevel fusions that are not only unnecessary but likely to leave the patient worse off.

The Impact of the Care of VIP Patients on the Health-Care System

One of the biggest concerns about the treatment of the VIP patient is that it may result in compromised care for other patients, which some have argued would be "morally unacceptable" [18, 19]. VIP patients can potentially utilize a significant amount of resources, which may then be unavailable to others in need. The bed (or hospital floor) taken by a VIP immediately on arrival to the hospital, for example, may result in less beds and hospital resources for others [18, 19]. In the authors' experience, physicians, nurses, administrators, and other clinical staff may similarly be less available due to high time demands involved in the care of the VIP.

On the other hand, VIP patients have often donated money or their influence and resources to the institution that takes care of them. In a study of emergency department medical directors, one physician commented how VIP patients "can be very influential in terms of projects, improvements, and the flow of capital dollars toward areas they appreciate" [9]. That is, treating a VIP patient may in the end result in more resources being available for other patients, which may improve their medical care.

Finally, the authors argue that patients being treated in the hospital simultaneous to VIPs have their own reactions to the VIP patient, all of which may impact their actual health-care outcome or their experience of receiving care. These reactions have been poorly characterized in the literature, but patients may feel overlooked or not cared for if they see a VIP patient being moved ahead of them in a line for a procedure, which may impact their mood and receptiveness toward care. At other times, encountering a VIP in the same health-care setting may be reassuring or even exciting and can potentially highlight that everyone shares the same struggles and resources.

Improving Treatment for VIPs

The VIP population, like other special populations, is heterogeneous, and the vulnerabilities in VIP care can be even more complex than one might expect. As discussed above, the authors of this chapter consider a VIP patient a patient in whom the health-care system has a special interest and has deemed important, for whatever reasons. The authors recommend that reducing the diverse VIP population to this definition allows one to approach the problem sensibly, rather than to redesign an individualized approach for scenarios that might have more in common than are first apparent.

With that in mind, HCPs and institutions should ideally have a strategic, simple, evidence-based plan in place for treating VIP patients in order to ensure that their care and the care of other patients are not compromised [1, 4, 8, 20]. The authors recommend several simple steps, which should be prepared ahead of time before starting care of a VIP patient. Such steps will provide focus and organization to the treatment plan. These include addressing "mechanical factors" [1], HCP's attitudes to VIP patients, and a plan for co-patient attitudes toward VIP patients in the event that the VIP's privacy is inadvertently not maintained, as well as providing guidance on the management of VIP patients to HCPs. These items are discussed below.

Addressing Mechanical Factors

HCPs and institutions may benefit from having a special code – which has, at times, been termed "Code Purple" – to address the mechanics of taking care of a VIP patient [1]. It should be a written procedure similar to what organizations have for catastrophes such as earthquakes [1]. This would result in less variability and more consistency in dealing with the VIP patient, especially upon the arrival of the VIP to the institution.

This "Code Purple" would deal with accommodations, safety and privacy, the media, gifts, etc. [1]. A wide variety of HCPs would ideally be a part of the "Code Purple" team to provide input. The code should also address the mechanics of caring for the other patients in the health-care setting at that time as well.

Addressing Attitudes of Health-Care Professionals

Numerous studies have looked at improving the attitudes of HCPs to a host of challenging patients [21–23]. It appears that increasing awareness of such attitudes through brief interventions, reflection exercises, and ongoing educational events is key [21–23]. These interventions can range from small-group interactive trainings to online modules [21–23]. Future work to develop such interventions for attitudes toward VIP patients may improve the care that these patients receive. As part of this training, the response of other patients toward a VIP patient should be addressed as well.

Management of VIP Patients

The authors strongly recommend that HCPs be prepared to dedicate more time toward VIP care than for the standard patient. It is likely that multiple other care providers and support staff will be present, including personal physicians, aides, and family members, and the care plan will need adequate time for collaborative discussion. At times, senior physicians who do not routinely work in the hospital setting may be called upon to consult in the care of VIP patients, and they may obstruct care and cause splitting among staff members if not integrated in a coordinated fashion as well [8].

VIP patients who are looking for immediate answers and treatment may challenge clinicians. They may express disappointment in the conservative, cautious answer, as in the case of back pain resulting in unnecessary surgery discussed above. The standard of care may require patience and observation. It is important to not overpromise results as the disappointment and anger from a VIP lead to embarrassment of the provider, blocking of further VIPs, and powerful litigious potential [4, 8].

Often, if multiple HCPs are involved, it is important to identify the leading medical expert who will take charge to prevent arguments or indecision leading to lack of progress in care [1, 8]. Sometimes an institution will assign the provider in the hospital who has extensive expertise in working with VIP patients; for example, a senior hospital physician may be called upon to coordinate and manage consultant care and ensure an open dialogue among physicians. It is important, especially in acute and more serious conditions, to have regular checkups from staff members to ensure proper compliance with treatment.

Conclusions

VIP patients are an unexpectedly vulnerable population and are at risk for stigma and prejudice in the health-care system. In this chapter, the authors provided an overview of the complex relationship between VIPs and the health-care system and discussed the effects of this relationship. The authors began by describing the VIP population. They then discussed the attitudes of health-care professionals (HCPs) toward VIPs and the impact of these attitudes on the VIP patient's health care. VIP patient and family expectations of health care were also discussed. Additionally, the authors outlined the impact of the care of the VIP patients on the health-care system. The chapter concluded with a discussion on ways to improve the treatment of VIPs. The authors argued that while more research is certainly needed on this topic, HCPs and institutions should have a plan in place for treating VIP patients in order to ensure that their care and the care of other patients is not compromised. This plan must attend to patient and provider expectations, a complex web of family and care-givers, and influence on the health-care system as a whole.

Future Directions

While there is a growing body of literature on the VIP patient, more research is needed to better characterize VIP patients, the impact of VIPs on the health-care system, HCP's stigma and prejudices toward VIP patients, and treatments that work for these individuals. Research into the interventions that improve the treatment of VIPs can focus on the structure of individual health-care settings, educating HCPs on their attitudes toward VIP patients, improving assessments of VIP patients, and how the treatment of VIP patients impacts others.

The impact of VIP patients is significant on HCPs and other patients, and further understanding this complex subset of patients may provide answers that benefit the whole health-care system. Specifically, it is important to figure out ways to provide care that is closest to the standard of care for all patients while still allowing for the flexibility which may be required for special populations. If this can be accomplished, the authors believe this will result in fewer stigmatizing attitudes and preju-dices toward special populations, like VIP patients, and provide the highest likelihood of effective and satisfying health care.

References

1. Groves JE, Dunderdale BA, Stren TA. Celebrity patients, VIPs, and potentates. Prim Care Companion J Clin Psychiatry. 2002;4:215–23.
2. Kucharski A. On being sick and famous. Polit Psychol. 1984;5:69–81.
3. Saari C, Johnson SR. Problems in the treatment of VIP clients. Soc Casework. 1975;576:599–604.
4. Weintraub W. "The VIP syndrome": a clinical study in hospital psychiatry. J Nerv Ment Dis. 1964;138:181–93.
5. Robbins GF, MacDonald MC, Pack GT. Delay in the diagnosis and treatment of physicians with cancer. Cancer. 1953;6:624–6.
6. Block AJ. Beware of the VIP syndrome. Chest. 1993;104:989.
7. Feuer EH, Karasu SR. A star-struck service: impact of the admission of a celebrity to an inpatient unit. J Clin Psychiatry. 1978;39:743–6.

8. Smith MS, Shesser RF. The emergency care of the VIP patient. N Engl J Med. 1988;319:1421–3.
9. Smally AJ, Carroll B, Carius M, Tilden F, Werdmann M. Treatment of VIPs. Ann Emerg Med. 2011;58:397–8.
10. Group for the Advancement of Psychiatry, Committee on Governmental Agencies. The VIP with psychiatric impairment. New York: Charles Scribner's Sons; 1973.
11. Stone MH. Treating the wealthy and their children. Int J Child Psychother. 1972;1:15–46.
12. Pinner M, Miller BF. When doctors are patients. New York: WW Norton; 1952.
13. Hahn RA. Between two worlds: physicians as patients. Med Anthropol Q. 1985;16:87–98.
14. Marzuk P. When the patient is a physician. N Engl J Med. 1987;317:1409–11.
15. Kucharski A. Medical management of political patients: the case of Dwight D. Eisenhower. Perspect Biol Med. 1978;22:115–26.
16. Breo DL. Pope's physicians redeem a request. Am Med News. 1981;24:1, 7, 14.
17. Park BE. The impact of illness on world leaders. Philadelphia: University of Pennsylvania Press; 1986.
18. Schenkenberg T, Kochenour N, Botkin J. Ethical considerations in clinical care of the "VIP". J Clin Ethics. 2007;18:56–63.
19. CCEP. Celebrities in the ED: managers often face both ethical and operational challenges. ED Manag. 2006;18:133–5.
20. Guzman JA, SAsidhar M, Stoller JK. Caring for VIPs: nine principles. Cleve Clin J med. 2011;78:90–4.
21. Avery J, Zerbo E. Improving psychiatry residents' attitudes toward individuals diagnosed with substance use disorders. Harv Rev Psychiatry. 2015;23(4):296–300.
22. Avery J, Zerbo E, Ross S. Improving psychiatrists' attitudes towards individuals with psychotic disorders and co-occurring substance use disorders. Acad Psychiatry. 2015. [Epub ahead of print] No abstract available. PMID: 25977100.
23. Haywood C, Williams-Reade J, Rushton C, Beach MC, Geller G. Improving clinician attitudes of respect and trust for persons with sickle cell disease. Hosp Pediatr. 2015;5(7):377–84.

Chapter 7
Stigma and Persons with Substance Use Disorders

Christina Brezing and David Marcovitz

Case Vignette
A 42-year-old man with a history of injection heroin use now in sustained remission on buprenorphine/naloxone presents to an emergency room with an injury sustained at a construction site. He fell one story off a ladder and landed on his back. He reports 9/10 pain on arrival and he reveals his history of opioid use disorder and medication-assisted treatment. He agrees to accept opiate analgesia while his work-up is ongoing given his significant pain. Trauma evaluation including CT scan does not reveal any significant traumatic injuries such as fractures or hemorrhage. He is diagnosed with a lumbar strain and shoulder contusion. He is able to ambulate and is ready for discharge. He continues to report 8/10 pain in his lumbar region following administration of a one-time dose of intravenous morphine. The ER physician explains the results of his imaging and his recommendation for analgesia with acetaminophen and ibuprofen only. The patient worries out loud that this will not be sufficient, and the physician responds, "Right, well, that may be all you will get because of your problem with these medications, but let me see what I can

C. Brezing, MD (✉)
Division on Substance Abuse, Columbia Department of Psychiatry,
Columbia University Medical Center, New York State Psychiatric Institute,
1051 Riverside Driver, Unit 66, New York, NY 10032, USA
e-mail: brezing@nyspi.columbia.edu

D. Marcovitz, MD
Department of Psychiatry, Massachusetts General Hospital, Harvard Medical School,
Boston, MA, USA

© Springer International Publishing Switzerland 2016   113
R. Parekh, Ed W. Childs (eds.), *Stigma and Prejudice: Touchstones in
Understanding Diversity in Healthcare*, Current Clinical Psychiatry,
DOI 10.1007/978-3-319-27580-2_7

do," leaving the room rather abruptly. The nurse returns to discharge the patient with a prescription for 7 days of oxycodone-acetaminophen 5/325 mg tabs, and nothing further is discussed. The patient leaves feeling he has done something wrong and wondering if adherence to his medication (buprenorphine/naloxone) is worth the reactions it generates from others.

Introduction

This case presentation unfortunately depicts a common scenario demonstrating the subtle and not so subtle stigma encountered by patients with substance use disorders (SUDs). Some physicians, nurses, and other healthcare providers are comfortable discussing issues of opioid prescribing with patients who have histories of addiction and working collaboratively with them to prevent relapse. However, many clinicians find such conversations stressful and/or simply lack education on how to approach these discussions, especially in cases where patients are receiving opioid agonist therapy. The resulting avoidance or negative affect directed at such patients can result in patients feeling unfairly stigmatized, in some cases simply based on the medication list they carry with them. Paradoxically, a compassionate but direct approach by clinicians where underlying concerns are raised about patient vulnerability, and outpatient providers are involved, can be more therapeutic and can minimize stigma. Such interventions take more time and skill but can be mutually satisfying for all parties. Given the substantial impact stigma toward SUDs has on quality of care and on the design and implementation of research studies, it is imperative that healthcare providers and researchers develop awareness of their biases and take steps to change their perspectives and management of these patients that is more in line with this latter approach. In this chapter, we will present the history of stigma toward SUDs in the United States, define stigma in terms of addiction, and then explore how the means by which various factors potentiate stigma toward addiction. We also propose ways in which we can think about the role of stigma in addiction treatment and how we can begin to combat it. We will look at how types of stigma, when conceptualized at a population level, can be used to benefit the greater good but run the risk of harming the individual (in other words, when the erosion of stigma can have unexpected, problematic consequences). We will conclude with some recommendations about future directions for individuals interested in this important issue.

History of Stigma and Addiction in the United States

Stigma toward addiction in the United States has far-reaching historical roots. Prior to the 1900s, drugs of abuse such as opiates, cocaine, cannabis, and alcohol were largely unregulated. However, beginning in the twentieth century, rates of problematic or dependent use of these substances were on the rise in America, and notable media sources, politicians, and academics began campaigns linking substance use with crime, insanity, minorities, and immigrants [1]. These campaigns fueled strong stigmatization against individuals with SUDs and led to the societal image of the "drug addict" and "alcoholic" who were unpredictable, unhealthy, dangerous, and socially rejected [2]. The idea of addiction as a failure of morals due to a poor personality or a lack of willpower was securely planted, and as a result, for the next century, the solution to this problem predominantly fell under the auspices of the legal system with the construct of laws that when broken lead to arrest and incarceration.

As a consequence of addiction being a moral problem solved by legal interventions, minimal investment was made to understand addiction's biological underpinnings, and it was seen as a distinct entity from health problems or diseases. "Treatment" or rehabilitation for SUDs developed separately from the traditional medical model. Individuals who overcame their own addictions provided the only options for care, resulting in "do-it-yourself" treatments. Grassroots organizations like Alcoholics Anonymous (AA), other 12-step programs, and therapeutic communities focused on character development, social sanctions, moral teachings, a sober community, and spirituality as a means to becoming "clean and sober." This segregated addiction treatment system was also separated financially from traditional medical care with most medical insurance payers not participating in reimbursement for substance abuse treatment or reimbursing at substantially lower rates compared to other medical treatments. Additionally, the facilities that provided addiction treatment were physically located outside of other healthcare settings, as opposed to being embedded within traditional medical clinics and hospitals. Patients and people with SUDs were viewed on many levels as "different" from others and, therefore, were kept separate, stigmatizing them only further.

Only over the last 40 years has there been a slow shift in how addiction is conceptualized and managed in the United States. During the time of the Vietnam War, many Veterans returning to the United States arrived home with substance use problems, specifically heroin dependence, and the US government developed interests in the factors associated with substance use. In the early 1970s, the National Institutes of Health (NIH) developed institutes separate from the National Institute of Mental Health (NIMH) that focused specifically on research of addictions including the National Institute on Drug Abuse (NIDA) and the National Institute on Alcohol Abuse and Alcoholism (NIAAA). By investing money in research to better understand addictive substances and people with addictions, the NIH accumulated more evidence supporting the conception of addiction as a chronic medical problem, influenced both by a patient's biology and environment. Subsequently, there have been gradual decreases in the perception of stigma associated with addiction [3]. With greater understanding, many have come to see addictions, or SUDs, as chronic diseases with complex psychosocial, cultural, and biological phenomena playing significant roles in how they develop, present, persist, and remit [4]. Like other chronic medical problems, SUDs are optimally treated with evidence-based approaches that incorporate medication, psychosocial support and/or therapy, and attention to environmental stressors that can contribute to morbidity and mortality.

Despite this greater understanding, implementation of this knowledge into wide-spread clinical practice and social perspective lags behind. While there are many reasons new information is delayed into practice, the significant history of stigma associated with SUDs and their associated stigmatizing factors play a substantial role in preventing up-to-date care of these patients.

Types of Addiction-Related Stigma

For the purposes of this chapter, three interacting levels of stigma are defined: (1) social stigma or public stigma enacted at the level of a group or individual against a stigmatized other group or individual; (2) structural stigma or institutional stigma that exists at the level of a system that includes the rules, policies, and procedures that restrict the rights of a stigmatized group; and (3) self-stigma or internalized stigma at the level of the individual and how they consider stigmatized stereotypes self-relevant [5].

With regard to social stigma toward patients with mental health disorders, those with addictions are the disorders that even when compared to schizophrenia, depression, anxiety, or eating disorders are the most severely judged [6]. People with drug and alcohol use disorders are rated as highly likely to be dangerous and to be kept socially distant [6]. People with SUDs are more likely to evoke negative opinions and disapproval as compared to other mental health diagnoses [7]. So why are alcohol and drug use associated with higher prejudice than other mental disorders? One consideration is the perceived degree of intentionality or control that an individual has over aspects of their mental health. Folk psychology has long held the view that use of addictive substances is under conscious, cognitive control, despite evidence from neuroscience that suggests more complexity be given to the topic [4]. Even in an informed population of psychology students, drug and alcohol use disorders were thought to be less likely causally determined by an individual's biology as compared to other mental health disorders since these same students' beliefs about causality were more highly weighted toward factors thought to be in control of the individual and intentional [6]. Indeed, health problems that are thought to be under greater control of the individual, such as SUDs or obesity, garner greater social stigmatization than disorders thought to be outside one's control such as genetic disorders like cystic fibrosis or certain kinds of cancer. As a result, people are less clear about appropriate treatments for SUDs given the prejudiced beliefs concerning etiology. Treatment of an SUD is thus thought to be a matter of an individual's "will" to stop engaging in the problematic behavior, which reinforces social stigma, particularly when few evidence-based treatments are thought to exist. In addition to this perception of control that leads to social stigma, individuals with SUDs tend to have a number of social and cultural factors that also predispose them to addiction, factors which themselves are highly stigmatized. These factors include poverty, marginalized, bleak environments, mental illness, prostitution, inability to care for self, inability to care for children, unemployment, legal problems and incarceration, injection drug use, and HIV.

Structural stigma against individuals with SUDs has infiltrated most major systems in the United States. People with SUDs encounter more obstacles in obtaining employment, accessing housing, accessing healthcare, and receiving support for treatment than almost any other group [8]. Many of these obstacles are a direct result of the current policies, rules, and regulations at the levels of state and federal governments, healthcare insurers, and healthcare treatment systems as demonstrated by strict laws leading to prosecution and incarceration for drug-related crimes at the level of the individual; inequality in terms of insurance coverage and reimbursement for SUDs; and separate treatment systems that often are not evidence-based.

Self-stigma is posited to develop out of the existence of public and structural stigma. Corrigan et al. propose that an awareness of stereotypical beliefs about a disorder as learned through public or structural stigma sets off a cascade of stigmatizing cognitions that in turn lead to an agreement about these stereotypes. These stigmatizing beliefs are then ultimately applied by the individual toward oneself if they later develop the disorder [9]. Applying this concept to SUDs, many individuals have developed strong, stereotypical beliefs about what it means to have a SUD long before they develop the disorder. In this context, once individuals develop SUDs and have internalized these stigmatizing views, they apply it to themselves, resulting in shame, diminished self-esteem, poor self-worth, and decreased self-efficacy [9, 10]. Their environments tend to validate these stigmatizing views, as individuals with SUDs commonly endorse experiences of rejection and regularly anticipate discrimination [8]. As a result, a vicious cycle is created, and ultimately propagates loss of status, marginalization, decreased help seeking from social supports, and avoidance of treatment and healthcare [11].

The Role of Language in Stigma

Just as persons with addictions are unique in the extent to which they are impacted by stigma, so too are they disproportionately stigmatized by our use of language itself. At issue here is the way in which language informs our notions of culpability and controllability around addictions. For example, there is no doubt that the use of the term *schizophrenic* to describe a person with schizophrenia is stigmatizing and diminishing of that individual's full personhood, but the term *substance abuser* adds yet another dimension: the very term *abuser* evokes the perception of willful, purposeful action. Indeed, a survey of clinicians at a gathering of mental health professionals found that, when reviewing vignettes alternately describing *persons with substance use disorders* and *substance abusers*, the clinicians reviewing the vignettes that employed the latter terminology tended to agree with notions of personal culpability and need for punitive measures [12]. The survey authors remind us that, a priori, this group of clinicians might have been expected to demonstrate greater sensitivity, suggesting that for society at large, these terms may carry even greater power to determine attitudes. To that end, in a neuroimaging study that did not select for clinician subjects, the authors were able to demonstrate decreased cerebral activation in participants in response to the words *drug addicts* compared with words representing other social groups, which could be interpreted to underscore the emotional disconnect that dehumanizing terminology can engender when applied to persons with addictions [13].

Any discussion on the impact of language should acknowledge its ability to alter attitudes for better or for worse. The field of positive psychology, for example, is in part predicated on the concept that we can alter our own attitudes and moods through emphasis—at times in writing—on the positive aspects of our daily lives [14]. Similarly, 12-step groups have long emphasized the ability of language to shape members' attitudes through the use of gratitude lists, slogans, and affirmations. Interestingly, these same groups have occasionally faced criticism for the tendency of members to self-label as *alcoholic* or *addict* in as much as such labeling can perpetuate a feeling of separation [15]. Could these members' use of language be furthering stigma, or is this a benign means to further a sense of identification and responsibility? Broyles et al. offer the compromise that we must consider the language-use needs and preferences of persons with addictions themselves—in the 12-step example, members may have different preferences internal and external to the group—and yet as clinicians, our choice to emphasize the biomedical aspects of addiction is more likely to open the door to often underutilized, evidence-based treatments. This approach acknowledges that the dehumanization caused by use in popular media of terms like *addict*, *junky*, and *drug pusher* and even the use in our own academic vernacular of the term *substance abuser* can only be remediated by deliberate and conscious efforts toward change. The DSM5 switch to the SUD nomenclature attempts to honor the personhood of individuals affected by addiction, even if we may temporarily err on the side of over-medicalization at the risk of emphasizing "pills over skills" [16, 17].

The present crafting of our clinical language around addiction offers an opportunity to highlight certain core principles, certainly including the principle of respect for personhood but also the principle of conceptualizing recovery as a holistic, long-term process rather than a binary transition from substance use to abstinence. Perhaps one day diagnostic specifiers like *in early remission* and *in sustained remission* will give way to even more nuanced stages of recovery that recognize this process in all its richness. Through these changes in language, we can slowly begin to alter a cultural narrative that has very real consequences for our patients' willingness to seek help, for our colleagues' willingness to treat all patients equally, and for society's willingness to embrace treatment and rehabilitation over condemnation and punishment.

See Table 7.1 for a list of common and preferred language related to clinical care for substance use disorders [18, 19].

In conjunction with the use of particular language, providers' styles of interaction with individuals around their substance use can either propagate or diminish stigma. Stigma, both on the part of the provider and the patient, can lead to discomfort, resulting in an additional barrier for patients to honestly and openly discuss

Table 7.1 Common and preferred language related to clinical care for SUDs

Commonly used term	Preferred term	Rationale
Addict, abuser, etc.	Person with a substance use disorder	Focuses on respect, dignity, and primacy of personhood
Substance abuse	Substance use disorder	Avoids implication of willful misconduct; also shift in emphasis to chronic disease model ("hazardous," "risky," or "unhealthy" use may be preferred for some who do not meet disorder criteria) [18]
Opioid substitution therapy/replacement therapy	Opioid agonist treatment	Avoids implication of "switching addiction"; pharmacologic classification more in line with other medications (i.e., angiotensin-converting enzyme inhibitors, serotonin reuptake inhibitors, etc.) [19]
Clean	Sober/abstinent	Avoids value-laden, nonclinical terminology
Dirty/clean urine	Positive or negative urine drug screen (for X)	Avoids value-laden, nonclinical terminology

their substance use. Healthcare providers should approach screening and intervention for identified substance use disorders as engaging in a collaborative partnership with their patients. Being compassionate, empathic, nonjudgmental, and nonconfrontational is preferred to assertive or oppositional styles of assessment and intervention. The conversations should focus on the patients' own goals and the obstacles that get in the way of accomplishing these goals as a result of direct or indirect consequences of substance use. Motivational interviewing (MI) is an efficacious, evidence-based approach to overcoming the ambivalence that keeps many people from making desired changes in their lives with regard to substance use and embodies this destigmatizing "spirit" of interaction. Providers interested in working with people who have substance use disorders should make it a priority to learn MI.

Healthcare Providers: Our Role in Stigma

Public attitudes that foster discrimination and devaluation toward people with SUDs are known barriers to the affected individual to acknowledging a problem and engaging in treatment [20]. But what happens to those individuals who, despite these barriers, access SUD treatment services? Are they met by healthcare providers and a healthcare system that foster an accepting, nonjudgmental environment that minimizes stigma? Generally, the answer appears to be no, as demonstrated in the case presented in the beginning of the chapter. Negative attitudes toward people with SUDs have been elicited from primary-care providers, psychiatrists, pharmacists, nurses, healthcare students in training, and physicians in other specialties [21]. Reasons for healthcare professional stigma (a type of social stigma) toward patients with SUDs include a perceived or actual lack of knowledge or skills in the treatment of substance use [22], lack of proper support structures in place to assist in appropriate care, and the association of unpleasant or unrewarding experiences in caring for these patients who are described by providers as "manipulative" and "dishonest" and perceived as violent and unmotivated [23, 24]. One study doing qualitative interviews of professionals in medicine, nursing, psychology, and social work found the following commonly held misbeliefs about individuals with illicit drug use: (1) people with illicit drug use cannot and do not wished to be helped, (2) "addicts" do not care for their own well-being, (3) harm reduction prevention efforts facilitate further substance use, and (4) people who use illicit drugs are a social burden [25]. Unfortunately, this kind of stigma leads to healthcare providers' unwillingness to treat patients with SUDs and non-evidence-based, biased, and lower quality of care when they do [21]. Stigma toward SUDs has been associated with decreased screening of substance use leading to a lost opportunity for intervention and referral for treatment, provider burnout, withholding of proper treatment (particularly in terms of pain control), and "zero tolerance" policies of cutting off care when a patient continues to use substances or relapses [25].

This stigma toward patients with SUDs is not limited to general medical settings but appears to also be present in SUD treatment settings. Patients receiving care in these specialized treatment settings also endorse a high level of perceived stigma by providers. These individuals' experiences with stigma-related rejection are shown to be directly correlated with the number of previous episodes of SUD treatment [8]. Two possible explanations are (1) people requiring more episodes of treatment have more severe SUDs that elicit more stigmatizing interactions and/or (2) greater experiences with stigma make it harder to succeed in treatment, thereby leading to more frequent relapses and reentry into treatment. There is some evidence for the latter explanation, as stigma-related attitudes of primary-care providers predicted poor adherence to psychiatric treatment and psychotropic medication in at least one study [26].

In contrast, what happens when more professional attitudes are implemented in treatment settings and stigma from healthcare professionals is decreased? Literature reviewed shows perceived stigma toward individuals with alcohol use disorders over a 20-year time period in Germany [20]. Notably, there was an erosion of stigma toward this group, particularly if they had undergone treatment for their alcohol use, which the investigators attributed to optimism with regard to treatment and recovery in alcohol use disorders [20]. Healthcare providers are often seen in the community as leaders and can have significant influence on how others perceive and treat socially oppressed populations of patients. Combatting stigma against substance use problems must start early on in the education of our healthcare professionals. There currently exist many opportunities for healthcare professionals to obtain accurate information and training in terms of evidence-based methods for screening, providing brief interventions, and referral for the many effective treatments (SBIRT—Screening, Brief Intervention, and Referral to Treatment) that exist across SUDs [27]. Educating our healthcare workforce and incentivizing implementation of evidence-based approaches to SUDs will empower both healthcare providers and patients as stigma is diminished.

Stigma Around Current Treatments

Stigma toward addiction itself inevitably extends its influence to how we as providers approach management and treatment. As we consider the various approaches currently employed, both psychosocial and pharmacologic, it quickly becomes apparent that choices between abstinence-based treatment and harm reduction, between agonist, antagonist, and other pharmacologic interventions, are sometimes influenced as much by evidence as they are by our conscious and unconscious biases. And as in other areas (psychodynamic psychotherapy comes to mind as one example), our best approach may be to improve our own awareness of these biases so we can help ourselves and our patients discuss our ambivalence and in some cases make wiser treatment choices than we would have otherwise.

In terms of global approaches to management, harm reduction and controlled use paradigms are frequently placed in opposition to abstinence-based treatments, though in practice we usually vary these approaches based on patient *stages of change* rather than viewing them as mutually exclusive [17]. Despite this clinical reality, non-abstinent recoveries and so-called self-change without treatment have been greeted in convenience surveys with skepticism, in contrast to studies showing that for many with alcohol use disorders, self-change is a common pathway to recovery [28, 29] and a significant percent of those with SUDs are able to moderate their use into the range of low-risk drinking [30]. While we would ideally approach any given intervention (in either camp) by assessing the evidence base, Robert MacCoun explains that from a policy standpoint, what he calls *symbolic psychological factors* often undermine more pragmatic evaluations of the evidence, and even self-described pragmatists can be driven by deep-seated retributive motives [31]. For example, he cites evidence that death penalty supporters offer *deterrence* as justification, while their views when surveyed are then impervious to nonsupportive research findings [32]. Macoun goes on to explain that we as humans prefer black and white as a rule inasmuch as it leads to predictability, and to that end, we want to view those around us in positions of trust as wholly abstinent or wholly dangerous. Further supporting this proposition is Tetlock's value pluralism model which says that people will go to great lengths to avoid explicit trade-off reasoning in favor of good-bad dichotomies [33]. Of course, media sensationalism only further exacerbates this perception of patients with SUDs as unpredictable and fear-inspiring [15]. All this may explain why needle exchange programs—well supported by a strong research base as both cost-effective and successful at reducing micro and macro harm [34]—have faced and continue to face opposition in certain policy arenas, while claims that harm reduction *sends the wrong message* find little evidence-based support [31].

Several specific treatments for addiction bring their own associated stigma, both psychosocial and pharmacologic. Simply initiating psychosocial treatment of any kind can represent an impasse for many patients; 40 % of survey respondents who had resolved an alcohol problem reported they had not sought treatment because of the stigma of being labeled an alcoholic [35]. The very anonymous nature of 12-step organizations was from the outset, in the words of AA's own literature, a protection against "public exposure" and "the social stigma of alcoholism" [36], and this continues to hold true, though this public understanding of anonymity is in many ways less important than internal understanding that anonymity levels the playing field among members so that they can place "principles before personalities" according to AA's 12th tradition. In any case, many patients have negative mental associations with 12-step groups and other psychosocial treatments—for example, that they cater to *only* people with severe substance use disorders, significant legal issues, family strife, or homelessness—any of which can prevent them from initiating engagement. In the realm of pharmacology, opioid replacement therapy, in particular methadone maintenance therapy (MMT), offers perhaps the most studied example where associated stigma is a well-identified barrier to treatment success [37]. Earnshaw et al. extensively interviewed patients receiving MMT and described numerous examples of stigmatizing interactions with family, employers, co-workers, and, perhaps most concerning, healthcare workers, in which patients felt they were viewed as untrustworthy or likely to steal [38]. These patients were acutely aware of shifts in attitude from nurses in the ER upon disclosing their use of MMT. The ways in which special dispensaries for MMT have engendered support as well as stigma have been discussed in literature [37], while patients' preference for dispensation from mainstream pharmacies has come up against reluctance by pharmacists to carry methadone for fear of robbery and alienation of other clientele. Buprenorphine/naloxone (BN) has been praised as a less stigmatizing alternative opioid replacement therapy with greater ease of use and expectation of privacy [39], though some patients have perceived stigma within 12-step groups when they disclose their use of BN to the group as a whole [40]. Stigma within treatment settings and, in this case, within mutual help organizations is indeed a challenge for patients as well as providers, but through greater education of our surrounding communities, and through self-reflection, we as providers can decrease barriers to care and help our patients integrate existing psychosocial resources (including mutual help) with newer treatments.

Special Populations

While it is difficult to do justice to all the ways in which stigma impacts the course and management of minority and vulnerable populations with addictions, we will use examples here of certain groups to illustrate several relevant concepts: intersectionality, social exclusion, stigma as a mediator of pathology, and stigma as a barrier to care. Intersectionality is a theoretical framework that helps us better understand how multiple social identities (race, ethnicity, gender, sexual orientation, socioeconomic status) intersect at the level of individual experience to reflect complex systems of privilege and oppression at the level of society [41]. To apply this framework here more directly, our patients with addictions have complex identities that can alter the extent to which they experience stigma and social exclusion, and this adjustment in the degree of stigma (often an increase) is not so much linear as it is a product of multiple interdependent aspects of their identity. A real life example illustrates this phenomenon: we noted earlier the unfortunate stigma specific to methadone maintenance treatment (MMT), and we also know that HIV-infected persons with SUD experience suboptimal highly active antiretroviral therapy (HAART) access, in part due to health professional prejudice; yet in spite of these findings, we have learned that patients with addictions who are HIV-infected *and* receiving MMT actually have better access to HAART [42]. Such complex intersections abound and caution us against nonempirical assumptions. Although we will use the expression "additive stigma," we acknowledge that the result is often more nuanced than the sum of its parts.

Another important theme in discussing additive stigma is that it not only results *from* multiple intersecting identities, but it also operates itself as a mediator of pathology. How precisely does this occur? Speaking specifically about sexual minorities, Hatzenbuehler explains that these minorities experience increased stress exposure due to stigma, and this stress in turn creates elevations in general emotional dysregulation, interpersonal problems, and cognitive processes conferring risk for psychopathology [43]. Underscoring this conclusion, Frischknecht et al. found a neurobiological correlate of such effects: they looked specifically at persons who use heroin and found that a higher perception of discrimination was associated on magnetic resonance (MR) spectroscopy with decreased N-acetylaspartate, a marker of energy utilization, in the anterior cingulate cortex, suggesting a malfunction in the neural system involved in cognitive control over emotionally relevant social stimuli [44]. Considering injection drug users specifically, Neale et al. found that these perceptions of discrimination are attributed to a range of healthcare providers including general practitioners, psychiatrists, pharmacists, and nursing staff [45], and the authors note that such patients are often labeled as "demanding" and "undeserving," evidently not without emotional costs for the clients whom they serve.

Though we have touched on sexual minorities and injection drug users, other special populations, including former prisoners, pregnant women, and persons infected with HIV, face important barriers to care resulting from stigma. Of the well over two million individuals incarcerated in the United States at present in local, state, and federal prisons, 668 thousand are released from prisons each year, exposing the extent to which our society demands that prison populations continually reintegrate with society at large [46]. The statistics related to substance use disorders among prisoners are quite remarkable: more than one half of federal inmates are incarcerated for drug law violations and roughly as many meet DSM4 criteria for drug dependence (this includes 13 % with a history of regular heroin injection). In a cross-sectional survey of men with SUD recently released from state prison,

42 % reported a history of criminal record discrimination by healthcare workers [47], and van Olphen et al. concluded from qualitative interviews with females with SUD recently released that incarceration-related stigma added further treatment barriers [48]. It should be noted, however, that in one study of a primary-care population receiving buprenorphine/naloxone, no difference was found in the post-incarceration subpopulation in terms of treatment outcomes [49], offering at least some reassurance that while stigma may prove a barrier to care, those who do receive SUD care may have similar success rates. Women with SUD who are pregnant or postpartum face greater stigma than women with SUD who are not, and such stigma may lead them to deny the harmful effects of their SUD and avoid seeking help [50]. Here again we can underscore the role of intersectionality theory by considering that while female felons are less stigmatized than male felons according to one survey [51], pregnancy may intersect with incarceration history in patients with addictions to yield a very different result (a question that could only be answered empirically). Finally, injection drug users infected with HIV were studied by Carrieri et al. who employed a novel study design meant to detect the presence of stigma as it impacted their HIV care: within the cohort, active users were divided into those the physician perceived as active, versus active users perceived as sober. Those active users perceived as using were considered less compliant than those perceived inaccurately of being in remission from their SUD, and active users as a group were less likely to receive HAART [52]. Just as management of these special populations will require awareness and sensitivity about stigma, our efforts to combat stigma and decrease barriers to care (discussed in the last section) will be that much more significant for these patients.

Stigma as a Public Health Tool: Is All Stigma Harmful?

As we discuss stigma, it is critically important to revisit at what level stigma is occurring and to what end. As mentioned earlier, historical propagation of stigma against addictions was linked to other characteristics that were highly stigmatized by society including poverty, race/ethnicity, and citizenship status, all leading to social oppression. In the early twentieth century, as cocaine came to be associated with Black Americans, marijuana with Mexican immigrants, and opium with Chinese immigrants, laws against drug use were passed that allowed perpetuation of discrimination. Social and structural stigmas, in this instance, were being used to capitalize on preexisting fears of "outsiders," fueling bigotry and mobilizing support for harsh consequences, ultimately leading to wide-scale self-stigma by the individuals affected. But what about the case of nicotine in the latter quarter of the twentieth century? Prior to strict regulations on advertising, labeling, and packaging of nicotine products, big tobacco companies portrayed smoking as healthy and glamorous, linking it to socially appealing factors that reflected high status. Attractive images of the Marlboro Man™ or women in Virginia Slims™ commercials conjured up positive associations that promoted initiation and continuation of smoking. These campaigns minimized negative stigma associated with smoking.

Smoking cigarettes was acceptable in restaurants, trains, planes, and even hospitals. For decades we saw rising numbers of cigarette smokers, particularly with women ultimately catching up and being equal in number to male smokers [1]. Lung cancer, cardiovascular disease, and other smoking-related ailments became the primary causes of death and medical morbidity. It was not until the landmark report by the surgeon general in 1964 that smoking was linked to ill health such as lung cancer and heart disease. As a result, public health campaigns, high-profile litigation against big tobacco companies, and policy changes (leading to broad-scale regulations on tobacco products) followed suit. With relentless efforts made by these public health pioneers, we have seen the stigmatization or denormalization of nicotine and tobacco products as a significant public health tool used over the last 50 years to create significant progress both in terms of primary prevention of nicotine use disorders and smoking cessation [53]. With these declines, significant decreases will continue to follow in smoking-related illnesses and death. These marked public health improvements come as a result of population-targeted social and structural stigma campaigns against nicotine and tobacco use.

Unfortunately, there is a double-edged sword to this population-level stigma campaign—person-level stigma against smoking cigarettes and being a "smoker." Now, in many settings, being a "smoker" is viewed in a highly stigmatized way, and people suffering from smoking-related illness like lung cancer are fraught with self-stigma, endorsing thoughts that they "deserve" and are judged for their consequential diseases [54]. Anyone who has seen people smoking alone or in groups on the outskirts of smoking-prohibited facilities can see the impact. The initial population-level stigma has trickled down to include the person. As a result, people who have nicotine use disorders are more likely to experience all types of stigma, high levels of shame, and barriers to seeking treatment out of fear of being judged. Additionally, people who initiate smoking cigarettes and develop nicotine addictions are now more disadvantaged and likely to have other stigmatizing characteristics such as poverty, lower education levels, and mental health disorders [4]. It is a critical challenge for healthcare providers, friends, colleagues, or family members of persons who smoke cigarettes to prevent population-level stigma from acting as a barrier to care at the individual level.

Is Erosion of Stigma Always Helpful?

In this same vein, what happens when a popular opinion campaign results in policy change that leads to de-stigmatization or normalization of a potentially harmful substance? The current state of affairs on medical and recreational marijuana legalization in the United States is one such example, and the outcomes are yet to be determined. At least within in the United States, legalized substances, such as alcohol and nicotine, are the most widely used with consequentially the greatest numbers of individuals with problematic and disordered use [55]. Marijuana is currently the most widely used illicit drug, with an estimated 14 million active users, 9 % of whom are dependent on marijuana [56]. The organized opposition to recreational use and legalization of medical marijuana worries that these numbers will increase with associated increases in the marijuana-related morbidity as legalization becomes more widespread. There is some preliminary evidence to substantiate these concerns. Recent data from Monitoring the Future 2013 shows that the perception of harm from marijuana has trended down, while adolescents' past year use of marijuana has trended up concurrently with a resurgence in popularity of marijuana since the 1990s [57]. However, the trajectories of these past-year users—who may become regular and chronic users, which groups are most at risk for poor outcomes and marijuana-associated harms—are not well known. Some large-scale national surveys in Australia and the Netherlands following decriminalization and depenalization of marijuana in conjunction with some early analyses in the United States with medical marijuana policies have not shown significant increases in the overall rates of marijuana use [58], with the caveat that it may be too early to tell the extent of the consequences of these policy changes. Potential benefits of destigmatizing marijuana through legalization, such as facilitating research on marijuana, decreased social and financial costs of incarcerating individuals for marijuana-related drug offenses, and economic gains for the states through taxation must also be considered. More longitudinal studies over a greater time period will be needed before we can fully appreciate the nuances and consequences of decreasing stigma associated with marijuana through legalization.

Thus far the authors have reviewed:

1. The historical factors including discrimination against marginalized and disenfranchised minority groups, the designation of SUDs as a "legal problem," and the development of separate treatment systems for SUDs from standard medical settings that contributed to the stigmatization of SUDs in the United States
2. The definitions of types of addiction-related stigma including social, structural, and self-stigma
3. The role of language around SUDs in creating and propagating stigma
4. The role of healthcare providers in continuing stigma toward individuals with SUDs and ways to create change that combat stigma
5. The role of stigma in impairing utilization of evidence-based treatments for SUDs
6. Stigma toward SUDs in special populations, specifically including prisoners, pregnant women, persons with HIV, sexual and racial minorities, and injection drug users
7. Nuances related to the possible risks and benefits of utilizing stigma or lack of stigma at various levels (population versus individual) in the cases of tobacco and marijuana

Combatting Stigma and Future Directions

The authors have discussed the extent to which the negative effects of healthcare-related stigma on persons with SUD are substantial and far-reaching, resulting in avoidance or non-completion of SUD-focused treatment and delayed recovery and reintegration processes [48, 59, 60]. We have also noted that stigma can be attributed variously to healthcare providers, society at large, and the individual with an addiction via self-stigma. With the tendency of social stigma to dampen initiation of tobacco and cannabis notwithstanding, we can reasonably deduce that efforts to combat stigma could improve patient outcomes, especially in the healthcare arena, in light of the aforementioned barriers stigma creates. Here we examine the theoretical and empirical basis for such a conclusion and then close with suggestions for how we might act on this evidence.

How might interventions to decrease stigma among healthcare workers actually achieve their aim? From a theoretical standpoint, this question can be divided into the impact of the intervention on the patient and on the provider. As we have discussed, stigma itself can exacerbate patient psychopathology by increasing stress exposure, which in an addiction model would likely amplify the negative reinforcement provided by the substance to further the addiction and avoidance of treatment. It follows that patients would find those providers who projected less stigma to be more approachable, less reinforcing of their negative self-image, and as a result, they would be more likely to engage in treatment. But by what mechanism would interventions aimed at providers decrease the stigma that they have internalized toward persons with SUD? Neale et al. discuss the analysis of social theorist Michel Foucault on power and knowledge as it relates to provider stigma. For Foucault, power is ubiquitous and is concentrated at local points called "micro-powers," of which the provider is one example. The provider's power results from the patient-provider dynamic (the provider possesses medical knowledge, makes diagnoses, and generates treatment plans, all of which creates an imbalance of power). Providers have the power to project stigma, but this power cannot be divorced from knowledge, which ultimately shapes *how* the power is used. In particular, the knowledge and awareness of stigma itself and how it functions in the larger context of barriers to recovery can allow providers to view patients with SUD differently [61]. For example, an emergency room physician with limited awareness of her own stigmatized attitude toward addiction is powerful inasmuch as she may discharge a patient presenting with a heroin overdose during a busy shift *without* involving social work because the patient appears "unready" to change. However, an awareness by that same physician of the barriers preventing the patient from accepting care—including perhaps the judgment the patient perceives from the ER staff—may allow the physician to use her power differently, perhaps to make an extra effort to connect the patient with treatment resources. In a similar vein, Livingston et al. note that often SUD-specific stigma serves as a loose but convenient proxy for stigma related to multiple identities (violent offender, criminal) but that education can help the provider disentangle these stereotypes and realize that such negative externalities of SUD are not applicable to all members of the group [62]. To integrate these models, a working knowledge on the part of the provider of both the impact of stigma and the intersectionality of related but nonequivalent identities can deepen their empathy for the patient with an SUD and ultimately function to combat stigma.

Of course, the question of whether educational interventions designed to reduce stigma can be effective is also an empirical one and can be subdivided into provider-centered and patient-centered outcomes (though as with any research question, the absence of evidence for changes in patient outcomes is not evidence of its absence).

One other caveat is that interventions to reduce societal and self-stigma are certainly important and have been reviewed elsewhere [63] but fall outside the scope of this section; the topic of reducing societal stigma toward substance use disorders is complex and necessarily would involve a larger discussion of our criminal justice system. Corrigan et al. have pointed out that the training period represents an ideal time for provider biases about certain patient populations to be addressed as stigma tends to calcify after the training years making them an ideal time for interventions [64]. Trainees across various disciplines are susceptible to projecting stigma, and even among psychiatric trainees—who one might hypothesize would hold less stigmatized attitudes (given both their specific addictions training and their training emphasis on self-examination)—a majority in one study responded that they would not like to work with this patient population [65]. Seven studies looking at interventions centered on medical trainees were reviewed by Livingston et al. who found overall that structured reflection techniques, additional contact with patients with SUD, and other stigma-related education interventions are likely to increase comfort with these populations and decrease stigmatizing attitudes [62]. In two more recent studies with similar interventions, one with physician-assistant students and another with nursing students, the authors noted limits in the potency of brief education interventions to alter stigmatized attitudes, while direct interaction with a person in longer-term recovery was one of the more potent aspects of their interventions [66, 67]. Of some interest was the phenomenon whereby trainees in the study by Crapanzano et al. felt their remaining stigmatized attitudes would not impact the care they ultimately delivered. Ultimately this literature is limited by lack of longer-term data regarding its impact on stigmatized attitudes, how patients experienced these providers, and ultimately whether it altered their disease course [63].

Does all this suggest a way forward? In the healthcare arena, we can focus on identifying the proverbial low-hanging fruit. Rasyidi et al. [68] point out that at present, the medical school accreditation bodies—the Association of American Medical Colleges (AAMC) and its Liaison Committee on Medical Education (LCME)—have no explicit requirement for medical education on the treatment of SUD. Residency (graduate medical education) witnesses similar limitations when one considers that psychiatry, representing 5 % of residents, is the only medical specialty for which the Accreditation Council for Graduate Medical Education (ACGME) mandates specific addiction training. Disciplines under the umbrella of primary care such as internal medicine or pediatrics, representing a quarter of medical school graduates, have required only that trainees be offered elective opportunities in addictions but have no specific mandates [68]. Certainly medical education has competing interests at all stages, but the enormous prevalence of SUD, its interaction with other diseases, and its uniquely stigmatized attributes would seem to demand a new era in medical education. While neuropsychiatric rotations in medical training may offer the most obvious focal points for adding the kinds anti-stigma-oriented reflection, patient encounters, and education described above, integrating addiction training within rotations or as intersession immersion programs for graduate trainees may also offer a path forward as described in promising small-scale efforts [69, 70]. As our larger healthcare system shifts its focus more and more toward value and quality, the need to break down silos of care and view patients holistically is greater than ever. We must help the providers of tomorrow to gain greater awareness into their explicit and implicit biases and stigmatized attitudes toward addiction so that they can deliver more compassionate care. Not only do patients with addictions deserve this kind of care, in many cases, their recoveries may depend upon it.

References

1. Fiore MC, Novotny TE, Pierce JP, Hatziandreu EJ, Patel KM, Davis RM. Trends in cigarette smoking in the United States. The changing influence of gender and race. JAMA. 1989;261(1):49–55. Epub 1989/01/06.
2. Dean JC, Rud F. The drug addict and the stigma of addiction. Int J Addict. 1984;19(8):859–69. Epub 1984/12/01.
3. Blazer DG, Wu LT. The epidemiology of substance use and disorders among middle aged and elderly community adults: national survey on drug use and health. Am J Geriatr Psychiatry Off J Am Assoc Geriatr Psychiatry. 2009;17(3):237–45. Epub 2009/05/21.
4. Bell K, Salmon A, Bowers M, Bell J, McCullough L. Smoking, stigma and tobacco 'denormalization': further reflections on the use of stigma as a public health tool. A commentary on social science & Medicine's stigma, prejudice, discrimination and health special issue (67: 3). Soc Sci Med. 2010;70(6):795–9. discussion 800-1. Epub 2010/01/02.
5. Livingston JD, Boyd JE. Correlates and consequences of internalized stigma for people living with mental illness: a systematic review and meta-analysis. Soc Sci Med. 2010;71(12):2150–61. Epub 2010/11/06.
6. Mannarini S, Boffo M. Anxiety, bulimia, drug and alcohol addiction, depression, and schizophrenia: what do you think about their aetiology, dangerousness, social distance, and treatment? a latent class analysis approach. Soc Psychiatry Psychiatr Epidemiol. 2015;50(1):27–37. Epub 2014/06/29.
7. van Boekel LC, Brouwers EP, van Weeghel J, Garretsen HF. Comparing stigmatising attitudes towards people with substance use disorders between the general public, GPs, mental health and addiction specialists and clients. Int J Soc Psychiatry. 2014. Epub 2014/12/17.
8. Luoma JB, Twohig MP, Waltz T, Hayes SC, Roget N, Padilla M, et al. An investigation of stigma in individuals receiving treatment for substance abuse. Addict Behav. 2007;32(7):1331–46. Epub 2006/11/10.
9. Corrigan PW, Rafacz J, Rusch N. Examining a progressive model of self-stigma and its impact on people with serious mental illness. Psychiatry Res. 2011;189(3):339–43. Epub 2011/07/01.
10. Link BG, Struening EL, Neese-Todd S, Asmussen S, Phelan JC. Stigma as a barrier to recovery: the consequences of stigma for the self-esteem of people with mental illnesses. Psychiatr Serv. 2001;52(12):1621–6. Epub 2001/12/01.
11. Ahern J, Stuber J, Galea S. Stigma, discrimination and the health of illicit drug users. Drug Alcohol Depend. 2007;88(2–3):188–96. Epub 2006/11/23.
12. Sacco P, Unick GJ, Kuerbis A, Koru AG, Moore AA. Alcohol-related diagnoses in hospital admissions for all causes among middle-aged and older adults: trends and cohort differences from 1993 to 2010. J Aging Health. 2015;27:1358–74. Epub 2015/04/24.
13. Harris LT, Fiske ST. Dehumanizing the lowest of the low: neuroimaging responses to extreme out-groups. Psychol Sci. 2006;17(10):847–53.
14. Seligman M. Flourish: a visionary new understanding of happiness and well-being. New York: Free Press; 2011.
15. Bhattacharyya S, Crippa JA, Martin-Santos R, Winton-Brown T, Fusar-Poli P. Imaging the neural effects of cannabinoids: current status and future opportunities for psychopharmacology. Curr Pharm Des. 2009;15(22):2603–14. Epub 2009/08/20.

16. Corrigan PW, Sokol KA, Rusch N. The impact of self-stigma and mutual help programs on the quality of life of people with serious mental illnesses. Community Ment Health J. 2013;49(1):1–6. Epub 2011/11/01.
17. Prochaska JO, DiClemente CC. Stages of change in the modification of problem behaviors. Prog Behav Modif. 1992;28:183–218.
18. Kelly JF, Wakeman SE, Saitz R. Stop talking 'dirty': clinicians, language, and quality of care for the leading cause of preventable death in the United States. Am J Med. 2015;128(1):8–9. Epub 2014/09/07.
19. Samet JH, Fiellin DA. Opioid substitution therapy-time to replace the term. Lancet. 2015;385(9977):1508–9. Epub 2015/05/02.
20. Schomerus G, Matschinger H, Lucht MJ, Angermeyer MC. Changes in the perception of alcohol-related stigma in Germany over the last two decades. Drug Alcohol Depend. 2014;143:225–31. Epub 2014/08/27.
21. Gilchrist G, Moskalewicz J, Slezakova S, Okruhlica L, Torrens M, Vajd R, et al. Staff regard towards working with substance users: a European multi-centre study. Addiction. 2011;106(6):1114–25. Epub 2011/02/16.
22. Siegfried N, Ferguson J, Cleary M, Walter G, Rey JM. Experience, knowledge and attitudes of mental health staff regarding patients' problematic drug and alcohol use. Aust N Z J Psychiatry. 1999;33(2):267–73. Epub 1999/05/21.
23. Baldacchino A, Gilchrist G, Fleming R, Bannister J. Guilty until proven innocent: a qualitative study of the management of chronic non-cancer pain among patients with a history of substance abuse. Addict Behav. 2010;35(3):270–2. Epub 2009/11/10.
24. van Boekel LC, Brouwers EP, van Weeghel J, Garretsen HF. Stigma among health professionals towards patients with substance use disorders and its consequences for healthcare delivery: systematic review. Drug Alcohol Depend. 2013;131(1–2):23–35. Epub 2013/03/16.
25. Kuerbis AN, Yuan SE, Borok J, LeFevre PM, Kim GS, Lum D, et al. Testing the initial efficacy of a mailed screening and brief feedback intervention to reduce at-risk drinking in middle-aged and older adults: the comorbidity alcohol risk evaluation study. J Am Geriatr Soc. 2015;63(2):321–6. Epub 2015/02/04.
26. Sher I, McGinn L, Sirey JA, Meyers B. Effects of caregivers' perceived stigma and causal beliefs on patients' adherence to antidepressant treatment. Psychiatr Serv. 2005;56(5):564–9. Epub 2005/05/06.
27. Babor TF, McRee BG, Kassebaum PA, Grimaldi PL, Ahmed K, Bray J. Screening, Brief Intervention, and Referral to Treatment (SBIRT): toward a public health approach to the management of substance abuse. Subst Abuse off Publ Assoc Med Educ Res Subst Abuse. 2007;28(3):7–30. Epub 2007/12/14.
28. Broadening the base of treatment for alcohol problems: hearing before the Institute of Medicine (US) Committee on Treatment of Alcohol Problems(1990).
29. Fillmore KM, Grant M, Hartka E, Johnstone BM, Sawyer SM, Speiglman R, et al. Collaborative longitudinal research on alcohol problems. Br J Addict. 1988;83(4):441–4.
30. Sobell LC, Ellingstad TP, Sobell MB. Natural recovery from alcohol and drug problems: methodological review of the research with suggestions for future directions. Addiction. 2000;95(5):749–64.
31. MacCoun RJ. Toward a psychology of harm reduction. Am Psychol. 1998;53(11):1199–208.
32. Ellsworth PC, Gross SR. Hardening of the attitudes – Americans views on the death-penalty. J Soc Issues. 1994;50(2):19–52.
33. Tetlock PE, Peterson RS, Lerner JS. Revising the value pluralism model: incorporating social content and context postulates. Ontol Symp Proc. 1996;8:25–51.
34. Ritter A, Cameron J. A review of the efficacy and effectiveness of harm reduction strategies for alcohol, tobacco and illicit drugs. Drug Alcohol Rev. 2006;25(6):611–24.
35. Sobel L. Recovery from alcohol problems without treatment. In: Heaher NM WR, Greeley J, editors. Self control and addictive behaviors. New York: Maxwell Macmillan; 1992. p. 198–242.

36. Alcoholics Anonymous. Understanding anonymity. New York: Alcoholics Anonymous World Services, Inc; 2011.
37. Anstice S, Strike CJ, Brands B. Supervised methadone consumption: client issues and stigma. Subst Use Misuse. 2009;44(6):794–808.
38. Earnshaw V, Smith L, Copenhaver M. Drug addiction stigma in the context of methadone maintenance therapy: an investigation into understudied sources of stigma. Int J Ment Health Addict. 2013;11(1):110–22.
39. Selzer J. Buprenorphine: reflections of an addictions psychiatrist. J Clin Psychiatry. 2006;67(9):1466–7.
40. Alford DP, Salsitz EA, Martin J, Renner JA. Clinical case discussion: treating opioid dependence with buprenorphine. J Addict Med. 2007;1(2):73–8.
41. Bowleg L. The problem with the phrase women and minorities: intersectionality-an important theoretical framework for public health. Am J Public Health. 2012;102(7):1267–73.
42. Malta M, da Costa MR, Bastos FI. The paradigm of universal access to HIV-treatment and human rights violation: how do we treat HIV-positive people who use drugs? Curr HIV/AIDS Rep. 2014;11(1):52–62.
43. Hatzenbuehler ML. How does sexual minority stigma "Get under the skin"? a psychological mediation framework. Psychol Bull. 2009;135(5):707–30.
44. Frischknecht U, Hermann D, Heinrich M, Hoerst M, Weber-Fahr W, Vollstadt-Klein S, et al. Experience of social discrimination correlates with neurometabolism: a pilot study in heroin addicts. Eur Arch Psychiatry Clin Neurosci. 2013;263(3):197–203.
45. Neale J, Tompkins C, Sheard L. Barriers to accessing generic health and social care services: a qualitative study of injecting drug users. Health Soc Care Community. 2008;16(2):147–54.
46. Wagner P, Sakala L. A prison policy initiative briefing. 2014. [cited 2014 Mar 12]. Available from: http://www.prisonpolicy.org/reports/pie.html.
47. Frank JW, Wang EA, Nunez-Smith M, Lee H, Comfort M. Discrimination based on criminal record and healthcare utilization among men recently released from prison: a descriptive study. Health Just. 2014;2:6.
48. van Olphen J, Eliason MJ, Freudenberg N, Barnes M. Nowhere to go: how stigma limits the options of female drug users after release from jail. Subst Abuse Treat Prev Policy. 2009;4:10.
49. Wang EA, Moore BA, Sullivan LE, Fiellin DA. Effect of incarceration history on outcomes of primary care office-based buprenorphine/naloxone. J Gen Intern Med. 2010;25(7):670–4.
50. Albright BB, Rayburn WF. Substance abuse among reproductive age women. Obstet Gynecol Clin North Am. 2009;36(4):891–906. xi–xii.
51. Steffensmeier DJ, Kramer JH. Differential impact of criminal stigmatization on male and female felons. Sex Roles. 1980;6(1):1–8.
52. Carrieri MP, Moatti JP, Vlahov D, Obadia Y, Reynaud-Maurupt C, Chesney M. Access to antiretroviral treatment among french HIV infected injection drug users: the influence of continued drug use. MANIF 2000 study group. J Epidemiol Community Health. 1999;53(1):4–8.
53. De Petrocellis L, Di Marzo V. Non-CB1, non-CB2 receptors for endocannabinoids, plant cannabinoids, and synthetic cannabimimetics: focus on G-protein-coupled receptors and transient receptor potential channels. J Neuroimmune Pharmacol off J Soc Neuroimmune Pharmacol. 2010;5(1):103–21. Epub 2009/10/23.
54. Lozovaya N, Min R, Tsintsadze V, Burnashev N. Dual modulation of CNS voltage-gated calcium channels by cannabinoids: focus on CB1 receptor-independent effects. Cell Calcium. 2009;46(3):154–62. Epub 2009/08/18.
55. Pacek LR, Mauro PM, Martins SS. Perceived risk of regular cannabis use in the United States from 2002 to 2012: differences by sex, age, and race/ethnicity. Drug Alcohol Depend. 2015;149:232–44.
56. Schutz CG, Rapiti E, Vlahov D, Anthony JC. Suspected determinants of enrollment into detoxification and methadone maintenance treatment among injecting drug users. Drug Alcohol Depend. 1994;36(2):129–38.

57. Johnston LD, Miech RA. Monitoring the future: national survey results on drug use, 1975–2013. Ann Arbor: Ann Arbor Institute for Social Research, University of Michigan; 2014.
58. Hall W, Weier M. Assessing the public health impacts of legalising recreational cannabis use in the USA. Clin Pharmacol Ther. 2015.
59. Brener L, von Hippel W, von Hippel C, Resnick I, Treloar C. Perceptions of discriminatory treatment by staff as predictors of drug treatment completion: utility of a mixed methods approach. Drug Alcohol Rev. 2010;29(5):491–7.
60. Town M, Naimi TS, Mokdad AH, Brewer RD. Health care access among U.S. adults who drink alcohol excessively: missed opportunities for prevention. Prev Chronic Dis. 2006;3(2):A53.
61. Substance Abuse and Mental Health Services Administration. Results from the 2012 national survey on drug use and health: summary of national findings. Rockville: Substance Abuse and Mental Health Services Administration; 2013. Contract No.: HHS Publication No. (SMA) 13-4795.
62. Livingston JD, Milne T, Fang ML, Amari E. The effectiveness of interventions for reducing stigma related to substance use disorders: a systematic review. Addiction. 2012;107(1):39–50.
63. Heijnders M, Van Der Meij S. The fight against stigma: an overview of stigma-reduction strategies and interventions. Psychol Health Med. 2006;11(3):353–63.
64. Corrigan PW, Penn DL. Lessons from social psychology on discrediting psychiatric stigma. Am Psychol. 1999;54(9):765–76.
65. Renner Jr JA, Karam-Hage M, Levinson M, Craig T, Eld B. What do psychiatric residents think of addiction psychiatry as a career? Acad Psychiatry J Am Assoc Dir Psychiatr Residency Train Assoc Acad Psychiatry. 2009;33(2):139–42.
66. Cadiz DM, O'Neill C, Butell SS, Epeneter BJ, Basin B. Quasi-experimental evaluation of a substance use awareness educational intervention for nursing students. J Nurs Educ. 2012;51(7):411–5.
67. Crapanzano K, Vath RJ, Fisher D. Reducing stigma towards substance users through an educational intervention: harder than it looks. Acad Psychiatry J Am Assoc Dir Psychiatr Residency Train Assoc Acad Psychiatry. 2014;38(4):420–5.
68. Rasyidi E, Wilkins JN, Danovitch I. Training the next generation of providers in addiction medicine. Psychiatr Clin North Am. 2012;35(2):461–80.
69. Alford DP, Bridden C, Jackson AH, Saitz R, Amodeo M, Barnes HN, et al. Promoting substance use education among generalist physicians: an evaluation of the Chief Resident Immersion Training (CRIT) program. J Gen Intern Med. 2009;24(1):40–7.
70. O'Connor PG, Nyquist JG, McLellan AT. Integrating addiction medicine into graduate medical education in primary care: the time has come. Ann Intern Med. 2011;154(1):56–9.

Chapter 8
Borderline Personality Disorder: From Stigma to Compassionate Care

Blaise Aguirre

Introduction: Why This Chapter?

I have been in the mental health field since 1990. I have worked predominantly with people with borderline personality disorder (BPD) since 2000 and almost exclusively with them since opening up a dedicated treatment unit since 2007. In that time, we have treated thousands of patients with BPD who have come from all over the world for a dedicated treatment approach. BPD is one of the stigmatized, if not *the* most, psychiatric disorders. Study after study, and my own clinical experience in the field, shows that people who carry the label of BPD receive more negative responses by my colleagues in the mental health profession than those with other labels. More than for other psychiatric disorders, people with BPD are thought to be more capable of controlling their socially "unacceptable" behavior, and yet often they cannot because they do not have the skill set to manage relationships and emotions. And so, and as research as well as my own professional experience shows, the mental health profession responds with less sympathy and optimism toward people who have this disorder. We, the mental health professionals, are to blame for the stigma attached to BPD, and it is up to us to repair the damage. We can do this through compassionate understanding, education, the removal of judgmental language, and the provision of evidence-based care. This chapter is an appeal to all mental health specialists to join in a concerted effort to stamp out the stigma.

In this chapter, I will delve into how the stigma got to be what it is and how it manifests in the clinical context and then suggest specific steps that our field can take in order to reduce the stigma. More specifically I will challenge the myths that

B. Aguirre, MD
3East DBT Continuum, 3East Mclean Hospital, 115 Mill Street,
Belmont, MA 02478, USA
e-mail: baguirre@partners.org

© Springer International Publishing Switzerland 2016   133
R. Parekh, Ed W. Childs (eds.), *Stigma and Prejudice: Touchstones in
Understanding Diversity in Healthcare*, Current Clinical Psychiatry,
DOI 10.1007/978-3-319-27580-2_8

have perpetuated the stigma, look at contemporary and compassionate evidence-based treatment approaches, and look at areas where we can improve psychoeducation. I will include the idea of educating, for instance, the legal and law enforcement professions which are not typically considered in such endeavors.

A Call to Action

"You will know that your patient has BPD when you feel like slapping her in the face at the end of a session" – Supervising Attending
   "When you walk onto your unit and your staff is at each other's throats you know you have a borderline on the unit" – Unit Medical Director
   These are direct quotes from senior psychiatrists and expressed in supervision while I was a young trainee. At the time I found the quips witty and succinctly didactic. Over the years of subsequent training, it was clear that only borderline personality disorder (BPD) was spoken about in this way. No other psychiatric illness was or remains as stigmatized by my colleagues in the mental health profession. How did this come to be?

Introducing Borderline Personality Disorder

Today BPD is known within the mental health profession as a common and serious mental illness that causes unstable moods, unstable behavior, unstable self-image, unstable cognitions, and unstable relationships. It typically begins in adolescence or early adulthood [1]. Those with the disorder experience significant suffering and distress due to the difficulty of trying to manage these difficulties, ones that impact all aspects of life. It is also a much stigmatized condition. Knowing the history of the diagnosis is an important step in understanding why it is so stigmatized and what we can do about it.

BPD: Back to the Past

Historically, the psychiatrist most responsible for introducing the label "borderline" was Adolphus Stern in 1938 [2]. He had identified what he termed as the tendency of certain patients to regress into "borderline schizophrenia" mental states in unstructured situations, and yet although distinct from schizophrenia, these patients were still categorized under the schizophrenia category. This construct remained essentially unchanged until 1967 [3], when Otto Kernberg, a psychoanalyst, defined "borderline" as the level of personality organization that was bookended on one side by sicker patients who were more psychotic and on the other side by those who were healthier or more "neurotic." In 1978 [4], psychiatrist John Gunderson published a seminal piece where the borderline syndrome became reliably assessable with discriminating criteria.

BPD: The Demographics

Depending on the survey used, BPD exists in approximately 2–6 % of the general population although the largest sample indicates that the number is closer to 6 % than 2 % [5]. It also appears in up to 20 % of all psychiatric inpatients and 15 % of all outpatients. Although the data show that BPD is distributed equally in females and males, females predominate (about 75 %) within psychiatric settings, while males predominate in substance abuse or forensic settings.

A Stigmatized Condition

How and Why Is This Population Stigmatized

The roots of stigma can be seen in early descriptions of BPD patients. They were termed "interpersonally needy." They were also considered to be "difficult" patients with considerable suicidal risk. Donald Klein [6] described them as "fickle, egocentric, irresponsible, love-intoxicated." John Houck [7] described women with BPD as "intractable, unruly" patients who used hospitals to escape from responsibilities.

These pejorative descriptions discouraged compassionate understanding for a condition that almost all who suffered from it would have wished it gone from their lives.

Stigmatized by the Profession

History is hard to erase from training, and as a consequence of these early descriptions, BPD is often viewed in negative terms by mental health specialists and consequently by the public. The disorder has a stigma that goes beyond that associated with other psychiatric illnesses and that is because the very nature of BPD is transactional and consequently affects how clinicians think, behave, and feel in the context of treating those with BPD. Further, people who struggle with BPD suffer in ways not obvious to clinicians, and so their symptoms are often minimized.

For instance, the misunderstood symptoms of self-hatred and intense emotional experiences are often difficult for clinicians to grasp. A few minutes of unrelenting suffering can feel like an eternity to the person suffering from BPD. Einstein once explained relativity as such: "Put your hand on a hot stove for a minute, and it seems like an hour. Sit with a pretty girl for an hour, and it seems like a minute. THAT'S relativity." And so is the experience of emotional pain for the person with BPD. And so it is that throughout history, society has distanced itself from misunderstood populations.

Just as for other stigmatized conditions, the misunderstanding has stemmed from lack of knowledge and research. Early descriptions of BPD by prominent authors used words like "manipulative," "needy," "clingy," "attention seeking," and "promiscuous" to describe people with BPD, making BPD a most undesirable condition to treat. Further, in the early days of the diagnosis, there was no reliably effective way to treat the condition, and without a therapy, many clinicians distanced themselves from their patients. The clinical perspectives by the leading thinkers of the time, members of my own mental health profession, had inadvertently laid the groundwork that created the most powerful stigma. As a consequence, it is our profession that needs to repair the damage.

The Interpersonal Dimension

As BPD is predominantly a problem of difficulty in interpersonal and emotional regulation, the distancing of therapist from patient worsens the suffering of people with BPD, because this group is particularly sensitive to rejection and abandonment. When the sensitivity is triggered, behaviors like self-harm and suicidality can manifest as attempts to deal with the abandonment or regulate intense emotions. The self-injury and suicidal behavior in turn push the clinician further way, and the cycle of rejection and self-destructive behaviors escalates and persists. It is not only these behaviors but also hurtful, devaluing statements by people with BPD and a clinician's sense of helplessness and hopelessness that lead to a sense of futility and ultimately a sense of personal failure on the part of the clinician.

It is understandable that therapists would withdraw in the face of the extreme behaviors of people with BPD, and yet this withdrawal from the symptoms of the disorder, the very behaviors that make it difficult to work with these patients, strongly contributes to the stigma of BPD. In clinical practice we see patients referred from therapists whose own emotional reactions to their patients have exacerbated the BPD symptoms of their patients. Because of the unpredictability and intensity of the emotions and behaviors of their clients, it becomes difficult for clinicians to see and maintain a perspective that their patient's problems are symptoms of the underlying brain pathology and are not the essence of the individual. Even expert clinicians can be taxed by the work, and when young supervisees see that the seasoned expert does not see their patient with compassion or neutrality, the roots of condemnation are planted.

For the person with BPD, the result of interactions with wary clinicians leads to a self-fulfilling prophecy and cycle of enduring stigmatization to which both patient and clinician contribute, a cycle that goes like this: The therapist predicts that the patient with BPD will be too hard to work with, increasingly withdraws from the patient who then behaves in ways that leads the therapist to terminate treatment; the patient predicts that they will be abandoned by their clinician, and when they are, hopelessness and worthlessness perpetuates. The disorder then becomes a self-stigmatizing condition as people with BPD then go on to develop similar judgments to those of their professional caregivers.

Further Stigmatized in Popular Culture: Myths and Misinformation

It is critical that our profession knows that the historical narratives have permeated all forms of available literature, and in particular in many circumstances, patients come into session having read misinformed, antiquated, or plain erroneous descriptions of BPD online. Perhaps worse is the experience of having been diagnosed by a non-clinician or by a mental health specialist whose understanding of BPD has not changed in decades.

Over the years since opening up our unit at McLean hospital, known as 3 East, one dedicated to the treatment of people with BPD, I have been asked to address the stigma associated with such representations at conferences all over the world. Although there is increasing acceptance as to the diagnosis and treatability of BPD, the nature of the questions asked at these lectures shows that many myths and misunderstandings persist and that these need to be addressed. There is plenty of misinformation available on the web and in online forums and blog posts, and the clinician who referred a patient with BPD needs to be ready to address these portrayals. The following widely accepted ideas have no basis in research:

1. BPD does not occur in people younger than 18.
2. People with BPD are manipulative and attention seeking.
3. BPD is a rare condition.
4. BPD is a form of bipolar disorder.
5. Bad parenting causes BPD.
6. People with BPD do not know how to love.
7. BPD only affects women.
8. There are high-functioning and low-functioning forms of BPD.
9. People with BPD are unbearable to be with.
10. People with BPD do not really want to kill themselves.
11. There are no treatments for people with BPD and they would not get better.
12. BPD is caused by trauma.

It is imperative that mental health experts not only know the latest research and neuroscience but further counter these myths and misrepresentations wherever they appear.

BPD: The Effect of the Stigma

In recent years, some research has focused on the lived experience of those diagnosed with BPD [8–14]. On our unit we find that an honest discussion about the condition without adding commentary about the historical perspective and stigma makes our patients' experience of the disorder no different from diagnosing any other mental health condition. Typically, on hearing the diagnosis and reviewing the symptoms, there is a sense of relief and appreciation that finally there is a diagnosis that makes sense. On the other hand, the research on the personal experience of being diagnosed with BPD shows that many women feel that it is a pejorative label.

Why the difference? On review of this research, we find that narratives include the idea that self-destructive behavior is perceived as manipulative, that there is no or limited help for the condition, and that health-care professionals consider the label with disdain [11]. The participants experienced being labeled rather than diagnosed. Some patients describe being terrified of disapproval or being rejected, particularly by the key people in their life including their therapist and as such will often withhold information to defend against this perceived rejection [10].

Private Misery

In terms of living with the BPD diagnosis, people with the disorder have described the hopelessness and misery they have felt and in particular the role of the behavior of self-harm as a short-term intervention used to reduce emotional suffering. There is also the suspicion that clinicians are not being totally honest with them, and in one study, two participants said that they were told of the BPD diagnosis only when they were recruited for the study [12].

Current Health-Care Treatment of BPD

Various psychotherapeutic approaches have been shown to have benefit in contemporary trials, and although the trials were considered "randomized controlled," it is important to remember that it is far more complicated to control for a psychotherapy than it is for a pill and a placebo in a medication trial. Nevertheless, the authors and treatment developers of the new psychotherapies have gone further in measuring adherence to their treatment models than other research has ever done before. The most robust findings are those showing the benefit of dialectical behavior therapy (DBT) [15] and then mentalization-based therapy (MBT) [16]. Other individual therapies that have been shown to be useful include cognitive behavioral therapy (CBT) [17], schema-focused therapy (SFT) [18], transference-focused psychotherapy (TFP) [19], cognitive analytic therapy (CAT) [20], and supportive psychotherapy [21]. Many of these treatments require dedicated training and many hours of specialist supervision. More recently, general psychiatric management (GPM) [22] blends elements of all of these treatments together including cognitive, behavioral, and psychodynamic interventions that are practical and simple to implement and have been developed as a way to reduce the complexity of some of the other therapies. The idea behind GPM is that although for many cases of severe BPD a dedicated psychotherapy in the hands of an expert is necessary, for the majority of cases of mild BPD, a basic knowledge of the condition and a pragmatic approach are easier to learn and appear to be as effective as more specialized treatments. In terms of dedicated group, therapy for treating BPD as Systems Training for Emotional Predictability and Problem Solving (STEPPS) (23) has been shown to be an effective approach.

Common Features

In looking at common features between the treatments, the following appear to be present in most: at least weekly meetings with an individual therapist, 1 or more weekly group sessions, and regular meetings of therapists for consultation or supervision. There is also a clear treatment framework that is explicit. Although not specifically stated, in meeting with practitioners of these various treatment modalities, one thing that they all have in common is a dedication to work with people with BPD, and so even though it is likely that the various therapeutic approaches have their own intrinsic utility, the effect of having a therapist who cares about people with BPD cannot be overestimated.

What About Medications?

No medications have been approved by the US Food and Drug Administration (FDA) to treat BPD. However, because other psychiatric disorders co-occur with BPD, many people with BPD are treated with medications together with psychotherapy. The target symptoms of medication include reducing anxiety, depression, and mood swings. On our unit we see patients coming in on polypharmacy despite there being very little evidence that the practice of multiple medications is either necessary or effective. Further there are serious health-care consequences of polypharmacy which are associated with high rates of obesity and in turn associated with elevated rates of osteoarthritis, diabetes, hypertension, and other illnesses. Mary Zanarini EdD has reported that in these circumstances, the health profile of a 30-year-old woman with BPD is comparable to that of a 60-year-old without BPD. Polypharmacy can be a subtle form of stigma due to the judgment associated with being on multiple medications, particularly if they are not effective in reducing the symptoms of the underlying condition.

Concluding Thoughts

In reviewing the chapter, it is easy to see how BPD became as stigmatized by the mental health profession as it is. It was never the intention of our field to stigmatize it so, but without our current understanding of BPD's neurobiology caused by genetic and environmental factors and without effective treatment options, the historical assumptions and interpretations of teachers and clinicians led to conclusions that compounded the suffering of people with BPD. These stigmatizing narratives can be undone by, firstly, the teaching of new clinicians using contemporary up-to-date material that relies on the latest research and, secondly, by openly, yet compassionately, challenging judgment, myth, and prejudice in the workplace and with the goal of opening a new dialogue and a new way of seeing the condition that will benefit both patient and clinician alike.

Future Directions

It is critical that clinicians know that people with BPD can and will recover. This information must be relayed to people with BPD, as all too often they picture a bleak future with little hope. Zanarini has been at the forefront of research that shows that a high proportion of people with BPD recover significantly and over time no longer meet diagnostic criteria for BPD. Specifically she found that over the 10 years of follow-up in her study, 78 % of people with the disorder attain or maintain broadly defined good psychosocial. Further that even among those who experience remission, only a minority relapse. It is also important to know that although most people with BPD will eventually achieve symptomatic recovery, some will still experience impaired psychosocial functioning. Some of the factors that predict recovery are:

1. Younger age
2. Good vocational record
3. No history of childhood sexual abuse
4. No family history of substance abuse

These factors lead to the recommendation that making the diagnosis of BPD should not be delayed and that there should be a strong focus on keeping the person with BPD either in school or in work.

BPD and Reducing Stigma: A Collective Responsibility

Tackling the stigma of BPD means better research, better clinical training of mental health professionals, and enduring education of those who struggle with the disorder as well as those who love them. Although there are various programs that attempt to target stigma in mental illness in general, there are very few that tackle the stigma associated with BPD specifically, even though the prevalence of the disorder is high. In order to make inroads into reducing the stigma associated with BPD, two broad approaches need be considered:

Training

Mental Health Clinicians Training interventions in multiple settings include ensuring that mental health trainees at all levels of education are using teaching materials that include the latest material. Ideally these materials would be reviewed for accurate content every 2 years.

Public As we, the experts, created the stigma in the first place, it is our moral obligation to undo the damage. We should take the ample opportunities to educate consumers, their families, and other non-mental health professionals about the various facets of BPD. Specifically the focus should highlight information on the causes, the neurobiology, the genetics, and the latest research on treatment of BPD. We need to highlight the experience of people with BPD by welcoming their voices with particular emphasis on the way in which they experience stigma. The National Education Alliance for Borderline Personality Disorder (NEABPD) has conferences that are the very model of such an undertaking.

Law Enforcement I have had the unfortunate situation of having to call 911 in situations where a person with BPD was so out of control that they were at risk of harming themselves or someone else. In order to keep the situation safe, law enforcement officials have, at times, needed to physically take control of the situation. From the perspective of an officer with no training in mental health, it is understandable that they perceive someone who is emotionally dysregulated, or who has self-injured with a blade or knife, as posing a threat. Experts in all mental health disorders including BPD should consider offering training opportunities to local community police departments to include psychoeducation.

Schools Given that emotion regulation problems can be an early indication of BPD and that BPD typically starts in adolescence, educational interventions that focus on explaining typical and disturbed brain development, without avoiding the discussion of all the major mental illnesses and including BPD, can lead to positive outcomes on attitudes and knowledge [22].

Individual Although there are no targeted interventions focused on reducing self-stigma or the promotion of feelings of empowerment and self-determination in people with BPD, conferences such as those by the National Education Alliance for Borderline Personality Disorder (NEABPD) include professionals, family members, and people with BPD and anecdotally help reduce stigma in individuals by providing psychoeducation including the latest findings in research and treatment.

Contact Strategies

Direct Interpersonal Contact Perhaps the most powerful of all interventions is
the practice of encouraging and fostering interactions with people with BPD. In
other mental illnesses, there is evidence that direct contact can have an even greater
impact on attitudinal changes than educational strategies in other mental illnesses.
These interpersonal contact strategies have been linked to behavioral change outcomes as well as to longer-term attitudinal changes.

A powerful example of direct contact was when Tami Green, a life coach, a
NAMI Peer-to-Peer educator, a NAMI Connections Peer Recovery and Support
Group facilitator, and a national spokesperson for BPD, addressed congress about
having BPD and said, "Twenty years ago, I walked these very halls, lobbying and
educating Congress. Why am I here? I am here because you don't know about this
illness. I would not be here, alive, if I had not been diagnosed with borderline
personality disorder and received the treatment I have been undergoing. This illness is highly treatable, and those of us who have it can have a life worth living."
In 2008, the US Congress resolved that May is Borderline Personality Disorder
Awareness Month.

Another example was when in 2010, soon after celebrity superstar NFL wide
receiver Brandon Marshall had landed a $50 million contract, he was diagnosed
with BPD. Since then, he and his wife Michi cofounded the Brandon Marshall
Foundation, an organization dedicated to end the stigma associated with mental
illness, advocate awareness, and paint the world lime green (which is the official
color for mental health awareness). This high-profile male athlete provided a res-
onant voice for BPD awareness. He teamed up with various groups including the
motorcycle company Harley Davidson, a group not typically thought of when
considering mental health awareness, to broaden the public scope of his
message.

The Borderline Horizon: The End of Stigma

We are moving in the right direction. We know *how* we got to stigma. Using science,
research, and new treatments, we know that people get better and are not destined to
lives of enduring suffering. With every new insight, there is an openness to name a
disorder that once upon a time did seem like a life sentence. The compassion of a
legion of therapists backed up by the force of the scientific method together with all
aforementioned ways we can tackle stigma will continue to chip away at the myths
and distortions that have underpinned the historical narrative. We are not there yet
and much work needs to be done. Nevertheless, as of the time of this writing, I am
excited as I notice a lessening in judgmental attitudes in lecture halls, clinical conferences, and patient and parent roundtables. As a DBT therapist, I see that two
things are true. We have come a long way and we cannot yet declare victory. Our
march is not over. Onward!

References

1. American Psychiatric Association. Diagnostic and statistical manual of mental disorders: DSM-5. Washington, D.C: American Psychiatric Association; 2013.
2. Stern A. Psychoanalytic investigation and therapy in the borderline group of neuroses. Psychoanal Q. 1938;7:467–89.
3. Kernberg O. Borderline personality organization. J Am Psychoanal Assoc. 1967;15:641–85.
4. Gunderson JG, Kolb JE. Discriminating features of borderline patients. Am J Psychiatry. 1978;135:792–6.
5. Grant BF, Chou SP, Goldstein RB, Huang B, Stinsin F, Saha T, Smith S, Damson D, Pulay A, Pickering R, Ruan J. Prevalence, correlates, disability, and comorbidity of DSM-IV borderline personality disorder: results from the wave 2 national epidemiologic survey on alcohol and related conditions. J Clin Psychiatry. 2008;69(4):533–45.
6. Klein D. Drug therapy as a means of syndrome identification and nosological revision. In: Cole J, Freeman A, Friedhoff A, editors. Psychopathy and Psychopharmacology. Baltimore: Johns Hopkins University Press; 1972.
7. Houck JH. The intractable female patient. Am J Psychiatry. 1972;129:27–31.
8. Kaysen S. Girl interrupted. London: Virago; 1993.
9. Nehls N. Borderline personality disorder: the voice of patients. Res Nurs Health. 1999;22(4): 285–93.
10. Miller CR, Eisner W, Allport C. Creative coping: a cognitive-behavioral group for borderline personality disorder. Arch Psychiatr Nurs. 1994;8(4):280–5.
11. Byrne P. Stigma of mental illness and ways of diminishing it. Adv Psychiatric Treat. 2000;6: 65–72.
12. Fallon P. Travelling through the system: the lived experience of people with borderline personality disorder in contact with psychiatric services. J Psychiatr Ment Health Nurs. 2003;10(4): 393–400.
13. Holm AL, Severinsson E. Struggling to recover by changing suicidal behaviour: narratives from women with borderline personality disorder. Int J Ment Health Nurs. 2011;20(3):165–73.
14. Rogers B, Dunne E. 'They told me i had this personality disorder… All of a sudden i was wasting their time': personality disorder and the inpatient experience. J Ment Health. 2011;20(3): 226–33.
15. Lynch TR, Trost WT, Salsman N, Linehan MM. Dialectical behavior therapy for borderline personality disorder. Annu Rev Clin Psychol. 2007;3:181–205.
16. Bateman A, Fonagy P. 8-year follow-up of patients treated for borderline personality disorder: mentalization-based treatment versus treatment as usual. Am J Psychiatry. 2008;165(5): 631–8.
17. Davidson K, Norrie J, Tyrer P, et al. The effectiveness of cognitive behavior therapy for borderline personality disorder: results from the borderline personality disorder study of cognitive therapy (Boscot) trail. J Pers Disord. 2006;20(5):450–65.
18. Giesen-Bloo J, van Dyck R, Spinhoven P, et al. "Outpatient psychotherapy for borderline personality disorder: randomized trial of schema-focused therapy vs transference-focused psychotherapy". Arch Gen Psychiatry. 2006;63(6):649–58.
19. Ryle A. The contribution of cognitive analytic therapy to the treatment of borderline personality disorder. J Pers Disord. 2004;18(1):3–35.
20. Aviram RB, Hellerstein DJ, Gerson J, Stanley B. Adapting supportive psychotherapy for individuals with borderline personality disorder who self-injure or attempt suicide. J Psychiatr Pract. 2004;10(3):145–55.
21. McMain SF, Guimond T, Streiner DL, Cardish RJ, Links PS. Dialectical behavior therapy compared with general psychiatric management for borderline personality disorder: clinical outcomes and functioning over a 2-year follow-up. Am J Psychiatry. 2012;169(6):650–61.
22. Essler V, Arthur A, Stickley T. Using a school-based intervention to challenge stigmatizing attitudes and promote mental health in teenagers. J Ment Health. 2006;15(2):243–50.

Chapter 9
Diagnosed with Breast Cancer: Stigmatized or Member of an Empowered Sisterhood?

Daleela G. Dodge and Andrew M. Jarowenko

In the emergency room I met an attractive, slim 57-year-old woman named Tina. We had been asked to consult in her care to discuss the surgical treatment options for her locally advanced cancer. Her two children, both in their early 20s, sat wide-eyed listening intently to my every word…they looked like any one of my son's friends. Their mom was lying on a gurney. One of her eyes was covered by a black pirate's patch. Beneath the sheet, a mass the size of her head distorted the right side of her chest. On the other side of her chest, her uninvolved left breast was not discernible beneath the white hospital sheet. If you had lifted the sheet, you would have seen her right breast was covered—first by a towel, then by a layer of saran wrap neatly taped along the sides to keep of the oozing cancer's drainage contained.

Tina had first been diagnosed with breast cancer five years earlier. As the cancer was then still small enough to be resectable, she had been offered a lumpectomy by one of my partners—a surgery that would have treated the

D.G. Dodge, MD, FACS (✉)
Department of Surgery, Lancaster General Hospital, Lancaster, PA, USA

LG Health Breast Service, Ann B Barshinger Cancer Center, Lancaster, PA, USA
e-mail: dgdodge@lghealth.org

A.M. Jarowenko
Undergraduate Student, School of Arts and Sciences, Tufts University,
Boston, MA, USA

© Springer International Publishing Switzerland 2016
R. Parekh, Ed W. Childs (eds.), *Stigma and Prejudice: Touchstones in
Understanding Diversity in Healthcare*, Current Clinical Psychiatry,
DOI 10.1007/978-3-319-27580-2_9

cancer while preserving her breast. She had declined. She had also refused to try any of the other standard cancer treatments; refusing both tamoxifen—an antihormonal pill—and the chemotherapy that had been offered. Instead she had chosen to seek and accept the counsel of a naturopath using only holistic treatments, including a macrobiotic diet. She had persisted with these alternative treatments though her breast cancer continued to grow, until the day she came to the ER coughing up blood.

On that day in the ER, Tina anxiously told me that she was now willing and ready to have surgery to remove her cancerous breast. Sadly, it was already too late. The cancer had progressed to invade the chest wall muscles and grown to involve the entire breast. In areas, the cancer had broken through the skin and was draining its fetid contents. Tina's eyepatch was used to control the double vision caused by a brain metastasis that was causing one of her eyes to shift permanently outward. I found it extraordinarily difficult to maintain the requisite emotional distance required of me as a physician. Tina was my age and her children looked so much like mine. I was frustrated that we as medical professionals had failed to gain the trust we needed in order to dispel her overwhelming fear of this disease and the consequences of its treatment while the cancer was still curable. Her perceptions of the shame and attendant stigma of cancer treatments would cost this woman her life and soon leave her son and daughter to navigate the world without their mom.

Cancer, symbolized by the crab with its destructive and menacing claws, has always been deeply feared and thus stigmatized. Writer Susan Sontag described cancer as "obscene—ill-omened and repugnant to the senses" [1]. Sontag in her book *Illness as Metaphor* also argued that societal myths surrounding disease could kill by instilling shame and guilt in the afflicted [2]. Cancer is a truly dreaded disease with a frequently silent presentation in which the body becomes a traitor, turning on itself in a particularly frightening way [3]. In 2015, an estimated 1,658,370 people will be diagnosed with cancer in the USA, and an estimated 589,430 people will die of it [4].

The magnitude of the impact of cancer on the population, especially of breast cancer due to its prevalence, is enormous. All healthcare providers in their practices will encounter breast cancer patients and thus should gain an understanding of the issues these women must confront and the sources of stigma that this group often experiences. The chapter will include several case presentations that, while de-identified for privacy, are based on actual patients in order to help illustrate the issues and complexity of this disease.

Breast cancer remains the most feared health condition affecting women today despite significant treatment advances with attendant improvement in survival and an open public discourse. The stigma associated with this disease is not simply emotionally taxing but can be so powerful that the consequences are lethal. The impact of this cancer is rooted in its attack on the breast, which is the symbol for both a woman's sexuality and her capacity to nurture. We will explore the fear this cancer evokes—rooted in its potential for leading to a painful and premature demise—and its treatment that still often includes the mutilation of mastectomy. The chapter will also highlight how the implications of a breast cancer diagnosis are especially unique because it develops in a paired and potentially expendable organ.

We will review the broad demographic of breast cancer that includes onset from early womanhood to the very last years of life. Despite modern treatment advances, breast cancer prognoses can still range from excellent to dismal in all demographics. As will be discussed, breast cancer is a spectrum of heterogeneous, biologically distinct cancers, each with unique characteristics that dictate the numerous and often confusing treatment choices that a woman diagnosed with breast cancer must make. The breast cancer patient's responsibility for choosing between these treatment options is far greater than in other health conditions, which adds significantly to the stress these patients experience.

The authors will explore how the historical evolution in the medical community's understanding of breast cancer biology has led to continually evolving treatment paradigms. These discoveries have been paralleled by the growth of a vigorous women's healthcare movement in which women have taken significant initiative in proactively working to protect their health. The consequence has been to open discourse and rally other women to help, both by urging other women to seek mammographic screening for early diagnosis and by creating enormously successful fundraising vehicles targeting breast cancer research.

The role of genetics and lifestyle factors in breast cancer causation will be reviewed while acknowledging that in the majority of cases, a woman diagnosed with breast cancer has few, if any, of the known risk factors. We will see that breast cancer remains a highly feared, stigmatized disease that strikes without warning at any time during a woman's lifetime. This chapter will highlight powerful emotional tools that can be utilized to modify the stigma of breast cancer, including the importance of "leaning in," by actually embracing the vulnerability caused by a cancer diagnosis. We will learn that many women have emerged from the breast cancer experience feeling empowered, even happier. Thus the factors determining an individual patient's journey and the degree of associated stigma are complex and unique. We will find that the degree of stigma experienced depends on a balance of the patient's internal coping mechanisms, as well as social and familial support, and also critically on the biology of her cancer and the subsequent treatments required.

The historical and contemporary contexts of breast cancer treatment will be reviewed to gain an understanding of the current challenges. We will also focus on the disproportionate anxiety or "misfearing" that breast cancer causes for women. This narrative will discuss the breast cancer risk as general population risk while also defining a special subset of women who are at significantly higher risk for the development of breast cancer. It will also highlight two important subgroups. The first cohort, black women with breast cancer, in whom there are outcome disparities across every stage and biologic variant of this disease. The second group discussed are the AYAs—an acronym for adolescents and young adults—who face unique challenges and for whom breast cancer-related survival has experienced little improvement over the last two decades.

Historically, the victims of breast cancer suffered in silence—ashamed, stigmatized, and closeted [5]. Currently the isolation for the majority of women has been replaced by "empowered pink" and a hyper-focused awareness of the threat of breast cancer. We will review how breast cancer advocacy has led to the formation of "pink sororities" and its status as the "media's darling among cancers" [6]. Because of this elevated status, breast cancer-focused charities are the recipients of more research funding than any other malignancy.

Finally we will explore how the necessary evolution in treatment options has had the unintended consequence of placing significant responsibility on the patient for her ultimate outcome. The patient's peers may view a cancer recurrence as her personal failure for having made a wrong choice. Women have characterized the currently rising rates of bilateral mastectomies for early-stage breast cancer as a choice that is made in an effort to "take control of cancer" and their lives [7]. In the current medical environment where physician compensation for services will be increasingly tied to patient satisfaction, the trend may move toward a new extreme—a consumerism-dominant model [8].

We will see that compared to several decades ago, there is no question that aspects of the stigma associated with breast cancer have been substantially reduced. Indeed, breast cancer has served to unite women in a common mission with accomplishments that have demonstrated the extraordinary powers of this demographic. However, as the story of Tina illustrated, perceptions of stigma are not universal or always rational. For these reasons, the specter of breast cancer treatment, as it can alter a woman's body image, her fertility, and role as a nurturer and her sexuality, can be powerfully stigmatizing, even lethal.

Epidemiology

Globally, breast cancer is the most frequently diagnosed cancer in women, regardless of age. Worldwide, breast cancer has a huge impact—in the year of 2012 alone, 1,700,000 cases were diagnosed [9]. In the USA, breast cancer is responsible for 14 % of all new cancer cases. In the USA in 2015, it is estimated that there will be 231,840 new cases of breast cancer in women and 40,290 will die of the disease [4]. It was estimated in 2012 that nearly three million women were living with breast cancer in the USA [10]. Incidence and mortality rates have been increasing in less developed countries, as compared with the USA and other Westernized countries. In Asian and Latin American countries, there is a younger age at peak incidence compared with Western countries [11]. According to the National Cancer Institute database, the national peak incidence of breast cancer is at age 61 [12].

Less than 1 % of breast cancers occur in men [13]. Male breast cancer is associated with conditions causing excess estrogen, such as cirrhosis and Klinefelter's syndrome, and with the BRCA2 mutation [13]. The onset of breast cancer in women occurs across the entire adult age spectrum, from the early 20s to 90s; in men the onset is generally later in life. Overall survival of breast cancer is the same in women and men, though breast cancer tends to present at a later stage in men [13, 14].

Approximately 10 % of the women who develop breast cancer have an identifiable genetic predisposition. These women carry one of the known breast cancer-associated genetic mutations in tumor suppressor genes, including the BRCA1 or BRCA2, PTEN (Cowden syndrome), TP53 (Li-Fraumeni syndrome), PALB2, CHEK2, or ATM mutations. In 2008, to protect genetic mutation carriers from discrimination, the Congress passed the Genetic Information Nondiscrimination Act (GINA). GINA prohibits the use of genetic information in making employment decisions and protects genetic mutation carriers against insurance discrimination [15]. Enforcement, however, can be difficult, and affected individuals are aware that employers may not want to hire them due to the higher anticipated costs of providing healthcare and the potential of frequent absences from the workplace for testing or treatment. Expected promotions have been denied after a breast cancer diagnosis and given to a "healthier" qualified candidate, so it is conceivable that high-risk genetic mutation carriers could be treated in a similar manner [16].

In May 2013, the actress, mother, and humanitarian Angelina Jolie published an editorial in the New York Times titled My Medical Choice, describing why she chose to have prophylactic mastectomies, after she learned that she carried a "faulty" breast cancer-associated gene, BRCA1. She began the editorial captivating her readers with the following narrative. "My mother fought cancer for almost a decade and died at 56. She held out long enough to meet the first grandchildren and hold them in her arms. But my other children will never have the chance to know her and experience how loving and gracious she was" [17]. The extraordinary fear that breast cancer inspires is based on the potential of causing a woman's premature death, especially while in her prime, and even more so if she is the mother of young children.

As the story of Julia told later in this chapter will illustrate, women who are BRCA mutation carriers are not only at an increased risk of developing breast cancer, but they also have an increased risk of developing other cancers. Ovarian cancer is the second most common malignancy in this population. Two years after having her prophylactic mastectomies, Angelina Jolie-Pitt also had her ovaries removed. BRCA carriers are advised to consider prophylactic oophorectomies after age 40 or when they have completed childbearing. Angelina emphasized in a subsequent editorial that the first step for those with a strong family history of cancer was to define their risk by having genetic testing. It is estimated that while only 60,000 women in the USA have been diagnosed as BRCA mutation carriers, the number of women affected approaches one million [18].

Alternatively, there are women who test negative for one of the known breast cancer-associated genetic mutations but still have a significantly elevated lifetime risk of breast cancer which is calculated based on family history and lifestyle factors. Lifestyle factors contributing to an increased breast cancer risk include not having born a child or delayed childbearing, not breast-feeding, taking a progesterone-containing hormone replacement therapy (HRT) after menopause, being overweight, smoking, or drinking alcohol in excess. Though these known risk factors aid in detection of individuals at high risk, the majority of patients who are diagnosed with breast cancer have minimal or no family history of breast cancer and few, if any, of the known risk factors.

The adolescents and young adults (AYAs) are a unique demographic, defined as individuals aged 15–39 years who develop cancer. Though only 6.6 % of breast cancer cases are diagnosed in women younger than 40 years of age, evidence suggests that the breast cancers in the AYAs may be clinically and etiologically distinct from breast cancer in older women. Cancer occurring in AYAs typically has a worse prognosis and a more aggressive phenotype, with higher proportions of high-grade and later-stage tumors and lower estrogen receptor positivity [11, 19]. Young women with an invasive breast cancer are also at a significantly higher risk for developing a second breast cancer. SEER data from 1976 to 2009 identified a disturbing increase in the incidence of metastatic cancer in those diagnosed between the ages of 25 and 39, without a corresponding increase among older women [20]. Hereditary breast cancer plays a role in some of these women, though surprisingly only 9.4 % of the women diagnosed with breast cancer at an age younger than 35 are found to harbor one of the BRCA mutations [11].

Among postmenopausal women, the rates of breast cancer are lower in black and Hispanic women compared to white women. However, under the age of 40, non-Hispanic black women have a higher risk of developing breast cancer. The lifestyle-associated protection gained by white women from early parity, multiple parity, and breast-feeding is not observed in young black women [21]. In this cohort, there is a higher preponderance of triple-negative cancers also observed, which are both the most difficult to treat and carry the worst prognosis. Triple-negative cancers have been observed to be more prevalent on the African continent, which suggests there may be a genetic predisposition for developing the most aggressive breast cancers that would account for some of the discrepancy [21, 22].

However, lower survival rates have been documented among black women across all age groups, for all stages of breast cancer, and recently for every biologic type of breast cancer [21, 23]. In a recent study of this demographic, black women were twice as likely to die of their breast cancer as white women [24]. Black women were diagnosed with lower percentages of the best-prognosis luminal A-type breast cancers and had a higher incidence of the worst-prognosis triple-negative basal subtype, when compared to white women. However, the worse outcomes were not due solely to a higher incidence of the more aggressive breast cancer subtypes. The data demonstrated that black patients were 2.3 times more likely to die from luminal A breast cancers, 2.6 times more likely to die with the luminal B subtype, 1.3 times more likely to die from the basal-like subtype, and 2.4 times more likely to die from the HER2-enriched subtype than their white counterparts [24]. Future research specifically targeting both non-Hispanic black women and the AYAs is needed to address and find how to modify these disturbing outcome discrepancies.

The Stigma and "Misfearing" of Breast Cancer

Despite comparatively high survival rates, breast cancer continues to be the most feared of all health threats facing women today [25]. This fear must be understood in context—as breast cancer attacks an organ that is fundamental to the female identity. A woman's breast conjures both her sexuality and her capacity to nurture. A woman's breast has come increasingly to signify danger, risk of disease, and especially the risk of death. As sociologist Maren Klawiter wrote in her book *The Biopolitics of Breast Cancer: Changing Cultures of Disease and Activism*—a work that provided the author pivotal perspectives in researching this complex topic—"Eroticism, motherhood, and death—breasts embody and inspire a heading brew of emotions" (p xx) [5].

Fear is a major contributing factor to the stigmatization of any condition, and cancer is feared more than any other disease [1]. Studies have demonstrated that an individual's sense of risk is based fundamentally on feelings. The term "misfearing" has been used to describe this human tendency to fear instinctively rather than logically [25]. Fear forms the foundation from which all stigma and prejudice arise. A death from cancer is often wretched [26], and after enduring mutilating treatments, a patient may spend her last days fraught with unbearable pain [27]. Many once believed that cancer was contagious. In developing nations, although cancer is no longer viewed as contagious, a cancer patient's appearance can cause others to think that the person has AIDS, a condition that is even more stigmatized than cancer in these societies.

Cancer treatments are uniformly dreaded. The treatments are by some felt to be worse than the disease; as our patient Tina demonstrated, as though she periodically interacted with medical professionals, she never agreed to treatment. As Dr. Kristen Bell has pointed out, individuals with a history of cancer do not rejoin the land of the well rather "they live in the ambiguous space between the well and sick" [28]. Cancer is viewed as such an undesirable fate that individuals often seek to distance themselves by attributing the disease to the victim, believing that the cancer has been caused by either their undesirable past behavior or personal characteristics [29].

There are three bases for the stigma that women battling breast cancer face. Each of these can be either real or perceived. External factors include societal perceptions and attitudes and can be tempered by key relationships and group allegiance. Internal factors, including perceptions and coping mechanisms unique to the given individual, exert a strong influence on a woman's view of her disease and the stigma associated with it. Finally, the extent and duration of the treatment, as well as a patient's prognosis and any resulting disability and disfigurement, will factor into the stigma that a patient faces.

Many breast cancer patients perceive that they are treated differently after people have learned that they have cancer. They often express feeling misunderstood, avoided, feared, or pitied. The perception of social stigma and discrimination may contribute to the transformation of a breast cancer survivor's self-concept into a "less preferred identity" [29]. Group activities can serve to modify these perceptions of stigma, by allowing survivors to share experiences and both receive and provide support [30]. The proliferation of breast cancer organizations and support groups has helped women with breast cancer find needed guidance, craft a post-cancer identity, and find validation and purpose both by supporting others with breast cancer and by rallying around early detection efforts, hoping to minimize the need for the most toxic treatments and save lives. For Tina, her perception of the stigma of breast cancer treatments was paralyzing and too overwhelming for her to agree to treatment until it was too late.

Historical Context

On a Thibodaux, Louisiana street, in the spring of 1968, a young woman, Mary, walked leaning on a cane and grimacing with pain. When her neighbors inquired what was wrong, she quickly told them she had been clumsy and fallen. To protect her family, Mary, who was battling metastatic breast cancer, hide the true reason for her disability from her neighbors. Mary's breast cancer had metastasized from her breast and was eating holes in this young woman's bones. A mother of four children and the wife of a surgeon, she had discovered the cancerous lump in her breast five years earlier. She and her family had been in Africa working as medical missionaries at the time. By her early 40s, Mary was dead. Mary's mother had met a similar fate in her mid 30s. It was only several decades later, in 1994, that the BRCA2 gene mutation that had caused Mary's breast cancer, and later would cause her daughter Julia to require cancer treatments, was finally identified.

Historically, women with breast cancer, indeed all cancer patients, had been deeply stigmatized. The word "cancer" was not verbalized. Instead cancer was referred to as the "C word"—a loathsome and hopeless disease [5]. Throughout most of the twentieth century, doctors were even more frightened and pessimistic about cancer than their patients [31].

With the advent of anesthesia, surgery could be performed to remove cancer, offering some hope of a cure. In 1913, the same month as the American Cancer Society (ACS) was founded, an article was published in the *Ladies Home Journal* entitled *What Can We Do About Cancer?* The premise was that if a cancer could be discovered at an early stage, the patient had a chance of being cured by an operation. In the 1920s, the ACS launched the "do not delay" campaign. By the 1950s, the campaign advertised an additional message, "every doctor's office is a cancer detection center" [31].

In the early 1930s, Clarence Cook Little, the director of the ACS, was looking for manpower to spread the message of early detection. He approached the General Federation of Women's Clubs, asking them to enlist their members in a public education campaign, which led to the formation of the Women's Field Army (WFA).

The WFA volunteers, dressed in brown uniforms, conducted door-to-door campaigns carrying the message of early detection and a promise of the potential for a cure through medical intervention. The WFA began the powerful ongoing legacy of women volunteers devoted to cancer awareness. The WFA volunteers, independently of the male ACS hierarchy, chose to target their efforts to also raising funds to aid the "needy," especially female cancer patients [5].

Women with breast cancer suffered in silence throughout most of the twentieth century. A woman was often left unaware of her diagnosis and prognosis [5]. In 1946, an article published in the *Annals of Internal Medicine* counseled physicians to avoid using the word "cancer" and to divulge as little information as possible to the patient about her condition. They were counseled, instead, to substitute vague terms as "tumor" or "lesion" for the word "cancer" [32].

A diagnosis of breast cancer was a deeply dreaded secret—a secret that women were expected to endure alone. Physicians advised women to use discretion in any communication about their condition, telling them that no one outside their immediate family needs to know about their diagnosis [32]. Author and cancer historian James Patterson wrote that by teaching a woman who underwent "the operation" to "hide the awful truth," a physician could help her avoid "crashing" into the public stigma and shame of having breast cancer [3].

Until the mid-1970s in the USA, there was only one treatment for breast cancer—the Halsted radical mastectomy. This operation removed the breast along with both chest wall muscles and all the axillary lymph nodes. After this surgery, a woman was left severely deformed, with only skin covering her ribs. Both lymphedema and permanent restriction of arm motion were very common, as a result of this surgery [33]. Before women left the hospital, the "mastectomees," as they were called, were given a prosthetic device and counseled that it "should be worn to maintain an appearance of normality every day" [34]. Women were then urged to resume "their normal lives" as quickly as possible. With the closet door tightly closed, these women lacked access to the psychological and social support services that are now key elements of contemporary breast cancer treatment.

During the 1950s, the "one-step" procedure—an excisional biopsy followed by immediate mastectomy if a pathologist confirmed the lesion was cancer—had been adopted as the standard of care for the treatment of breast cancer. The woman only learned of her cancer diagnosis after awakening from anesthesia and discovering that her breast was gone.

When I was a medical student, we were tasked with starting intravenous (IV) lines on these women, the night before surgery. Most were relatively young and had not been previously ill, so accessing their veins was "easy" - a good place for a beginner to learn this skill. Though I was concentrated on my assigned task, the deep fear, even terror, that these women were experiencing as they waited for the next day when they would learn their fate was palpable. These women I had met on "IV rounds" remain forever vividly ingrained in my memory.

The sole positive of the Halsted era was that breast cancer treatment was over quickly. Surgery was only rarely followed by any other treatment—these women did not face the contemporary daunting spectrum of therapeutic choices. Indeed the responsibility for treatment decisions was firmly in the hands of the sovereign surgeon. With the advent of patient participation in treatment, choice has come a sense not only of empowering shared decision-making but also of frightening personal responsibility for the ultimate outcome.

Breast Cancer Biology and Heterogeneity

Before continuing our exploration of the history of the evolution of breast cancer treatment, I will pause to review our contemporary understanding of breast cancer biology. Over the last several decades, it has become clear that there are several biologically distinct variants of breast cancer that are broadly categorized as the luminal A, luminal B, Her2-positive, and triple-negative cancers [35]. As will be illustrated by the following examples, as a consequence of the heterogeneity of breast cancer presentations and biology, an individual patient's treatment and experience may vary widely:

Nancy, a 50-year-old, underwent a screening mammogram, which detected a stage I HER2+ cancer.

For treatment of this small (6 mm), node-negative cancer, her treatments continued for a full year—a lumpectomy with sentinel lymph node biopsy, radiation, and chemotherapy including Herceptin (trastuzumab), a HER2-targeted agent.

Susan, a 65-year-old, had not had a mammogram in 4 years. She found her cancerous lump, which was a stage IIB, moderately large (4 cm), node positive, and strongly ER/PR-positive cancer with a low-risk Oncotype DX recurrence score of 10.

She was advised that she would not benefit from chemotherapy because of the low Oncotype DX recurrence score. After her surgical treatment and radiation, she received an aromatase inhibitor—a pill, which she will take daily for the next 10 years.

Megan, a 35-year-old with a strong family history of premenopausal breast cancer but negative genetic testing, was diagnosed with a triple-negative (ER/PR/HER2-negative) cancer that was found on a screening breast MRI—a small (10 mm), stage I, node-negative, and triple-negative cancer.

She was advised that after completing surgical treatment, she needed to have 4–6 months of chemotherapy. After completing chemotherapy, there was no other treatment, only surveillance visits with her physicians monitoring for recurrence.

Of the three patients presented, Megan's prognosis was the worst but her treatment the shortest. Of concern is that AYAs, like Megan, have experienced little improvement in breast cancer-related survival over the past two decades as compared with other age groups. In addition to incurring more biologically aggressive variants of breast cancer, these young women face many additional potential stresses and sources of stigma. Young women diagnosed with breast cancer report steeper decline in mental health, as well as social and sexual functioning using standardized QoL parameters and depression measures compared to older women with breast cancer [30, 36]. Breast cancer diagnosed in young women also potentially disrupts childbearing. Treatments can result in infertility and early menopause. These stresses are compounded by the fact that a cancer diagnosis can also significantly alter opportunities for employment and advancement outside the home [11, 29].

Dr. Siddhartha Mukherjee elucidates in his book *The Emperor of All Maladies* that cancer is not a single disease but rather a dynamic entity that has the power to transform itself [37]. Currently, we know that the biology of a breast cancer trumps the cancer's stage as the key determinant of treatment. Stage is still used to compare cancer treatment outcomes. The stage of a breast cancer is based on the tumor size, presence or absence of lymph node involvement, any secondary signs of cancer, and the presence/absence of spread to other sites. Today multispecialty teams of physicians treat breast cancer by tailoring scientifically based treatment plans. The treatment plan is based on an assessment of the cancer's biologic characteristics, determined by its histology—ductal versus lobular, tumor grade, estrogen and progesterone receptor status (ER/PR), HER2 receptor status, and the assessment of tumor genetics, with tests such as the Oncotype DX. The ultimate goal is to provide the best possible outcome while minimizing any toxicity [38].

The Dawn of Alternative Treatments

In the 1970s, the medical establishment's view of breast cancer began to evolve. The scientific dogma changed from the belief in sequential progression of cancer—embraced by Halsted and his contemporaries—to a conviction that by the time cancer could be diagnosed, it had already become a systemic disease [5, 39]. The pioneers who changed the character and substance of the breast cancer treatment dialogue came from both the medical community and women advocates.

One of the great medical pioneers, Dr. George Crile, Jr., learned during his military service to question prevailing dogma, such as a belief, held at that time, that it was lifesaving to perform emergency appendectomies aboard a submarine. Dr. Crile realized that while these surgeries were courageous, they often did more harm than good. During this era of medical treatment, the prevailing belief among physicians was that only those with the technical prowess to perform the most radical of surgeries could cure cancer. Dr. Crile challenged that entrenched dogma when in

1972 he published a review of the results of breast cancer treatment with lumpectomy or simple mastectomy compared to those treated with radical mastectomy. His comparative review of these procedures found equivalent survival rates [40, 41]. Dr. Crile also published two truly revolutionary books, *What Women Should Know About the Breast Cancer Controversy* [42] and *Surgery, Your Choices, Your Alternatives* [43], in which he included a "Patient's Bill of Rights" [42]. These titles by this pioneer surgeon are what we might expect to find on Amazon.com today, but not in the bookstores of the 1970s.

In 1969, an Italian surgeon Dr. Umberto Veronesi, now considered the father of breast conservation, proposed to the World Health Organization (WHO) a randomized trial of breast-conserving surgical treatment. This trial, with multiple centers participating, was designed as an ultimate challenge to the necessity of radical surgery for treatment of breast cancer. The results demonstrated that surgical treatment with quadrantectomy followed by radiation was equivalent to mastectomy for the treatment of early-stage breast cancer [44, 45]. Then further dispelling any superiority of radical surgery for breast cancer, in 1979 Dr. Bernard Fisher reported preliminary follow-up results of NSABP B-04, one of the first randomized clinical trials. This trial demonstrated that there was no improvement in the outcome for patients who underwent the Halsted radical as compared to mastectomy with preservation of the chest wall muscles, either with or without lymph node removal [39, 46].

In response to these findings, in 1979, the first cancer consensus conference was held by the National Institutes of Health (NIH) to review the primary treatment of breast cancer. Rose Kushner, a pioneer activist, was the only woman invited to serve on the panel. The NIH conference delegates concluded that there was no data supporting better clinical outcomes in women treated with the Halsted radical mastectomy when compared to the less debilitating and disfiguring modified radical mastectomy [47]. With physician acceptance of the results of these pivotal clinical trials, an era of patient participation in therapeutic choice commenced.

Advocacy

By the mid-1970s, physicians had stopped shielding women from knowing of their cancer. However, patients were still being informed only after their breast had already been removed. In 1974, Rose Kushner, today considered the mother of breast cancer activism, was working as a freelance medical journalist when she discovered a lump in her breast. Kushner found and read Dr. Crile's first book and, after completing additional research at the NIH library, decided to refuse to have the standard one-step procedure [5]. With great difficulty and after many inquiries, Kushner found a surgeon willing to perform just the biopsy, and she drew up her own surgical consent, confirming the plan [48]. After learning she had breast cancer, Rose Kushner had to search again to find a surgeon willing to perform only a modified radical mastectomy, leaving her with her chest wall muscles intact, rather than the Halsted radical mastectomy.

Kushner described her experiences in her book, *Breast Cancer: A Personal History and an Investigative Report*, published in 1975. Kushner wrote, "this book is to show that we women should be free, knowledgeable, and completely conscious when the time comes for decision, so that we can make it ourselves" [48]. It was Kushner and other like-minded women who also helped pass the first legislation requiring preoperative, informed consent. This formal consent process ensured that there would be shared decision-making between patient and physician, weighing options together before treatment [5]. Kushner's politics paralleled the rise of feminism in the USA. As she pointed out, at that time, the entire breast cancer establishment was male. Her activism was foundational in the burgeoning women's health movement.

In 1974, during her tenure as our nation's First Lady, Betty Ford was diagnosed with breast cancer. Ford's cancer, unlike Kushner's, was not palpable at the time of diagnosis. Rather, her cancer was identified as the result of a screening mammogram. The use of radiation for diagnostic imaging of the breast began in 1913. During the first half of the twentieth century, X-rays were used as a therapeutic treatment for breast cancer, rather than as a technology for the diagnosis and viewing of breast lesions. By the 1950s, radiology units designed explicitly for breast imaging became available. In 1967, the first dedicated mammography machines entered the market [49].

While Betty Ford did not question her doctor's recommendations and underwent a "one-step" procedure, she did choose to eschew the tradition of silence and isolation. When Betty Ford shared with the world the news of her breast cancer diagnosis and treatment, she pushed open the closet door.

> Though at the time I was well aware of her disclosure, I was naïve and unaware that a woman could face prejudice for undergoing treatment of a life-threatening disease.

Betty Ford's motivation was based on her deep commitment to helping other women. She became a lifelong advocate for preventive health, especially urging other women to have screening mammograms. After the closet door opened, in the 1970s, women began immediately to work together to form what would become the strongest healthcare advocacy movement in history. The movement encouraged women to network and to question their doctors [5]. These women lobbied and advocated for laws protecting patient rights and for a woman's right to participate in her treatment choices.

In 1982, Nancy Brinker founded Susan G. Komen for the Cure, named after her sister who died in her 30s from breast cancer. To date, Komen has raised $1.5 billion and currently receives over $55 million a year from more than 200 corporate sponsors [50]. As an author and political activist, Barbara Ehrenreich described in her

2001 Harper's Magazine essay, *Welcome to Cancerland*, "breast cancer has blossomed from the wallflower to the most popular girl at the corporate charity prom" [6]. Komen volunteers have lobbied for insurance coverage for baseline mammograms and transformed the issue of mammography for low-income, uninsured, and underserved demographics, especially women of color, into a moral imperative [5]. The message of the Komen movement has been that the solution to breast cancer lies in early detection and continued medical research.

The annual Komen Race for the Cure features stories of individual triumph and self-determination, focusing on redemption and survivorship. At these events, successful survival has been depicted as a matter of personal choice. The Komen women embraced wearing the color pink to show their support in the fight against breast cancer [51]. At Komen events, bright pink visors with corporate logos and the message "I'm a survivor" were worn. These pink visors have been described by sociologist Maren Klawiter as highly symbolic, "an act of social disobedience—a collective coming out, a rejection of stigma and invisibility, an appropriation of the traditional color femininity by the survivor identity" (p. 143) [5].

The empowered pink breast cancer movement has been criticized for both an over-feminization and infantilization of breast cancer [6]. Some have described the movement as a "pinkwashing," where corporate marketers donate to Komen while promoting products that are not healthy, such as KFC fried chicken. Barbara Ehrenreich also criticized the "tyranny of the positive" espoused by Komen and other breast cancer groups, which demands that women with breast cancer should maintain an appropriate upbeat attitude. Breast cancer survivors have been saddled with expectations to quickly rebound and celebrate their blessings—gratitude with no room for negative thoughts, which Ehrenreich calls a "relentless brightsiding" [52]. With these demands for perpetual optimism, some groups have stigmatized and even targeted the women with breast cancer who chose to openly express anger, pain, or negative feelings. The traditional emphasis on survivorship by organizations like Komen has affectively excluded women with recurrent or metastatic cancer.

With National Breast Cancer Awareness Month (NBCAM), an annual ritual started in 1985, a powerful connection was formed between the breast cancer advocacy movement and image-conscious corporations engaged in cause-related marketing philanthropy. Original major sponsors of NBCAM included IHI, a British firm whose pharmaceutical division held the patent for *tamoxifen*, as well as General Electric and Kodak, corporations which had a major role in the manufacture of the equipment and film used in mammography [5].

Breast cancer philanthropy has deeply resonated for businesses, as its constituents are predominantly middle-aged women, a key consumer demographic. Breast cancer became a powerful "feel-good" selling tool, a "sexy cancer" [51]. As columnist Lisa Belkin wrote in the New York Times in 1993, "Breast cancer is not hot just because Nancy Brinker, Ralph Lauren, Ron Perelman and Evelyn Lauder willed it to be hot. Breast cancer is hot because it resonates" (p. 45) [53]. The Komen Foundation's greatest accomplishment extended beyond just raising awareness or money; it was that the Komen women served to transform the "discourses of breast cancer from images of death, deformity and victimization to images of feminine triumph, strength and beauty" (p. 138) [5].

Alternative Breast Cancer Initiatives and Support Organizations

In the 1990s, San Francisco's Women and Cancer was founded. The organization used tactics that were inspired by the successful AIDS activism of the gay community, seeking to be multicultural and to encourage a more raw and personal community that praised service over survival. Many of the women chose not to wear a breast prosthesis after mastectomy. The Women and Cancer organization avoided any corporate sponsorship, and at events individual women were singled out for their activism, not for their survival [5]. This group avoided using the term "survivor" with its implicit shunning of those women whose cancer had progressed. Members were also encouraged to openly display anger. At their events, stories of emotional devastation, economic hardship, and profound loss were told. They fought for access to be provided for all patients to expensive cancer treatments as was demonstrated when they rallied against Genentech to win "compassionate use" access to *Herceptin*, a highly effective but extraordinarily expensive new breast cancer treatment. At the demonstration, participants dressed in black and carried signs reading "Don't go quietly to the grave! Scream for compassionate use!" [5].

These organizations also expanded the discussion by demanding investigation of potential environmental carcinogens in breast cancer causation. They challenged the cancer establishment by bringing attention to what they believed were false promises and misrepresentations—the ineffectiveness of mammographic screening, the unreliability and toxicity of treatments, and the inadequacy of research into the chronic nature of breast cancer. They emphasized the low priority that was being given to cancer prevention research and education [5].

These later groups have continued to express feelings of deep stigmatization as a consequence of breast cancer. In contrast, many of the women who participate in the "empowered pink" movement express feeling strengthened by their cancer journey. Both responses should be acknowledged as valid expressions of the breast cancer experience.

Breast cancer activists were also aware of and sensitive to cross-cultural differences. The Komen strategies had failed to engage significant participation in screening by minority women, so federal and state Breast Cancer Early Detection Programs (BCEDP) employed new tactics in an effort to engage a broader demographic of women. Their campaign targeted especially African American, Asian American, and Latina women by insisting that mammography screening saved not only a woman's life but also the family. The BCEDP campaign included the distribution of Mother's Day cards telling the recipient that because I love you, please "do something important for both of us" and call to get information about obtaining a free breast exam and mammogram [5].

Breast Cancer Screening Guidelines

The breast cancer screening guidelines are currently being debated both within professional medical specialty organizations and pervasively through the media. Cancer screening is now being scrutinized through a lens that evaluates not only the benefits of screening—lives saved—but also looks at the costs and potential harms of the screening test, such as the additional imaging, biopsies, and anxiety due to false-positive results, in the case of mammography. Mammograms are not a perfect screen as they miss some cancers. This risk is heightened for women with dense breast tissue. Changes are being proposed both for the age at which an average risk woman starts to get mammograms, suggesting beginning at 50, instead of 40, and also decreasing the frequency of breast cancer screenings, moving from an annual to a biannual schedule [54].

Simultaneously, a contradictory message has been sent to those women who live in states where dense breast legislation has been passed. The legislation mandates that women must be informed, in writing, if they have dense breast tissue found on their mammogram. It is estimated that 40–60 % of women in the USA have dense breast tissue [55, 56]. The risks facing these women are twofold. They face both increased higher risk of developing breast cancer and decreased efficacy of standard mammography screening [57]. Furthermore, in most states where legislatures have passed these laws, the lawmakers have failed to either address what additional testing should be performed or to mandate insurance coverage for any additional imaging.

Highlighting an equally powerful opposing force was the 2011 editorial in the journal of the NCCN by its Editor-in-Chief Dr. Harold Burstein. Dr. Burstein cited the huge variation nationally in the median cost for a diagnosis of breast cancer, ranging from $17,319 to $27,233. He emphasized that this cost differential had not demonstrated any bearing on the long-term survival results. Dr. Burstein suggested that new guidelines with strong "do not do this" recommendations could make cancer care less expensive, without making it less effective [58].

Many breast cancer survivors credit a screening mammogram with saving their lives and are thus disturbed by the recent discourse criticizing the costs and benefits of the traditional screening guidelines. Promoting the routine use of mammography for early detection had been the mantra and a primary focus of the breast cancer advocacy movement. As a consequence of the current debate and contradictory messaging, women are becoming increasingly confused about what they should be doing to decrease their personal risk of dying of the health threat they fear most.

Conclusions

Mary's daughter Julia, when she was in medical school, felt a lump in her breast. Her biopsy demonstrated severe atypia of the breast tissue. Julia's family history and the abnormal biopsy results served as catalysts for taking action. A decade before any of the BRCA mutations were discovered, Julia chose to undergo prophylactic mastectomies—a choice which proved to be wise, as years later, Julia would learn that she was a BRCA2 mutation carrier. In the early 80's, her decision was viewed as far too radical by most of the medical community, including her surgeon who advised her that "no man will chose to marry a woman who has lost her breasts." Julia, using a degree of personal initiative and effort reminiscent of Rose Kushner's story, found a team of surgeons willing to treat her.

However, Julia was destined to fight cancer. Four years after finishing her surgical training, she was diagnosed with lung cancer. In addition to having a significant risk of breast and ovarian cancer, BRCA mutation carriers are also at an elevated risk of developing many other types of malignancy. Julia's lung cancer was found to be Stage III, suggesting a dismal prognosis— less than a 10 % chance of long-term survival. Julia beat the odds through carefully chosen treatments and intervention and was cured., The chemotherapy, however, left Julia with a permanent neuropathy affecting her hands and feet that caused a premature end to her surgical career.

During the two decades since her lung cancer treatment, Julia and her husband, John, have raised a blended "yours, mine and ours" family of six beautiful children. A few years ago after John developed breast cancer, they both underwent genetic testing. They learned then that they are both BRCA2 mutation carriers. Julia uses her medical expertise to work in a clinic that provides indigent women access to mammograms, biopsies and counseling. Julia and John, generally with several of their kids, have run in the Komen Race for the Cure every year since Julia completed her cancer treatments. The genetic "curse" has so far not limited their children's opportunities, as just this year their family has celebrated a wedding, the birth of their first grandchild and two engagements!

As Julia's story illustrates, remarkable progress has been made in our understanding of the causes and treatment of cancer. Gone are the days when Julia's mother had to bear the burden of her illness alone, cloaked in silence. With proactive, vigilant healthcare, even BRCA mutation carriers can live long, healthy, and fulfilling lives. It is the "wholehearted," as described by researcher and author Brené Brown—those who are capable of embracing their own vulnerability and seeking connection, who are best suited to overcoming the inherent prejudice that still accompanies a diagnosis of breast cancer [59]. Tina, our first patient, was tragically unable to surmount her fears before the cancer had become eminently lethal and incurable.

In this narrative, we have seen how the woman's health movement and breast cancer advocacy have evolved in parallel. Women have overcome the deep historical stigma that existed, emerging from the silence in which this disease was once shrouded, to becoming advocates—an organized force seeking to help educate and rally their "sisters" to be proactive. Cancer support groups have urged women to follow screening mammography guidelines and to seek early care for any sign of breast cancer, believing that through early intervention lives will be saved [5].

Transformations in breast cancer treatment have been ushered in by an evolution in the medical profession's understanding of the complex biology of this cancer [38]. Highlighting the extent of this transformation, we have seen how breast cancer treatment evolved from the days of the "one-step procedure" and mutilating Halsted radical mastectomy to the current paradigm where women are integrally involved in treatment decision-making, requiring them to weigh the pros and cons of myriad confusing treatment pathways and options. We have seen that a once paternalistic model, in which treatment was determined unilaterally based solely on the physician's expertise, transformed into one of informed, patient-centered choice. Quoting a recent patient.

> I had to make my own decisions, because only I know myself and my own body.

As an individual agonizes over hard choices, she will naturally turn inward, comparing and contrasting the alternatives. This process can provide many opportunities for self-discovery and become a key to future happiness, resulting in self-realization, joy, and empowerment [60]. How a woman responds is strongly influenced by her self-esteem and her self-concept, which is determined by a balance of her perceptions of stigma, vulnerability, and mastery [61, 62]. If sufficient time and counseling are invested upfront, patients treated for breast cancer will rarely express regret over their choice of treatments [7]. Under the right circumstances, many women with breast cancer are able to redraw their future life path, shifting priorities and focus to become the person they have always wanted to be.

However, the inherent emotional journey that comes with the detection and subsequent treatment of breast cancer can also cause patients to feel changed from within and alienated from those who have not lived through the same experience. Women often express feeling judged or blamed by others who expect them to return to their pretreatment level of function immediately after treatment is completed. Today, a woman who develops breast cancer is also increasingly likely to be held at least partially accountable for her illness by those around her. This is especially true for those women who are diagnosed at an advanced stage. They may be held culpable for failing to have a screening mammogram, for failing to perform breast exams, or for making unhealthy lifestyle choices. Breast cancer treatment for early-stage breast cancer can require 10 years to complete. Treatment for women who develop stage IV metastatic breast cancer can span decades. Women who have had breast cancer express feeling that they continue being treated as a walking time bomb, with others expecting that they will eventually succumb to this deeply feared disease. The women who develop metastatic breast cancer are an important and highly stigmatized group who could not be discussed adequately in this chapter due to the immense scope of the subject. In the future, one hopes that these patients will be treated more like others with chronic diseases as many with treatment are now seeing prolonged remissions and surviving for years, even decades.

There remain expectations for women who have had breast cancer to become active members of the pink "sorority," participating in outreach and fundraising events. Women who decline often express feeling stigmatized for their failure to meet the expectations of others or for failing to give back by joining the "fight" [63, 64]. The breast cancer movement has successfully taught women that when they unite, they can be extraordinarily powerful advocates. For many women, the breast cancer movement has become truly sacred. Undeniably, the movement represents a remarkable example of female solidarity that has substantially changed the stigma that once kept those with breast cancer isolated. The movement has also demonstrated to women the benefits of constructive activism and their newly recognized economic power.

While some women can seize the opportunity that a breast cancer experience provides to create a new life canvas, for women of lower socioeconomic status, there may be little time for making life changes, as both economic and personal consequences are often out of their control [65]. The lower survival rates we discussed earlier found among black women cannot be solely attributed to a higher incidence of the biologically more aggressive variants of breast cancers [21]. These discrepancies in outcome warrant future investigation. Any role of overt or more occult prejudice within the medical community that may contribute to this substantially worse outcome need to be identified and eradicated. Issues of unequal access to healthcare need to be addressed. Some of the solutions to these disparities will likely be found outside the realm of traditional treatments.

The stigma of breast cancer, while less than it once was, persists on multiple levels. Society has high expectations for women, both to prevent breast cancer and to participate in its early detection. Women are expected to continue to function normally with their usual roles and especially to maintain a positive and "sunny" attitude, which differs from the expectations of other cancer patients. To a greater degree than in any other cancer or disease, a woman diagnosed with breast cancer is asked to make crucial treatment decisions. Consequently, a woman with breast cancer becomes accountable for her recovery and survival or relapse. The continual evolution in breast cancer treatments, while promising, has also added to often conflicting information from friends, the Internet, and their healthcare team, and patients may worry, wondering whether they have been offered or chosen the most current, effective treatment options available.

We have evolved into an era in which women are held responsible for the choices they make. Recently, this has had the effect of reversing the historic trend toward treatment with breast conservation. Instead, there are increasing rates of bilateral mastectomies, including the prophylactic removal of an uninvolved breast. This choice may be based on women's desire for symmetry and the improved results with breast reconstruction, or it may be the result of an overwhelming desire to do everything possible to avoid ever having to undergo treatment for another breast cancer. In the future, it remains to be seen whether patients will feel either more, or perhaps less, stigmatized and conflicted, as some of the current choices, especially for the frequency of cancer screenings or the ability to electively undergo prophylactic breast removal, are being challenged and may become increasingly limited. Although the advances in breast cancer treatment over the last several decades have significantly improved outcomes across most demographics, the persistent stigma associated with breast cancer still keeps some women, like Tina, from accessing treatment, while they are still curable.

The cases presented in this chapter are based on actual clinical scenarios seen by the author though the details and names were altered to protect the individual's privacy.

References

1. Sontag S. Illness as metaphor. New York: Vintage Books; 1979.
2. Nowinski J. Rethinking societal attitudes about people who get cancer. Huffington Post. 3 Nov 2011.
3. Patterson JT. The dread disease: cancer and modern American culture, vol. xii. Cambridge: Harvard University Press; 1987. p. 380.
4. NCI. 2015. Available from: http://www.cancer.org/research/researchprogramsfunding.
5. Klawiter M. The biopolitics of breast cancer: changing cultures of disease and activism, vol. xxxi. Minneapolis: University of Minnesota Press; 2008. p. 397.
6. Ehrenreich B. Welcome to cancerland. Harper's Magazine. November, 2001:43–53.
7. Covelli AM, Baxter NN, Fitch MI, McCready DR, Wright FC. 'Taking control of cancer': understanding women's choice for mastectomy. Ann Surg Oncol. 2015;22(2):383–91.
8. Tuttle TM, Burke EE. Surgical decision making for breast cancer: hitting the sweet spot between paternalism and consumerism. Ann Surg Oncol. 2015;22(2):351–2.
9. WCRF. Available from: http://www.wcrf.org/int/cancer-facts-figures/data-specific-cancers/breast-cancer-statistics.
10. National Cancer Institute, 1 May 2015. Available from: http://www.seer.cancer.gov.
11. Tichy JR, Lim E, Anders CK. Breast cancer in adolescents and young adults: a review with a focus on biology. J Natl Compr Canc Netw. 2013;11(9):1060–9.
12. American Cancer Society. Cancer facts and figures 2015. Atlanta: American Cancer Society; 2015; [April 1, 2015].
13. Gomez-Raposo C, Zambrana Tevar F, Sereno Moyano M, Lopez Gomez M, Casado E. Male breast cancer. Cancer Treat Rev. 2010;36(6):451–7.
14. Agrawal A, Ayantunde AA, Rampaul R, Robertson JF. Male breast cancer: a review of clinical management. Breast Cancer Res Treat. 2007;103(1):11–21.
15. Genetic Information Nondiscrimination Act (GINA) of 2008, 1 July 2015. Available from: http://www.genome.gov/24519851.
16. Denieffe S, Gooney M. A meta-synthesis of women's symptoms experience and breast cancer. Eur J Cancer Care. 2011;20(4):424–35.
17. Jolie A. My medical choice. The New York Times. May 14 2013;14(05):2013.
18. King MC, Levy-Lahad E, Lahad A. Population-based screening for BRCA1 and BRCA2: 2014 Lasker Award. JAMA. 2014;312(11):1091–2.
19. Bleyer A, Barr R, Hayes-Lattin B, Thomas D, Ellis C, Anderson B, et al. The distinctive biology of cancer in adolescents and young adults. Nat Rev Cancer. 2008;8(4):288–98.
20. Johnson RH, Chien FL, Bleyer A. Incidence of breast cancer with distant involvement among women in the United States, 1976 to 2009. JAMA. 2013;309(8):800–5.
21. Dehal A, Abbas A, Johna S. Racial disparities in clinical presentation, surgical treatment and in-hospital outcomes of women with breast cancer: analysis of nationwide inpatient sample database. Breast Cancer Res Treat. 2013;139(2):561–9.

22. Dookeran KA, Silva A, Warnecke RB, Rauscher GH. Race/ethnicity and disparities in mastectomy practice in the Breast Cancer Care in Chicago study. Ann Surg Oncol. 2015;22(1):66–74.
23. Wray CJ, Phatak UR, Robinson EK, Wiatek RL, Rieber AG, Gonzalez A, et al. The effect of age on race-related breast cancer survival disparities. Ann Surg Oncol. 2013;20(8):2541–7.
24. Abstract: Women had worse breast cancer mortality regardless of cancer subtype [press release]. AACR, 15 May 2013.
25. Rosenbaum L. "Misfearing" — culture, identity, and our perceptions of health risks. N Engl J Med. 2014;370(7):595–7.
26. Day E. The patient with cancer and the family. N Engl J Med. 1966;274(16):883–6.
27. Hinton J. Bearing cancer. Br J Med Psychol. 1973;46(2):105–13.
28. Bell K, Ristovski-Slijepcevic S. Cancer survivorship: why labels matter. J Clin Oncol. 2013;31(4):409–11.
29. Peters-Golden H. Breast cancer: varied perceptions of social support in the illness experience. Soc Sci Med. 1982;16(4):483–91.
30. Carter BJ. Surviving breast cancer: a problematic work re-entry. Cancer Pract. 1994;2(2):135–40.
31. Ross WS. Crusade: the official history of the American Cancer Society, vol. xx. New York: Arbor House; 1987. p. 283.
32. Lund CC. The doctor, the patient, and the truth. Ann Intern Med. 1946;24:957–8.
33. Cotlar AM, Dubose JJ, Rose DM. History of surgery for breast cancer: radical to the sublime. Curr Surg. 2003;60(3):329–37.
34. Maxine D. "After breast surgery". Good housekeeping. Sept 1954.
35. Sorlie T. Molecular portraits of breast cancer: tumour subtypes as distinct disease entities. Eur J Cancer. 2004;40(18):2667–75.
36. Waljee JF, Ubel PA, Atisha DM, Hu ES, Alderman AK. The choice for breast cancer surgery: can women accurately predict postoperative quality of life and disease-related stigma? Ann Surg Oncol. 2011;18(9):2477–82.
37. Mukherjee S. The emperor of all maladies: a biography of cancer. Large print ed. Waterville: Thorndike Press; 2010.
38. Sorlie T. How to personalise treatment in early breast cancer. Eur J Cancer. 2011;47 Suppl 3:S310–1.
39. Fisher B, Ravdin RG, Ausman RK, Slack NH, Moore GE, Noer RJ. Surgical adjuvant chemotherapy in cancer of the breast: results of a decade of cooperative investigation. Ann Surg. 1968;168(3):337–56.
40. Crile G. A biological consideration of treatment of breast cancer, vol. xii. Springfield: Charles C. Thomas; 1967. p. 189.
41. Crile Jr G. Low incidence and morbidity of local recurrence after conservative operations for cancer of the breast. Ann Surg. 1972;175(2):249–53.
42. Crile G. What women should know about the breast cancer controversy, vol. x. New York: Macmillan; 1973. p. 179.
43. Crile G. Surgery: your choices, your alternatives, vol. xvi. New York: Delacorte Press/S. Lawrence; 1978. p. 175.
44. Veronesi U. Conservative treatment of breast cancer: a trial in progress at the Cancer Institute of Milan. World J Surg. 1977;1(3):324–6.
45. Veronesi U. Rationale and indications for limited surgery in breast cancer: current data. World J Surg. 1987;11(4):493–8.
46. Fisher B. Biological and clinical considerations regarding the use of surgery and chemotherapy in the treatment of primary breast cancer. Cancer. 1977;40(1 Suppl):574–87.
47. Online NCS. The treatment of primary breast cancer: management of local disease. NIH Consens Statement Online 5 Jun 1979 [Cited year month day] 1979;2(5):29–30.
48. Kushner R. Breast cancer: a personal history and an investigative report, vol. xiii. 1st ed. New York: Harcourt Brace Jovanovich; 1975. p. 400.
49. Kevles BH. Naked to the bone: medical imaging in the twentieth century. New Brunswick: Rutgers University Press; 1997.

50. Komen SG. 2015. Available from: http://ww5.komen.org/uploadedFiles/_Komen/Content/About_Us/Financial_Reports/Susan. G Komen 2013 Annual Report.pdf.
51. Bell K. The breast-cancer-ization of cancer survivorship: implications for experiences of the disease. Soc Sci Med. 2014;110:56–63.
52. Ehrenreich B. Bright-sided: how the relentless promotion of positive thinking has undermined America. 1st ed. New York: Metropolitan Books; 2009. p. 235.
53. Belkin L. How breast cancer became this year's hottest charity. New York Times Magazine. 22 Dec 1996,
54. Warner E. Clinical practice. Breast-cancer screening. N Engl J Med. 2011;365(11):1025–32.
55. Rabin RC. Dense breasts may obscure mammogram results. NY Times. 16 Jun 2014.
56. Gard CC, Aiello Bowles EJ, Miglioretti DL, Taplin SH, Rutter CM. Misclassification of Breast Imaging Reporting and Data System (BI-RADS) mammographic density and implications for breast density reporting legislation. Breast J. 2015.
57. Yeh VM, Schnur JB, Margolies L, Montgomery GH. Dense breast tissue notification: impact on women's perceived risk, anxiety, and intentions for future breast cancer screening. J Am Coll Radiol. 2015;12(3):261–6.
58. Burstein HJ. The fifth "C" is cost: highlights from ASCO 2011. J Natl Compr Canc Netw. 2011;9(7):691.
59. Brown B. Power of vulnerability. [Internet]. 3 Jan 2011. Podcast. Available from: https://www.ted.com/speakers/brene_brown.
60. Chang R. How to make hard choices. [Internet]. June 2014. Podcast.
61. den Heijer M, Seynaeve C, Vanheusden K, Duivenvoorden HJ, Vos J, Bartels CC, et al. The contribution of self-esteem and self-concept in psychological distress in women at risk of hereditary breast cancer. Psychooncology. 2011;20(11):1170–5.
62. Vodermaier A, Esplen MJ, Maheu C. Can self-esteem, mastery and perceived stigma predict long-term adjustment in women carrying a BRCA1/2-mutation? Evidence from a multi-center study. Fam Cancer. 2010;9(3):305–11.
63. Ehrenreich B. Smile or die: how positive thinking fooled America and the world. London: Granta; 2009. p. 235.
64. Ehrenreich B, English D. Complaints and disorders: the sexual politics of sickness. 2nd ed. New York: Feminist Press; 2011. p. 173.
65. Graves KD, Jensen RE, Canar J, Perret-Gentil M, Leventhal KG, Gonzalez F, et al. Through the lens of culture: quality of life among Latina breast cancer survivors. Breast Cancer Res Treat. 2012;136(2):603–13.

Chapter 10
Stigma and Prejudice in Patients with HIV/AIDS

Hermioni N. Lokko and Valerie E. Stone

Introduction

An abundance of advances related to pharmacology, diagnostics, patient education, management, and biomedical research over the past three decades has resulted in a dramatic decrease in the morbidity and mortality from HIV/AIDS. However, suffering remains high among those who are affected with HIV and their families as a result of negative mental health and quality of life consequences due to stigma. HIV stigma exists worldwide; its common drivers are recognized across different settings [1]. Stigma continues to be one of the greatest challenges in the fight against HIV/AIDS [2]. The goal of this chapter is to highlight stigma and prejudice as it pertains to patients with HIV/AIDS. We will set the stage with regard to stigma and HIV in this chapter by giving a historic overview of the HIV/AIDS epidemic from the 1980s; summarize the biology of HIV, transmission of the virus, course of illness and how they impact stigma; and discuss the implications of HIV detection and diagnosis on stigma.

This chapter also provides an overview of the literature on stigma and medicine, emphasizing that stigma in patients with certain medical illnesses predates the HIV epidemic. We will then review the theoretical framework and forms of stigma in

H.N. Lokko, MD, MPP (✉)
MGH/McLean Adult Psychiatry Residency Training Program,
Harvard Medical School, Massachusetts General Hospital, Boston, MA, USA

McLean Hospital, Belmont, MA, USA
e-mail: hlokko@partners.org

V.E. Stone, MD, MPH
Department of Medicine, Mount Auburn Hospital, Cambridge, MA, USA

Charles S. Davidson Professor of Medicine, Harvard Medical School, Boston, MA, USA

© Springer International Publishing Switzerland 2016   167
R. Parekh, Ed W. Childs (eds.), *Stigma and Prejudice: Touchstones in Understanding Diversity in Healthcare*, Current Clinical Psychiatry,
DOI 10.1007/978-3-319-27580-2_10

patients with HIV/AIDS. The last four sections of the chapter then focus on the causes of stigma in HIV/AIDS patients, the impact of stigma and prejudice in HIV/AIDS, and the ongoing efforts to address stigma and prejudice in HIV/AIDS. We finally conclude the chapter by highlighting the key themes in each section of the chapter and provide some recommendations for future directions on how to continue to address stigma and prejudice among patients with HIV/AIDS.

Historic Overview of HIV/AIDS

The US Centers for Disease Control (CDC) first suggested the name acquired immunodeficiency syndrome (AIDS) in 1981 to describe the disease responsible for the high mortality of young homosexual men – who died from unusual opportunistic infections such as Pneumocystis jiroveci (formerly carinii) pneumonia and rare malignancies such as Kaposi's sarcoma [3]. Stigma and prejudice surrounding the cause and etiology of the virus stemmed from the high prevalence among intravenous drug users and the gay community. People quickly attributed the cause of AIDS to certain lifestyles such as having multiple sexual partners and the use of amyl nitrite (poppers) or injection drugs. Before the name AIDS was coined, people referred to the cause of these unusual infections as "gay cancer," "gay compromise syndrome," or "community-acquired immune dysfunction" [4]. However, with reports of AIDS in children who have received blood transfusions and in heterosexual adults, it became clearer that AIDS was caused by an infectious agent and not just related to certain stigmatized lifestyles. In an attempt to adequately care for those infected with AIDS, the first AIDS clinic was opened in San Francisco in 1982, and a year later, several cases of AIDS were also observed (not only in homosexual men but in individuals who engaged in heterosexual sex) in various European and African countries.

In 1983, Dr. Robert Gallo of the National Cancer Institute identified the human T-lymphocytic virus III (HTLV-III) as the causative agent of AIDS [5]. In Europe, the French insisted the same virus was called the lymphadenopathy-associated virus (LAV) [6]. The conflict surrounding the name of the virus was eventually resolved in 1986 when the International Committee on Taxonomy of Viruses coined the name human immunodeficiency virus (HIV). With little evidence about treatment for AIDS and the rising number of deaths among those infected, medications such as ribavirin which were thought to be active against HIV were smuggled from Mexico into the USA by HIV activists who felt it was unreasonable for patients with AIDS to wait for the US Food and Drug Administrative (FDA) processes for drug testing [7]. The discovery of HIV helped scientists to research effective ways of testing for the virus, and in 1985, FDA approved the first sensitive blood test, enzyme-linked immunosorbent assay (ELISA), for AIDS [8]. Almost two decades after the first HIV test, the FDA approved the first at-home HIV test (which was 99.6 % accurate) kit in 2002 [9].

Evidence from clinical trials using azidothymidine (AZT) showed a significant improvement in symptoms and less mortality during the drug arm of the study with one death among patients on AZT compared to 19 deaths for patients on placebo. AZT also slowed down the progression to AIDS for HIV-infected individuals which greatly impacts stigma because it is easier for individuals to identify someone who had AIDS compared to a person infected with HIV which has not progressed to AIDS. In 1995, the FDA approved the first protease inhibitor to target HIV, which resulted in this so-called highly active antiretroviral therapy (HAART) becoming the standard of care for HIV and AIDS. Individuals with HIV/AIDS living in high-income countries have benefited (with respect to mortality and morbidity) the most from HAART because of the cost of therapies and the inefficient healthcare delivery systems in many affected countries [10]. Early treatment with HAART controls the replication of the virus and its destruction of the immune system, resulting in less opportunistic infections and associated illnesses which results in the AIDS stigmata which include cutaneous lesions, wasting syndrome, hair loss, swollen lymph nodes, oral ulcers, or persistent diarrhea. Hence HIV stigma is less overt in high-income countries where affected individuals do not often acquire AIDS-related illnesses.

The Biology of HIV

A good understanding of the basic biology of the HIV is essential to appreciating the sophisticated nature of the virus and how it causes the stigmata of HIV/AIDS. HIV is part of the family of human retroviruses (*Retroviridae*) and the subfamily of lentiviruses [11]. There are ·two distinct human immunodeficiency viruses, HIV-1 and HIV-2. The most common cause of HIV in the USA is HIV-1 (which is a likely primate virus, with little evidence on how it was transmitted to humans), and there are currently four identified groups of HIV-1 (M, N, O, P) with the HIV-1M primarily responsible for the AIDS pandemic [11]. HIV-2 is not easily transmitted and is mostly prevalent in West Africa [12]. The HIV virion is an icosahedral structure covered by two major envelope proteins (external gp120 and transmembrane gp41), which form several external spikes. Although HIV is an RNA virus, it can transcribe its RNA to DNA with its reverse transcriptase, after which the viral DNA is eventually integrated into the host cell DNA. The virus replicates by binding to its host (such as a CD4+ lymphocytes, macrophages) via several receptors, which catalyzes a complex replication cycle influenced by a variety of viral and host regulatory gene products [11]. An HIV infection therefore causes cellular immune deficiency characterized by the depletion of helper T lymphocytes (CD4+ cells) which result in the development of AIDS-associated opportunistic infections and neoplastic disease in infected individuals. As HIV-infected individuals progress to AIDS, their risk of experiencing stigma becomes dramatically increased.

Transmission and Course of Illness

HIV/AIDS-related stigma experienced by patients can be impacted by how they contracted the virus or by how people around them perceive they contracted the virus. Patients with HIV/AIDS also experience various forms of stigma depending on where they are in the course of illness after infection. The three primary modes of transmission of the HIV are sexual, parenteral, and mother to child [10]. The most common mode of transmission is via sex with an infected individual, and the stigma experienced by patients who were perceived to have contracted the virus via sex is somewhat different from those who contracted it from their mothers at childbirth or parenterally. The probability of infection with one sexual encounter depends on many factors including: there is a higher chance of infection from male to female than from female to male and receptive anal sex also has a high probability of transmission than vaginal sex [13, 14]. Ulcerative sexually transmitted diseases (such as herpes) as well as higher viral loads usually during seroconversion or at later stages of the disease also increase the likelihood of transmission during sexual activity [15]. Shared needles among intravenous drug users and contaminated needle stick injuries among healthcare workers constitute parenteral transmissions. About 66 % of mother-to-child transmissions occur in utero, while 33 % occur from breastfeeding [10]. Commercial sex workers, intravenous drug users, and men who have sex with men are ostracized by many communities, and their infection with HIV/AIDS is automatically attributed to their lifestyles, further increasing their risk of stigma. HIV transmission therefore highlights the culturally sensitive issues of sexuality, commercial sex, intravenous drug use, and homosexuality which often drive HIV stigma [10].

The progression of HIV infection and illness, outlined in Table 10.1, can vary among individuals although the overall course of the infection is relatively the same if effective antiviral therapy is not initiated to interrupt the process [16]. Each stage of HIV disease progression to AIDS is associated with a different level of stigma as the physical manifestations of the disease become more obvious with disease progression. Patients at the early stages of disease right after infection only experience flu-like symptoms and experience no stigma associated with the virus because most patients are not even aware they have the virus and the infection does not impact their level of functioning or relationships with others. However, as the disease progresses to AIDS, the marked weight loss and other physical symptoms become visible and increase their risk for stigma.

HIV Detection and Diagnosis

Over the past three decades, diagnostic tests for HIV have evolved from the first FDA-approved enzyme immunoassay and Western blot tests [17]. The newer diagnostic tests have significantly advanced HIV screening because they are faster and

Table 10.1 Time course of HIV infection

Approximate time from infection	
1–2 weeks	HIV virus replicates and spreads to various tissues and organs
	Viral loads are not detectable and there is no immune response or symptoms observed
2–4 weeks	This acute phase where high viral loads are detected with large numbers of infected CD4+ T cells in the blood and lymph nodes
	Some individuals will experience flu-like symptoms characterized by fever and enlarged lymph nodes
	As viral levels peak, infected cells begin to express antibodies for all viral proteins
	There is transient decrease in the number of CD4+ T cells in the blood and viral levels also decline rapidly
1–20 years	Individuals are asymptomatic although viral levels are slowly increasing, infecting CD4+ T cells
20+ years	Continuous decline of CD4+ T cells results in a weakened immune system which allows opportunistic infections to flourish
	Acquired immunodeficiency syndrome (AIDS) characterized by CD4 cells less than 200 cells/μL and the presence of any AIDS defining condition including Kaposi's sarcoma, encephalopathy, or lymphoma

can sometimes be carried out in nonclinical settings [17]. The FDA has approved six rapid tests for the detection of HIV antibody, four of which can be completed in nonclinical settings. The HIV-1 RNA assay detection test has been useful for diagnosing HIV infection in individuals who are unaware of the infection. Advances in the diagnostic tests impacts HIV stigma because the newer tests are easier to perform and individuals do not have to return for test results or they can test themselves in the privacy of their homes [18]. Also, the evolved state laws and policies regarding HIV testing procedures (i.e., informed consent and pretest counseling) have also increased the number of tested individuals as well as decreased HIV stigma surrounding testing. The 2006 Center for Disease Control and Prevention (CDC)'s study provided support for routine testing and recommended that a separate written consent and prevention counseling for HIV testing not be required. This helped to reduce the existing stigma associated with HIV testing [19].

Conceptual Framework of Stigma and Medicine and How It Informs HIV Stigma

Stigma in patients with medical illness is not unique to patients with HIV infection. Over the past few decades, patients with a variety of medical conditions, including leprosy, tuberculosis, sexually transmitted disease, dwarfism, and mental illness, have also been faced with significant stigma. Sociologist Erving Goffman's conceptualization of stigma as a discrediting attribute that creates a "spoiled identity"

which removes the stigmatized individual "from himself and from society" forms
the foundation of HIV and stigma research [20]. He suggested that negative attitudes toward undesirable behaviors arise from the perceptions that "out-groups"
exhibiting these unacceptable behaviors have violated a community's set of values
or norms [21].

A community usually determines and defines what is ordinary and natural for
different physical, psychological, and social features of a person, and any deviation
from being ordinary results in a person being consciously or unconsciously discounted by other people in the society. This socially constructed identification forms
the foundation for subsequent disqualification of membership from the group in
which that person was initially accepted [22]. Goffman's work dates back to his
work in psychiatric hospitals in the late 1950s where he developed what has become
the benchmark social theory of the association between stigma and disease.

In some societies, the mere fact of having a disease or illness symbolizes a deviation from the ordinary and leads to negative attitudes from others. The cause of
stigma varies by the manifestation of the illness, its history, specific symptomatology, the nature of the population perceived to carry the illness, ease of contagion,
treatment modalities or the lack thereof, and societal perceptions of mortality. For
example, a patient with leprosy is stigmatized because of the associated disfigurement and how easily it is transmitted, while individuals with tuberculosis are stigmatized because of the lack of knowledge regarding modes of transmission and
perceived risk of transmission [23]. Historically, misconceptions about the etiology,
prognosis, and treatment of mental illness produce stigma, in addition to the symptoms and disabilities associated [24]. Society's perception of HIV/AIDS being contracted through promiscuity, prostitution, and unconventional sexual practices and
lack of knowledge about treatment options and modes of transmission have heavily
fueled HIV/AIDS-related stigma.

Some scholars challenge the static and unidimensional nature of Goffman's formulations on stigma emphasizing that stigma is more dynamic and complex than
has been previously perceived [25–27]. In essence, stigma and discrimination are
characterized by cross-cultural diversity and complexity [25]. With the increasing
understanding of HIV infection and AIDS, novel conceptual frameworks have
arisen from Goffman's definition [21, 28]. The societal and structural nature of
stigma further articulates the process of stigmatization [25, 28, 29]. Stigma is a
harmful societal phenomenon which is enabled by underlying social, political, and
economic powers; it usually begins when a difference is labeled and linked to negative stereotypes, leading to separation of "us" from "them" and finally status loss and
discrimination for those carrying the trait [29]. Stigma should therefore be analyzed
by drawing on concepts of power, dominance, hegemony, and oppression which
calls for interventions that have deeper social, political, and economic roots [22].

Although many interpretations of stigma have focused on the individual and
have been separated from broader social processes (especially relations of power),
some anthropologists have focused their interpretations of stigma by lived experiences of those who suffer from HIV [30–32]. In some societies, HIV stigma is
influenced by the contribution the individual makes to society (whether he or she is

a drain to societal resources), and this material symbolism of stigma in some cultures is pertinent as the life expectancy of people with HIV is prolonged [33–35].

The stigmatization process can be divided into specific domains (drivers, facilitators, intersecting stigmata, and manifestations of stigma) each of which can be addressed through programmatic and policy efforts [36]. Drivers are individual factors that negatively influence the stigmatization process, such as lack of awareness of stigma and its harmful consequences and fear of HIV infection via casual contact. Facilitators are societal- or policy-level factors, such as those of countries with laws that ban harm reduction initiatives for IV drug users or the prosecution of individuals who pass on the virus even without intent, which influence the stigmatization process (either negatively or positively including protective or punitive laws). Intersecting and layered stigmata refer to the multiple stigmata that people often face due to HIV status, gender, profession, migrancy, drug use, and poverty [36].

Forms of Stigma

HIV stigma experienced by infected patients can be categorized as felt stigma, enacted stigma, perceived stigma, and self-stigma [37]. Felt stigma refers to a patient's feelings about his or her condition and the expectations about others' reactions to them. Felt stigma damages the mental well-being of patients and the fear of discrimination destroys confidence to seek help and the necessary medical care for treatment. Felt stigma also results in the fear of a negative community reaction that bolsters the walls of silence and the shame surrounding contracting the disease.

Enacted stigma is the actual experiences of stigma, which is manifested when patients are discriminated against because they have, or are thought to have, HIV infection. Enacted stigma also refers to the discrimination based on the attribute that is ascribed to the stigmatized group [38, 39]. The story of Ryan Wayne White (1971–1990), an American teenager from Kokomo, Indiana, who contracted HIV from a blood transfusion to treat his hemophilia, clearly depicts the impact of HIV enacted stigma on a patient and his family [40]. Despite physician's report stating that he posed no risk to other students and that Ryan could return to school after treatment, school officials denied his return to school; many teachers and parents rallied against his attendance. Ryan was finally able to resume school after a court ruling; it is reported that he had few friends, was required to eat with disposable utensils, used a separate bathroom, and was forbidden to interact with other students. In his book, *My Own Story*, Ryan reported on how people would leave restaurants or refuse to sit near him in public or in church [41]. Enacted stigma experienced by individuals with HIV in 2014 may look a bit different from what Ryan experienced considering the advances in medicine for treatment options and an increased awareness of modes of transmission of HIV.

Perceived stigma is the fear of enacted stigma and the shame associated with the stigmatized attribute [42]. Perceived stigma is quite prevalent among patients in the asymptomatic phase of HIV infection; this consciously and unconsciously fuels a desire to conceal the diagnosis. Concealing a diagnosis of HIV infection not only harms the infected individual as delayed diagnosis and progression to AIDS increases mortality, but it also poses a major public health threat as more people become infected. Perceived stigma can also manifest as self-blame and depreciation [43].

Very often, patients with HIV infection experience more than one form of stigma. The kind of stigma a patient may experience could evolve over the course of their illness especially if they receive no treatment and they develop AIDS. Little scholarly work exists on whether the specific form of stigma experienced by a patient has a differing impact on antiretroviral medication adherence, disclosure of HIV status, support-seeking, testing or prevention, mental health, or quality of life.

Causes of HIV Stigma

The etiology of stigma experienced by HIV/AIDS patients is dynamic and universal. The complexity ingrained in the etiology of HIV stigma reflects how multidimensional stigma can be. Several factors including socioeconomic status (mostly poverty), gender (especially in women), sexuality (men who have sex with men), level of education, age, religious beliefs, and culture, just to name a few, influence the causes of HIV stigma.

HIV stigma is perpetuated by reduced social capital [44]. Stigma and poverty are woven in a reciprocal and mutually reinforcing relationship. Poor people have more HIV-related stigma; the lower the socioeconomic status, the greater the stigma. Poorer communities typically tend to also have limited access to healthcare. Hence poorer patients with HIV have less access to treatment which results in a faster progression of the disease to AIDS, and its associated opportunistic infections, stigma, and discrimination. Some poor communities also consider patients with HIV to be less productive members of the society who draw on community resources and all these perceptions feed into the stigmatization process.

Ignorance and misinformation about how HIV is transmitted, the prognosis of the disease, and its treatment options also contribute to stigma [45]. The mystery of HIV/AIDS and how the disease progresses was a major contributor to stigma in the 1980s when much was not known about the transmission of the virus. With efficacious treatment options to control the virus, the decrease in morbidity and mortality of patients with HIV and the increased awareness of HIV infection has dramatically reduced HIV stigma.

Some patients with HIV/AIDS are also stigmatized because HIV is associated with "deviant behavior" with the individual responsible for the illness as compared to other diseases, which can be contracted independent of a person's behavior. In these contexts, the HIV/AIDS is tainted by cultural beliefs that the disease is a result of a morally sanctionable behavior which introduces a contagious disease that is threatening to the community and is associated with an undesirable form of death [21].

In many situations, social norms intensified HIV stigma as it was layered on top of preexisting inequalities, such as those related to sexual minority status, poverty, and injection drug use [46, 47]. Historically, HIV/AIDS was first recognized as a new disease in the USA in young homosexual men who presented with opportunistic infections typically seen in immunosuppressed individuals [4]. Although we know that there is great diversity in the demographics of patients infected with HIV/AIDS, some cultures around the world still hold the notion that the disease mostly affects gay men. Despite the efforts to reduce stigma, prejudice, and discrimination against gay men over the past few decades, it still remains a commonplace in many cultures. Hence, in societies where homosexuality is not widely acceptable, individuals with HIV infection are stigmatized because of suspicions that they practice homosexuality [48].

Structural violence can also determine in large part who suffers from AIDS-related stigma and discrimination [22]. Observations in Haiti and other low-income countries assert that racism, sexism, stigma, and prejudice are worsened when there is political violence and social inequalities. In essence, structural violence creates the environment that predisposes certain people to the risk of infection and also determines those who have access (or do not have) to quality healthcare for effective treatment of their diseases [49]. Being a victim of violence in itself predisposes one to stigma, which is often worsened after a person contracts HIV and has limited access to care.

HIV-related stigma can be damaging within healthcare facilities. HIV-related stigma is a key barrier to both the effective delivery of quality services by clinicians and the utilization of services by the community. Increased morbidity and mortality results when HIV-related stigma causes clinicians to delay, deny, or avoid the provision of healthcare to patients with HIV [50]. HIV-related stigma also results in patients receiving differential treatment characterized by emotional harassment, avoidance by clinical staff, and the use of gloves by clinicians regardless of physical contact and public designation of HIV status on charts [50]. At the start of the epidemic and in some countries, factors associated with stigma among healthcare providers included a lack of knowledge, fear related to incurability of AIDS, fear of being infected, lack of certainty of how it was contracted, and prejudice toward marginalized behaviors [51].

The perceived stigma in healthcare settings results in late detection of the HIV infection, reduced utilization of prevention services, and rejection of care and medication nonadherence among patients with HIV/AIDS.

Impact of HIV Stigma

HIV-related stigma is a multilayered phenomenon which has been shown to impact many aspects of the disease on patients and their communities [52]. Stigma inflicts hardships and suffering on patients living with HIV infection both in resource-rich and resource-constrained settings [53]. The impact of HIV stigma affects individuals, families, societies, and healthcare systems.

For affected patients, HIV stigma causes physical, psychological, social, and economic burden. It remains one of the most challenging barriers to maintaining overall health (e.g., physical, mental, and emotional well-being) in those living with HIV/AIDS. Physically, stigma serves as a barrier to timely testing, to participation in prevention measures, and to adherence to antiretroviral treatment. Having HIV infection and mental illness, both of which are stigmatized in many communities, poses a higher risk of morbidity for individuals. The lack of access to needed medical care and assistance with daily functions breeds discouragement, which hastens the patient's demise. Socially, HIV stigma discourages self-disclosure due to the threat of being ostracized. Stigmatized patients are often isolated with minimal social interactions resulting in decreased communal support and social networks. Isolation from friends and family, as well as employment loss, causes psychological pain and fosters depression, low self-esteem, and anxiety. Stigma also undermines adaptive coping strategies and promotes maladaptive coping strategies like regression and avoidance. The possible economic impact of HIV on individuals is multifaceted. The disease itself could deprive the individual of stamina and motivation to work; at the beginning of the HIV epidemic and much less today, stigma created a barrier for job opportunities due to incorrect perceptions of contagion. Patients with HIV infection also have to deal with stigma from their coworkers and employers, including social isolation or ridicule and in some cases discrimination. Overall, HIV stigma not only worsens the course of disease for patients but also contributes significantly to poor quality of life to those affected.

The impact of HIV stigma extends to the family of affected individuals. The impact can be economic, psychological, or social. An HIV-infected person who was the breadwinner of the family or the primary care giver for children is less likely to function adequately in their role as a result of the progression of the disease, resulting in a disruption in the family structure. Financial instability becomes a problem from lack of gainful employment to inability to work due to the physical toll of the disease on the body. The psychological drain on family members results from caregiver burden experienced by family members who are primarily responsible for the needs of the patient depending on the stage of their condition. Seeing a loved one slowly deteriorate from medical complications resulting from untreated HIV/AIDS can be traumatic for family members who feel helpless because they are unable to deter impending demise of their loved one. The shame experienced by an HIV-infected individual is often shared by the family who may be ridiculed by their community. The superstitious beliefs held in some communities about the etiology of the AIDS (with regards to immoral behavior) can be extended to family members even if they do not have the virus. Socially, the isolation of individuals infected with HIV is also extended to their family and those who come into contact with them.

The impact of HIV stigma on healthcare systems is complicated and multidimensional, affecting both medical resources (both human and physical asset) and service delivery. An increased burden of HIV/AIDS can greatly increase healthcare costs, stretch the existing healthcare services, and cause disparities in healthcare delivery especially in areas where the facilities and resources needed to adequately manage these patients are lacking. Healthcare-related stigma has changed over the past three decades with the increased knowledge about the pathophysiology of HIV infection and advancements in treatment options. In the 1980s and 1990s, the burden of HIV/AIDS caused a strain on healthcare providers. Stigma further exacerbated disparities in healthcare access in populations that already struggle to access quality healthcare.

At the beginning of the HIV epidemic, many physicians and other healthcare providers were fearful for their physical well-being as very little was known about how the virus was spread. Brave and dedicated healthcare providers who specialized in infectious diseases served as the primary consultants for HIV patients. These made a huge impact on reducing stigma by dedicating their careers to understanding how the virus affects the immune system and how its impact can be curtailed. Governmental financial support and generous individual donors who set up foundations dedicated to understanding the virus really advanced HIV research in the 1990s, resulting in effective therapeutics and treatment options that have tremendously helped to reduce stigma. Advances in diagnosis, treatment, and management of HIV/AIDS in western countries have minimized the stigma in healthcare facilities. However, in low- and middle-income countries with limited access to treatment of HIV, the stigma in healthcare facilities remains prevalent.

The complicated and substantial nature of HIV-related stigma exists outside the healthcare system and actually impacts an entire economy as evidenced in many African countries. Over the past two to three decades, several million people died from AIDS, and majority of the people with HIV/AIDS reside in Africa [54]. The burden of disease in sub-Saharan Africa reduced labor supply and productivity, resulting in exponential increases in imports and decreases in exports, stifling Africa's economic development. The stigma created by the disease also impacted foreign investors' choices to work in Africa and other low-income countries that could not cope with the pandemic. Unfortunately, poorer communities and countries who were most plagued by the virus lost human resources which further worsened the unfavorable economic conditions required to promote economic growth [55].

Efforts to Address HIV and Stigma

Many unanswered questions remain, as do gaps in HIV stigma research; there are no fully powered randomized controlled trials on HIV stigma prevention strategies [27, 56, 57]. Doubling research efforts on HIV stigma would not only expand the peer-reviewed literature with evidence for stigma interventions, but it would also motivate healthcare workers to actively engage their patients on issues related to HIV stigma.

Interventions with the goal of reducing HIV/AIDS-related stigma must reflect the multidimensional and layered nature of the stigmatization process of the disease [58] which acknowledges community contexts and uses culturally appropriate intervention strategies [50, 59–61]. Currently, very few interventions exist for reducing stigma at the intersection of HIV infection and key population variables [52, 56]. However, there are several intervention categories as follows [56]:

- Information-based approaches (e.g., brochures)
- Skill-building and hands-on learning approaches
- Counseling and peer support approaches
- Contact with affected groups
- Media (e.g., radio, TV, play, movies) and printed information

Information-based approaches include the use of brochures and other educational materials, which are disseminated in communities. Skill-building and hands-on learning approaches (via workshops for both individuals with HIV infection and the general public) usually target negative attitudes. Counseling and peer support approaches are effective because collective participation in livelihood activities provides skills to cope with external stigma and confidence to overcome self-stigma via pooling of labor and resources [62–65]. Although the natural tendency of individuals with HIV infection is to hide their disease from their communities because of stigma, studies have shown that meaningful engagement of people living with HIV and their communities can contribute to interventions to mitigate HIV stigma. Testimonials from individuals with HIV/AIDS usually empower other infected individuals and their families to engage their communities and to educate people around them.

The American media, public figures, and the entertainment industry via radio, TV, plays, and movies have been powerful tools in the campaign to address HIV and stigma over the past couple of decades. Celebrities, like Magic Johnson, made a huge impact on awareness about HIV in the early 1990s by announcing that they had the virus [66]. It is reported that Magic Johnson's announcement encouraged people, especially, heterosexuals, to get tested for the virus and changed perceptions that HIV was mostly contracted by men who had sex with men [66].

HIV stigma has been successfully subverted in resource-limited settings by strengthening social support and livelihoods of HIV-positive individuals since the economic impacts of HIV typically exacerbate the symbolic aspects of stigma [67, 68]. When an individual has HIV and is unable to work, addressing community-level social economic status inequality reduces HIV stigma [44]. However, economic strengthening strategies as a way to reduce HIV stigma have not been formally tested [27, 56].

Establishing peer support groups has been shown to be an effective way to address HIV stigma [69]. In sub-Saharan Africa, increasing the availability of anti-retroviral therapy (ART) and counseling alone did not reduce HIV stigma, but ART coupled with support groups that teach coping strategies and resiliency to people living with HIV was thought to be more effective [69, 70].

Ignorance and lack of knowledge about the causes of HIV, testing, modes of transmission, and treatment modalities have been primary sources of stigma in several communities around the world. Hence, increasing awareness and community education interventions about the virus can result in reduced HIV-related stigma as reported by Logie and Vyas [71, 72].

Conclusion

Well-known sociologists like Erving Goffman, PhD, described stigma as a discrediting attribute and identity, which removes the stigmatized individual from himself and society. Inherently, an individual's societal norms define what is acceptable and normal, impacting which attributes are considered stigmatized. For centuries patients with several medical conditions including leprosy, tuberculosis, and mental illness have been stigmatized in many societies. Patients with HIV/AIDS similar to historically stigmatized populations became stigmatized because of limited knowledge about how the disease is transmitted and how it can be cured. Therefore, the manifestation of an illness, historical causes, specific symptomatology, ease of contagion, and limited treatment modalities usually influence stigma associated with disease. The causes of stigma in patients with HIV/AIDS are dynamic and universal, including socioeconomic status, gender, sexuality, and education level. The impact of stigma is as complex and multidimensional as the causes of the stigma and it impacts both individuals and their communities alike.

Stigma in patients with HIV/AIDS has evolved over the past three decades, as pharmacology and medical technology has advanced to elucidate more about the pathophysiology and treatment to control the effect of the virus on the immune system. As we become more educated about HIV/AIDS, patients with the infection and disease experience a different kind of stigma today than existed three decades ago at the start of the epidemic. Furthermore, the issues of stigma and prejudice surrounding HIV/AIDS have different implications for younger generations of healthcare providers today than providers caring for patients with HIV/AIDs three decades ago.

Celebrities, organizations, foundations, and governmental policies in some heavily affected countries have helped to reduce stigma by public health education efforts and educating people about modes of transmission with hopes of treatment of the virus. However, there are many gaps and unanswered questions about HIV stigma, which call for a collaborative effort by experts in medicine, sociology, anthropology, and policymakers to work on creative ways to eradicate stigma.

References

1. Thomas BE, Rehman F, Suryanarayanan D, Josephine K, Dilip M, Dorairaj VS, Swaminathan S. How stigmatizing is stigma in the life of people living with HIV: a study on HIV positive individuals from Chennai, South India. AIDS Care. 2005;17(7):795–801.
2. Wolfe WR, Weiser SD, Leiter K, Steward WT, Percy-de Korte F, Phaladze N, Iacopino V, Heisler M. The impact of universal access to antiretroviral therapy on HIV stigma in Botswana. Am J Public Health. 2008;98(10):1865–71.
3. Greene WC. A history of AIDS: looking back to see ahead. Eur J Immunol. 2007;37 Suppl 1:S94–102.
4. Altman LK. New homosexual disorder worries health officials. The New York Times. May 11 1982.
5. Broder S, Gallo RC. A pathogenic retrovirus (HTLV-III) linked to AIDS. N Engl J Med. 1984;311(20):1292–7.

6. Laurence J, Brun-Vezinet F, Schutzer SE, Rouzioux C, Klatzmann D, Barre-Sinoussi F, Chermann JC, Montagnier L. Lymphadenopathy-associated viral antibody in AIDS. Immune correlations and definition of a carrier state. N Engl J Med. 1984;311(20):1269–73.
7. Kwitny J. Bad medicine. American Journalism Review Features. 1993. http://ajrarchive.org/Article.asp?id=1411. Accessed 31 Aug 2015.
8. Busch MP, Lee LL, Satten GA, Henrard DR, Farzadegan H, Nelson KE, Read S, Dodd RY, Petersen LR. Time course of detection of viral and serologic markers preceding human immunodeficiency virus type 1 seroconversion: implications for screening of blood and tissue donors. Transfusion. 1995;35(2):91–7.
9. Kahn JO, Walker BD. Acute human immunodeficiency virus type 1 infection. N Engl J Med. 1998;339(1):33–9.
10. Morison L. The global epidemiology of HIV/AIDS. Br Med Bull. 2001;58:7–18.
11. Fauci AS, Lane HC. Chapter 189: Human immunodeficiency virus disease: AIDS and related disorders. In: Longo DL, FA, Kasper DL, Hauser SL, Jameson J, Loscalzo J, editors. Harrison's principles of internal medicine. 18th ed. New York: McGraw-Hill; 2012: http://accessmedicine.mhmedical.com.ezp-prod1.hul.harvard.edu/content.aspx?bookid=331&Sectionid=40726947. Accessed 3 Sep 2015.
12. De Cock KM, Adjorlolo G, Ekpini E, Sibailly T, Kouadio J, Maran M, Brattegaard K, Vetter KM, Doorly R, Gayle HD. Epidemiology and transmission of HIV-2. Why there is no HIV-2 pandemic. JAMA. 1993;270(17):2083–6.
13. Bouvet E, De Vincenzi I, Ancelle R, Vachon F. Defloration as risk factor for heterosexual HIV transmission. Lancet. 1989;1(8638):615.
14. de Vincenzi I. A longitudinal study of human immunodeficiency virus transmission by heterosexual partners. European Study Group on Heterosexual Transmission of HIV. N Engl J Med. 1994;331(6):341–6.
15. Vernazza PL, Eron JJ, Fiscus SA, Cohen MS. Sexual transmission of HIV: infectiousness and prevention. AIDS. 1999;13(2):155–66.
16. Coffin J, Swanstrom R. HIV pathogenesis: dynamics and genetics of viral populations and infected cells. Cold Spring Harb Perspect Med. 2013;3(1):a012526.
17. Branson BM. State of the art for diagnosis of HIV infection. Clin Infect Dis. 2007;45 Suppl 4:S221–5.
18. Hutchinson AB, Branson BM, Kim A, Farnham PG. A meta-analysis of the effectiveness of alternative HIV counseling and testing methods to increase knowledge of HIV status. AIDS. 2006;20(12):1597–604.
19. Prevention CfDCa. State HIV testing laws: consent and counseling requirements. HIV/AIDS. 2015. http://www.cdc.gov/hiv/policies/law/states/testing.html. Accessed 31 Aug 2015.
20. Goffman E. Stigma: notes on the management of spoiled identity. New York: Simon & Schuster Inc: 1986.
21. Alonzo AA, Reynolds NR. Stigma, HIV and AIDS: an exploration and elaboration of a stigma trajectory. Soc Sci Med. 1995;41(3):303–15.
22. Castro A, Farmer P. Understanding and addressing AIDS-related stigma: from anthropological theory to clinical practice in Haiti. Am J Public Health. 2005;95(1):53–9.
23. Courtwright A, Turner AN. Tuberculosis and stigmatization: pathways and interventions. Public Health Rep. 2010;125 Suppl 4:34–42.
24. Corrigan PW, Watson AC. Understanding the impact of stigma on people with mental illness. World Psychiatry. 2002;1(1):16–20.
25. Parker R, Aggleton P. HIV and AIDS-related stigma and discrimination: a conceptual framework and implications for action. Soc Sci Med. 2003;57(1):13–24.
26. Deacon H, Inez S, Sandra P. Understanding HIV/AIDS Stigma A theoretical and methodological analysis. Cape Town: Human Sciences Research. 2005.
27. Sengupta S, Banks B, Jonas D, Miles MS, Smith GC. HIV interventions to reduce HIV/AIDS stigma: a systematic review. AIDS Behav. 2011;15(6):1075–87.
28. Aggleton P. Barcelona 2002: law, ethics, and human rights. HIV/AIDS-related stigma and discrimination: a conceptual framework. Can HIV AIDS Policy Law Rev. 2002;7(2–3):115–6.
29. Link BG, Phelan JC. Conceptulaizing stigma. Annu Rev Socio. 2001;27:363–85.

30. Kleinman A, Wang WZ, Li SC, Cheng XM, Dai XY, Li KT, Kleinman J. The social course of epilepsy: chronic illness as social experience in interior China. Soc Sci Med. 1995;40(10):1319–30.
31. Whittaker AM. Living with HIV: resistance by positive people. Med Anthropol Q. 1992;6(4):385–90.
32. Farmer P, Kleinman A. AIDS as human suffering. Daedalus. 1989;118(2):135–60.
33. Campbell C, Skovdal M, Mupambireyi Z, Madanhire C, Robertson L, Nyamukapa CA, Gregson S. Can AIDS stigma be reduced to poverty stigma? Exploring Zimbabwean children's representations of poverty and AIDS. Child Care Health Dev. 2012;38(5): 732–42.
34. Hontelez JA, de Vlas SJ, Baltussen R, Newell ML, Bakker R, Tanser F, Lurie M, Barnighausen T. The impact of antiretroviral treatment on the age composition of the HIV epidemic in sub-Saharan Africa. AIDS. 2012;26 Suppl 1:S19–30.
35. Reidpath DD, Chan KY, Gifford SM, Allotey P. 'He hath the French pox': stigma, social value and social exclusion. Sociol Health Illn. 2005;27(4):468–89.
36. Stangl AL, Brady L, Fritz K. Technical Brief: Measuring HIV stigma and discrimination, tackling the structural drivers of HIV. International Center for Research on Women, Washington DC. 2012.
37. Gray AJ. Stigma in psychiatry. J R Soc Med. 2002;95(2):72–6.
38. Earnshaw VA, Chaudoir SR. From conceptualizing to measuring HIV stigma: a review of HIV stigma mechanism measures. AIDS Behav. 2009;13(6):1160–77.
39. Jacoby A. Felt versus enacted stigma: a concept revisited. Evidence from a study of people with epilepsy in remission. Soc Sci Med. 1994;38(2):269–74.
40. Evans T. Retro indy: ryan white (1971–1990). IndyStar. April 8, 2010.
41. White R, Cunningham AM. Ryan white: my own story. New York: Signet; 1992.
42. Herek G. Beyond "Homophobia": thinking about sexual prejudice and stigma in the twenty-first century. Sexual Res Soc Pol. 2004;1(2):6–24.
43. Bharat SAP, Tyrer P. India, HIV and AIDS-related discrimination, stigmatization and denial. Geneva: UNAIDS; 2001.
44. Lim T, Zelaya C, Latkin C, Quan VM, Frangakis C, Ha TV, Minh NL, Go V. Individual-level socioeconomic status and community-level inequality as determinants of stigma towards persons living with HIV who inject drugs in Thai Nguyen, Vietnam. J Int AIDS Soc. 2013;16(3 Suppl 2):18637.
45. Valdiserri RO. HIV/AIDS stigma: an impediment to public health. Am J Public Health. 2002;92(3):341–2.
46. Edwards LV. Perceived social support and HIV/AIDS medication adherence among African American women. Qual Health Res. 2006;16(5):679–91.
47. Konkle-Parker DJ, Erlen JA, Dubbert PM. Barriers and facilitators to medication adherence in a southern minority population with HIV disease. J Assoc Nurses AIDS Care. 2008;19(2):98–104.
48. Anderson M, Elam G, Gerver S, Solarin I, Fenton K, Easterbrook P. HIV/AIDS-related stigma and discrimination: accounts of HIV-positive Caribbean people in the United Kingdom. Soc Sci Med. 2008;67(5):790–8.
49. Ramin B. Anthropology speaks to medicine: the case HIV/AIDS in Africa. Mcgill J Med. 2007;10(2):127–32.
50. Nyblade L, Stangl A, Weiss E, Ashburn K. Combating HIV stigma in health care settings: what works? J Int AIDS Soc. 2009;12:15.
51. Rutledge SE, Abell N, Padmore J, McCann TJ. AIDS stigma in health services in the Eastern Caribbean. Sociol Health Illn. 2009;31(1):17–34.
52. Grossman CI, Stangl AL. Editorial: global action to reduce HIV stigma and discrimination. J Int AIDS Soc. 2013;16(3 Suppl 2):18881.
53. Obermeyer CM, Osborn M. The utilization of testing and counseling for HIV: a review of the social and behavioral evidence. Am J Public Health. 2007;97(10):1762–74.
54. Dixon S, McDonald S, Roberts J. The impact of HIV and AIDS on Africa's economic development. BMJ. 2002;324(7331):232–4.

55. Barnighausen T, Bloom DE, Humair S. Human resources for treating HIV/AIDS: needs, capacities, and gaps. AIDS Patient Care STDS. 2007;21(11):799–812.
56. Brown L, Macintyre K, Trujillo L. Interventions to reduce HIV/AIDS stigma: what have we learned? AIDS Educ Prev. 2003;15(1):49–69.
57. Hong Y, Li X. HIV/AIDS behavioral interventions in China: a literature review and recommendation for future research. AIDS Behav. 2009;13(3):603–13.
58. Jain A, Nuankaew R, Mongkholwiboolphol N, Banpabuth A, Tuvinun R, Oranop NA Ayuthaya P, Richter K. Community-based interventions that work to reduce HIV stigma and discrimination: results of an evaluation study in Thailand. J Int AIDS Soc. 2013;16(3 Suppl 2):18711.
59. Bernal G, Jiménez-Chafey MI, Domenech Rodríguez MM. Cultural adaptation of treatments: a resource for considering culture in evidence-based practice. Prof Psychol Res Pract. 2009;40(4):361–8.
60. Gearing RE, Schwalbe CS, MacKenzie MJ, Brewer KB, Ibrahim RW, Olimat HS, Al-Makhamreh SS, Mian I, Al-Krenawi A. Adaptation and translation of mental health interventions in Middle Eastern Arab countries: a systematic review of barriers to and strategies for effective treatment implementation. Int J Soc Psychiatry. 2013;59(7):671–81.
61. Li L, Lin C, Guan J, Wu Z. Implementing a stigma reduction intervention in healthcare settings. J Int AIDS Soc. 2013;16(3 Suppl 2):18710.
62. Stangl AL, Lloyd JK, Brady LM, Holland CE, Baral S. A systematic review of interventions to reduce HIV-related stigma and discrimination from 2002 to 2013: how far have we come? J Int AIDS Soc. 2013;16(3 Suppl 2):18734.
63. Mburu G, Ram M, Skovdal M, Bitira D, Hodgson I, Mwai GW, Stegling C, Seeley J. Resisting and challenging stigma in Uganda: the role of support groups of people living with HIV. J Int AIDS Soc. 2013;16(3 Suppl 2):18636.
64. Roopnaraine T, Rawat R, Babirye F, Ochai R, Kadiyala S. "The group" in integrated HIV and livelihoods programming: opportunity or challenge? AIDS Care. 2012;24(5):649–57.
65. Pulerwitz J, Michaelis A, Weiss E, Brown L, Mahendra V. Reducing HIV-related stigma: lessons learned from horizons research and programs. Public Health Rep. 2010;125(2):272–81.
66. Specter M. How magic Johnson fought the AIDS epidemic. The New Yorker. 2014. http://www.newyorker.com/news/daily-comment/how-magic-johnson-fought-the-aids-epidemic.
67. Seeley J, Russel S. Social rebirth and social transformation? Rebuilding social lives after ART in rural Uganda. AIDS Care. 2010;22 Suppl 1:44–50.
68. Tsai AC, Bangsberg DR, Weiser SD. Harnessing poverty alleviation to reduce the stigma of HIV in sub-Saharan Africa. PLoS Med. 2013;10(11):e1001557.
69. Midtbø V, Shirima V, Skovdal M, Daniel M. How disclosure and antiretroviral therapy help HIV-infected adolescents in sub-Saharan Africa cope with stigma. Afr J AIDS Res. 2012;11(3):261–71.
70. Campbell C, Skovdal M, Madanhire C, Mugurungi O, Gregson S, Nyamukapa C. "We, the AIDS people…": how antiretroviral therapy enables Zimbabweans living with HIV/AIDS to cope with stigma. Am J Public Health. 2011;101(6):1004–10.
71. Logie C, Gadalla TM. Meta-analysis of health and demographic correlates of stigma towards people living with HIV. AIDS Care. 2009;21(6):742–53.
72. Vyas KJ, Patel GR, Shukla D, Mathews WC. A comparison in HIV-associated stigma among healthcare workers in urban and rural Gujarat. SAHARA J. 2010;7(2):71–5.

Chapter 11
Commercially Sexually Exploited and Trafficked Minors: Our Hidden and Forgotten Children

Wendy Macias-Konstantopoulos and Miri Bar-Halpern

Introduction

Slavery has existed across civilizations since the beginning of human history. Dating as far back as 4000 B.C., clay drawing depictions of slave practices in ancient Sumer have survived the test of time, and so too, slavery itself. In early colonial times, the United States participated in the transatlantic slave trade that ultimately enslaved millions of Africans across the Americas. Following the US prohibition of the international slave trade in 1808, internal slave trading of imported slaves and their descendants became a major economic activity in the United States and the predominant form slavery.

The trafficking of persons, also known as human trafficking, is a form of modern day slavery. Much like historical slavery, human trafficking is an egregious human rights violation and a reprehensible crime. As in centuries past, trafficked persons are brought under control through threats and violence—their rights denied and their labor exploited for profit. An estimated 20.9 million persons worldwide are trapped in forced labor or forced sexual exploitation in today's age [1]. Though laws outlawing slavery have been in place since the Thirteenth Amendment of 1865, the practice of controlling, trading, and economically exploiting human beings

W. Macias-Konstantopoulos, MD, MPH (✉)
Division of Global Health and Human Rights, Department of Emergency Medicine,
Massachusetts General Hospital, 55 Fruit Street, Boston, MA 02114, USA

Harvard Medical School, Boston, MA, USA
e-mail: wmacias@mgh.harvard.edu

M. Bar-Halpern, PsyD
Adolescent Acute Residential Program, McLean Hospital, Boston, MA, USA

Harvard Medical School, Boston, MA, USA

© Springer International Publishing Switzerland 2016
R. Parekh, Ed W. Childs (eds.), *Stigma and Prejudice: Touchstones in Understanding Diversity in Healthcare*, Current Clinical Psychiatry,
DOI 10.1007/978-3-319-27580-2_11

continues to thrive in the United States. The forced exploitation of persons in labor industries (labor trafficking) and in the commercial sex industry (sex trafficking) are the two major US forms of human trafficking.

With profoundly detrimental short- and long-term health effects, the commercial sexual exploitation of children remains a significant public health problem worldwide. Moreover, the cumulative effects of complex trauma and stigma place victims and survivors at a disadvantage in a number of health metrics. Trafficked minors are challenged by unfavorable social determinants of health, high-risk health behaviors, poor health outcomes, numerous barriers to health care, and retraumatization in the health care setting. Through education and training, health care providers knowledgeable about sex trafficking and the experiences of trafficked minors can provide culturally sensitive trauma-informed care, thus helping to break the cycle of trauma and stigmatization, lessen health care disparities, and contribute to the healing and recovery of victimized minors.

The following chapter will review the current state of knowledge about commercial sexual exploitation and sex trafficking of minors in the United States, including a brief overview of definitions; prevalence; risk factors; recruitment and control mechanisms; physical, sexual, and mental health outcomes; and cumulative effects leading to complex trauma. The historical underpinnings of stigma are explored, as well as the impact of stigma on the response to this vulnerable group. Finally, the authors discuss formal education and training of health care providers, a culturally sensitive and trauma-informed approach to patient care, and a multidisciplinary response to minor victims identified in the health care setting as essential preliminary steps to a more effective health sector response.

The Epidemiology of Commercial Sexual Exploitation and Sex Trafficking

Definitions

Though the commercial sexual exploitation of children (CSEC) in the United States has garnered much attention in the last decade, CSEC is not a recent occurrence. The term *commercial sexual exploitation of children* is a broad term that comprises a range of sexually exploitative "criminal practices that demean, degrade, and threaten the physical and psychosocial integrity of children" [2]. The US Department of Justice Office of Juvenile Justice and Delinquency Prevention (OJJDP) defines the commercial sexual exploitation of children as "crimes of a sexual nature committed against juvenile victims for financial or other economic reasons" [3]. Trafficking for sexual purposes, or sex trafficking, is one of the primary forms of CSEC [2]. Other forms of CSEC include survival sex, sex tourism, mail-order brides, pornography, and stripping or performing in sexual venues [2–4].

US federal law against human trafficking has been in effect since the start of the millennium, and as of the year 2013, all 50 states have passed anti-trafficking legislation. Similar to the United Nations' *Protocol to Prevent, Suppress and Punish Trafficking in Persons, especially Women and Children* signed in 2000, the US federal law known as the *Victims of Trafficking and Violence Protection Act of 2000* (TVPA) defines *sex trafficking* as the "recruitment, harboring, transportation, provision, or obtaining of a person for the purpose of a commercial sex act" and defines "sex trafficking in which a commercial sex act is induced by force, fraud, or coercion, or in which the person induced to perform such act has not attained 18 years" as a severe form of human trafficking. This piece of federal legislation further defines a *commercial sex act* as "any sex act on account of which anything of value is given to or received by any person" [5], and remuneration may take many forms including money, drugs, food, shelter, and any other need or desire. The TVPA was reauthorized in 2003, 2005, 2008, and 2013 and is currently titled the *Trafficking Victims Protection Reauthorization Act of 2013* [6].

Prevalence

Minors under the age of 18 years are at considerably high risk for human trafficking and, in particular, sex trafficking. According to UNICEF's State of the World's Children 2006 report, approximately 2 million children worldwide are commercially sexually exploited [7]. In the United States alone, an estimated 100,000–300,000 children are at risk for commercial sexual exploitation each year. The average age at time of exploitation is 11–13 years for boys and transgender youth and 12–14 years for girls [8, 9]. To be clear, the prevalence of minor sex trafficking in the United States is difficult to accurately determine due to the clandestine nature of this criminal activity, the barriers to disclosure for victims of this crime, and the lack of a centralized and systems-integrated tracking database.

Risk Factors

Factors that heighten a minor's risk for commercial sexual exploitation (CSE) and sex trafficking can exert their influence at the individual, interpersonal (family), community, and societal levels of the social ecological model [10]. Unfortunately, the very factors that place minors at increased risk for commercial sexual exploitation and sex trafficking are also those elements that contribute to stigmatization in early life and give rise to a trajectory of progressively more profound social isolation, risk, polyvictimization, and poor health outcomes.

One of the most salient risk factors for commercial sexual exploitation and sex trafficking is child abuse and neglect. Childhood sexual abuse, in particular, has been cited as highly correlated to an increased risk for CSE or sex trafficking by the professionals who work closest with survivors of these sex crimes [11]. Research has found that survivors of CSE often report rape as their first sexual encounter, that minors with a history of childhood sexual abuse are significantly more likely than their non-abused counterparts to become involved in commercial sex, and that between 33 and 90 % of sex crime victims report this type of early childhood abuse [12–15]. Theories of mechanisms for this correlation are widely based on the disruptive effects of sexual abuse—a type of complex trauma—on children's ability to develop self-esteem, forge healthy relationships, and maintain appropriate boundaries [16]. Individuals involved in commercial sex are more likely to engage in sexual self-denigration, to report initiation of sexual activity by the age of 13, and to perceive sexual activity as a viable means for securing affection, intimacy, and material goods [13, 17, 18]. Unfortunately, such "sexually deviant" behaviors also give rise to the early stigmatization that, in turn, further damages their self-esteem.

Family dysfunction—including factors such as domestic violence, lack of parental involvement, parental prostitution, and parental substance use—has also been identified as an important risk factor [15]. Such harmful exposures in the home affect children's perception of normality, disrupt their sense of safety, and may result in the development of similar behaviors. Overall, these complex traumatic experiences contribute to poor health outcomes and heighten future risk for experiencing polyvictimization such as CSE and sex trafficking.

Family dysfunction may also provoke runaway and throwaway episodes and out-of-home residential placements in foster homes or group homes [4, 8]. Housing instability occurring when minors run away or are thrown out of their homes may entail "couch surfing" in the homes of friends or even virtual strangers, as well as homelessness and the need to survive on the streets. Lack of stable housing abruptly heightens minors' vulnerability to predators who would sexually assault, rape, and/or exploit them for economic gain. In fact, child advocacy groups estimate that as many as one in every three youth is lured by a sex trafficker within the first 48 h of running away or being thrown out of the home [19].

Similarly, minors who self-identify as lesbian, gay, bisexual, transgender, and queer or questioning (LGBTQ) may also experience housing destabilization and increased risk for CSE and sex trafficking after coming out as a result of being forced out of their homes or running away to escape ensuing abuse and violence [4, 8, 20]. Indeed, in a national survey of homeless youth providers, 48 % of providers felt that family rejection is one of the most important factors leading to LGBTQ youth homelessness [20]. Additionally, homeless LGBTQ adolescents are more likely to report sexual victimization on the streets than their homeless non-LGBTQ counterparts (58.7 % vs. 33.4 %), with LGBTQ youth reporting an average of seven more perpetrators [21, 22]. However, LGBTQ adolescents' risk for commercial sexual exploitation and sex trafficking may also be heightened in the process of seeking affection and acceptance outside their homes even if they never physically leave their homes of origin. In fact, research estimates that LGBTQ youth are up to five times more likely than heterosexual youth to be trafficked due to the increased vulnerability conferred by their feelings of difference, alienation, and rejection [23]. According to the Young Men's Project, LGBTQ youth do not receive enough information from their surroundings about their sexual feelings and thoughts. They often feel that they do not have an accepting environment to talk about their feelings, and therefore, they remain at an increased risk of sexual exploitation as they might engage in risky behavior while exploring their sexuality [24].

Other risk factors for commercial sexual exploitation and sex trafficking of minors include substance use, gang affiliation, and commonly cited social determinants of health such as poverty, lack of education, and exposure to violent crime, police corruption, and adult prostitution in their communities [4, 25]. Learning, cognitive, and physical disabilities, as well as language barriers and immigrant status, may also increase minors' risk for forced commercial sexual exploitation.

Unfortunately, complex traumatic experiences such as personal childhood trauma and exposure to family and community violence may also result in mental health disorders and give rise to "mal"-adaptive behaviors that heighten minors' social isolation, stigmatization, and risk for CSE and sex trafficking. Moreover, these personal, family, and community risk factors all collide with societal risk factors, such as high demand for commercial sex and media-driven sexualization of minors, to exponentially heighten the vulnerability of minors in the United States [26].

Recruitment and Control Mechanisms

Predators capitalize on the vulnerabilities of youth in order to recruit or lure them for CSE and sex trafficking. As previously described, these vulnerabilities are profound. The personal histories of minors at heightened risk of CSE and trafficking are riddled with neglect, trauma, stigma, and yearning for unfulfilled needs/desires, including safety, happiness, and affection. Such powerfully negative experiences facilitate the efforts of exploiters to recruit or lure a minor by means of pretense and deception. Perpetrators may lure a minor away from their current circumstances and into a life of commercial sex with pretenses of love and affection and false promises of safety and happiness [4, 9, 11, 27, 28].

After successfully luring a minor into commercial sexual exploitation, the exploiter will use any means possible to maintain control over the recruited minor. Physical, sexual, psychological, and emotional violence are inflicted with or without instigation. Physical assaults, forced substance use, sleep deprivation, rape, gang rape, verbal abuse, threats of harm to family or friends, isolation, restriction of movement, stalking, and economic control through confiscation of all monies are common tactics used by perpetrators to establish controlling power dynamics [4, 9, 11, 27, 28].

Having lost trust in the adults in their lives (and in some cases, entire systems of protection), minors with histories of trauma rely heavily on themselves to stay out of harm's way. As a result, minors who are successfully tricked by an exploiter may also lose trust in their own judgment and ability to keep themselves safe. This loss of self-trust, along with the threats and violence wielded by the perpetrators, effectively disarm minors of the confidence and courage they need to seek help, leaving them feeling powerless to change their circumstances. Failing to have recognized the danger they were facing and subsequently staying with their exploiter—typically due to a combination of fear, intimidation, violence, and other psychological means of control and subordination—can be a source of immense guilt and shame that further damages their self-esteem and potentiates the stigma they bear [28].

Importantly, health care providers should be aware that traumatic events during childhood and during recruitment into exploitation may impact a minor's experience of the health care setting. These powerful experiences result in minors becoming distrustful of others. The fact that the adults in their lives failed to protect them—or were themselves the perpetrators of abuse and violence—results in a distorted perception of adults in general, particularly those who may use their positions of authority to hurt or exploit them. They may view the power differential in their relationships with adults as threatening, and this in turn influences their interactions with health care providers and other adults who may try to gain their trust to help them. This concept will be explored further in the Sect. on 11.4.

The Pathology of Commercial Sexual Exploitation and Sex Trafficking

With profound physical and mental health effects, the commercial sexual exploitation of minors violates a child's right to freedom from all forms of violence—including physical, sexual, and mental abuse—and thus represents a significant public health problem worldwide. Trafficked minors are challenged by unfavorable social determinants of health, high-risk health behaviors, poor health outcomes, numerous barriers to health care, and retraumatization in the health care setting. Though not an exhaustive list, Table 11.1 contains common health problems encountered among victims and survivors of commercial sexual exploitation and sex trafficking.

Physical and Sexual Health Effects

Commercial sexual exploitation of children results in a wide range of poor short-term and long-term physical and sexual health outcomes [4, 11, 27–34]. Due to the nature of their exploitation, one of the most obvious health risks leading to poor health outcomes is the unrelenting exposure to unprotected sex with large numbers of clients willing to pay higher prices for unprotected sex. Rarely able to negotiate condom use, commercially sexually exploited minors are at high risk for recurrent sexually transmitted infections (STIs) that may progress to their long-term disease

Table 11.1 Health problems associated with the commercial sexual exploitation and sex trafficking of minors [4, 7, 11, 27–34, 37–41]

Physical health	Assault injuries
	Branding tattoos
	Poor dentition
	Communicable diseases
	Malnutrition
	Chronic pain syndromes (i.e., somatization)
	Substance use
	Physical addiction
	Harmful physical effects (e.g., cardiac arrhythmias, malignant hypertension, seizures, cardiopulmonary arrest)
Sexual health	Recurrent STIs
	Diseases resulting from untreated STIs
	Infertility
	Cervical/anal cancers
	Chronic liver disease
	HIV/AIDS
	Genitourinary/anorectal injuries
	Unwanted pregnancies
	Lack of prenatal care
	Unsafe abortions and complications
Mental health	Anxiety
	Panic attacks
	Depression
	Post-traumatic stress disorder
	Dissociation
	Sleep disturbances
	Lack of impulse control
	Pathologic self-soothing behaviors (e.g., self-injury)
	Substance use
	Psychological addiction
	Harmful mental effects (e.g., high-risk or bizarre behaviors, hallucinations, psychosis)
	Complex trauma effects
	Insecure attachments
	Dysregulation of emotions, including emotional numbing
	Poor self-concept and negative future orientation

states such as infertility, cervical cancer, chronic liver disease, hepatocellular cancer, and HIV/AIDS if left untreated.

In addition to sexually transmitted infections and diseases, the following health outcomes are also particularly alienating and stigmatizing for commercially sexually exploited minors: poor dentition, branding tattoos, eating disorders, physical signs of assault (broken teeth, cigarette burns, chemical burns), genitourinary and anorectal injuries and foreign bodies, unwanted pregnancies, high-risk pregnancies in the case of very young girls, complications of unsafe abortions, and substance use disorders [4, 9, 11, 27–34]. Many of these become chronic painful reminders of the physical and sexual violence endured.

Physical health effects may also result from chronic stress and psychological distress. When children are chronically exposed to stress, their body's stress response and immune systems may not develop normally. Indeed, studies have found a link between chronic stress and the occurrence of high blood pressure and atopic disorders such as asthma [35, 36]. A study of 192 women and girls entering post-trafficking services in Europe found that 63 % reported more than ten concurrent physical health symptoms with the most common being headaches (82 %), fatigue (81 %), dizziness (70 %), back pain (69 %), abdominal pain (61 %), and pelvic pain (59 %) [29]. These particular symptoms may result from repeated head injury, long work hours, lack of sleep, limited access to nutritious foods, dehydration, prolonged muscle contraction and strain, blunt abdominal trauma, and untreated pelvic infections. However, it is also possible that minors experiencing the traumatic effects of exploitation in the commercial sex industry will develop chronic physical symptoms without a true organic cause (psychosomatization). Furthermore, exploited minors may also engage in self-cutting behavior, develop eating disorders, and suffer the harmful physical effects of self-medicating with one or more substances.

Mental Health Effects

Alongside the physical and sexual health problems, mental health comorbidities are common among victims of commercial sexual exploitation and sex trafficking [4, 9, 11, 12, 23, 25, 27, 28, 30, 31, 37, 38]. Although not every victim will meet full criteria for the diagnosis of a mental health disorder, it is safe to assume that all of them will suffer from emotional reactions and symptoms related to their traumatic experiences. Studies have demonstrated that the violence and abuse endured while sex trafficked are associated with an increased risk of high levels of symptoms of anxiety, depression, and post-traumatic stress disorder (PTSD) [37]. In fact, one study found that survivors of human trafficking reported feeling depressed/very sad (95 %), nervous (91 %), fearful (85 %), hopeless about the future (76 %), and terror/panic (61 %) when asked about their mental health symptoms [30]. Other symptoms may include dissociation, sleep disturbances, difficulty regulating emotions, self-injurious behaviors, and substance use disorders. Substance-related disorders may be due to adaptive coping mechanisms or, in many instances, forced drug and/or alcohol use by the traffickers [9, 28, 39].

In the National Survey of Adolescents, teenagers who had experienced physical or sexual abuse/assault were three times more likely to report past or current substance use than those without a history of trauma [40]. Similarly, in surveys of adolescents receiving treatment for substance use disorders, more than 70 % of patients had a history of trauma exposure. Furthermore, studies indicate that up to 59 % of young people with PTSD subsequently develop substance use disorders [40, 41]. It is not surprising that victims of sex trafficking who did not previously use any substances may start using—or be forced to use—substances as a way of managing the intense emotional distress associated with their exploitation.

It should be noted that mental health problems are highly influenced by culture. Cultural beliefs may lead to discrimination against individuals seeking mental health services, thereby inciting stigma and affecting readiness for treatment. Culture, inclusive of religion, may not only impact one's perception of the source and severity of mental illness, and the need for treatment, but also the type of symptoms manifested. Moreover, symptoms may change across the lifespan or may be attenuated by varying degrees of coping skills and coping mechanisms such as self-medication. In addition, health care providers' general cultural knowledge and insights into specific populations may lead to stereotyping based on appearance and cultural background while ignoring the diversity within the population. In such situations wherein culture obscures the diagnosis and treatment of specific mental health disorders, it is important to consider the cumulative effects of chronically undiagnosed, misdiagnosed, or untreated mental illness as well.

Cumulative Effects: Complex Trauma and Stigma

Childhood trauma, traumatic events that cause physical, emotional, or psychological distress or harm, may have a profound effect on the cognitive, behavioral, and socio-emotional development of children. While some children recover from a traumatic event by integrating the experience into their lives, others may develop a variety of symptoms and impairments in response to the trauma. Multiple factors influence the outcome including characteristics of the child (age, stage of maturity, culture), characteristics of the trauma (type of trauma, what or who causes the trauma, duration of the trauma, single or recurrent events), and the reaction of those in the surrounding environment. As an example, a traumatic event that occurs during adolescence can influence personality and identity development and may lead to symptoms such as avoidance, isolation, flashbacks, sleep disturbances, anxiety, depression, substance use, risky behavior, impulsivity, and self-harming behavior. Furthermore, children exposed to trauma, particularly trauma of an interpersonal nature, are at greater risk of re-experiencing similar future traumatic events [42]. For example, children who are victims of sexual abuse are at increased risk for sexual re-victimization, and this recurrent exposure to similar interpersonal traumatic events across the developmental years can result in a psychological injury known as complex trauma.

Complex trauma refers to a type of trauma that is repetitive and cumulative and occurs during periods of heightened vulnerability, most often childhood, and within specific enduring social contexts [43]. Complex traumatic exposures include physical and sexual abuse, emotional abuse, neglect, and witnessing violence [44]. The types of impairments found in survivors of complex trauma can be somewhat different than those caused by a single traumatic event, and an understanding of these is crucial in the care of minor victims of commercial sexual exploitation.

Attachment and Relationship Impairments

Commercially sexually exploited minors may hold a distorted view of what constitutes a healthy relationship and may have difficulty maintaining healthy boundaries. As a result, they may perceive their relationship with their exploiter as "normal" and, under such circumstances, would be less likely to seek or accept help or participate in treatment [44]. On the other hand, particularly if they were previously sexually abused or if they were lured into sexual exploitation by someone they trusted, commercially sexually exploited minors may become fearful and distrusting of others, perceiving relationships as unpredictable and experiencing interpersonal closeness as a threat. They may develop a fragile and distorted sense of safety, causing a perception of danger or "false alarm" even when none exists. As a result, these minors have difficulty trusting and opening up to health care providers or other adults trying to help them.

Emotional and Behavioral Regulation Impairments

Children who have suffered complex trauma may experience difficulty with describing feelings and internal experiences, recognizing internal states, and communicating wishes and desires. Complex trauma survivors commonly react to a reminder of a traumatic event with trembling, anger, sadness, or avoidance and have difficulty calming down when upset. Reminders of traumatic events (i.e., trauma triggers) may include loud noises, specific scents, touch, and other stimuli. Unfortunately, they learn to "tune out" to their triggers and other threats in their environment (i.e., emotional numbing), making them vulnerable to re-victimization.

Minors who experience complex trauma may also struggle with impulse and behavioral control. They may exhibit aggression, poor impulse modulation, pathological self-soothing behaviors, oppositional behaviors, and difficulty understanding and complying with rules. They often behave in ways that appear unpredictable, oppositional, volatile, and extreme—all of which may exacerbate their social stigma. Their inability to regulate their emotions and impulses may lead to self-destructive and risky behaviors. Self-injurious behavior such as cutting is one method used by complex trauma survivors to regulate their emotions. However, numbing the emotional pain by self-inflicting acute physical pain may effectively increase their risk for escalating severity of physical injuries and suicidality [44].

Self-Concept and Self-Esteem Impairments

For minors in commercial sexual exploitation, their emotional dysregulation is potentiated by the experience of chronically having their feelings disregarded or invalidated by traffickers, solicitors, and adults who are quick to pass judgment. The resultant sense of worthlessness, in addition to any shame or guilt they harbor over their circumstances, can damage their self-concept, interfere with future orientation, and prevent them for seeking help. Thus, children who experience complex trauma are at significantly greater risk for re-victimization and hence, polyvictimization (i.e., repeated victimization in other contexts).

When working with this unique population, it is important to take the time to build rapport and develop an understanding of their core beliefs. Additionally, it will be important to understand the background and events leading to victimization without judgment or blame. Understanding the origins of their deep-rooted fear and distrust of others can assist health care providers to anticipate and accept their reactions with the patience and compassion necessary to avoid potentiating these negative feelings. Although isolated patient encounters without continuity of care may be a barrier to any single provider gaining their trust, a concerted effort across the health care sector could potentially help these minors to see health care providers as professionals they can trust.

Stigma: A Historical "Victim-Blaming" Frame of Reference

Historically, society has failed to recognize minors entangled in the commercial sex industry as victims and has instead labeled them *child* or *juvenile prostitutes*—morally culpable *sexual deviants*, deserving of their hardships and in need of discipline. Boys entangled in commercial sex—whether straight, gay, bisexual, or transgender—have been particularly vulnerable to such stigmatizing labels in part due to stereotypes that contend the male gender as strong, always in control, always capable of self-preservation, and always having a choice [23, 45].

This deprecating position is based on several ill-conceived assumptions about the abilities of minors, mainly, that minors possess the ability to (1) understand and consent to their own exploitation, (2) act of their own accord and negotiate their own terms during their exploitation, and (3) disengage at will from the exploiters who manipulate and control them. Such an ill-conceived frame of reference not only fails to recognize the victimization of minors but to some extent absolves exploiters of their role in this victimization, thereby further blaming and victimizing the minor for his or her predicament. In fact, child victims of sex trafficking live under the control of their traffickers, enduring threats, abuse, violence, and the denial of human rights.

The pervasive view of "troubled" or "deviant" minors who "willfully" engage in commercial sex is painfully stigmatizing as it has influenced societal attitudes and limited the response of social systems—such as the juvenile justice, child welfare, and health care systems—to one that may perpetuate stigma and may even be punitive. The TVPA of 2000 represents, in effect, one of the first US legislative attempts to debunk this victim-blaming frame of reference and shift societal mindset to one that recognizes the child as the victim of a heinous crime. Indeed, while this law requires that the use of force, fraud, or coercion as a means of inducing a person to perform a commercial sex act be established in cases involving adults, this requirement is obviated in cases involving minors under the age of 18 years [5]. This legal exception essentially affirms that any minor involved in a commercial sex act is a victim of a sexually exploitative crime regardless of whether force, fraud, or coercion was used to exploit them. It also represents a legal acknowledgment of what child psychologists already knew; mainly, that while children may seemingly "voluntarily" engage in such commercial sex acts, their psycho-cognitive development has not reached the level of maturity necessary to fully understand and consent to their own commercial sexual exploitation.

Yet unfortunately, despite the TVPA, there continues to be an absence of a shared language regarding commercial sexual exploitation and sex trafficking of minors across all jurisdictions. A minor exploited in the commercial sex industry may be identified as a "prostitute" and face criminal charges and juvenile detention in one jurisdiction, or he/she may be identified as a "victim" of commercial sexual exploitation and be referred for treatment and protective services. Though progress has been immense, comprehensive efforts to educate state legislators, law enforcement officers, legal representatives, and court officials are still needed.

Health Care Disparities

Hampered by a lack of awareness and, perhaps, the same ill-conceived stigmatizing assumptions that permeate societal attitudes toward minors ensnared in the commercial sex industry, the response of the health care system to the complex health care needs of this vulnerable population has similarly lagged. Victims' access to health care services may be limited by a multitude of factors including restrictions imposed by the trafficker, fear of punishment from the trafficker, fear of the involvement of legal or immigration authorities in the health care setting, shame over their exploitation, logistical barriers (e.g., transportation, health insurance, language), and avoidance due to prior traumatic experiences in the health care setting [11, 28].

Notwithstanding the numerous barriers to care, studies have found that up to 87.9 % (range 28–87.9 %) of trafficking survivors report receiving medical care from a health care professional during their exploitation on at least one occasion [46–48]. Yet despite being one of the professions that may routinely interact with trafficking victims, health care professionals have infrequently identified or intervened in cases of child trafficking. Indeed, sex trafficking of minors has been cited as the most underreported and undertreated form of child abuse [49].

According to the Institute of Medicine and National Research Council's report *Confronting Commercial Sexual Exploitation and Sex Trafficking of Minors in the United States*:

> These crimes may be overlooked, as they often occur at the margins of society and behind closed doors; victims may not come forward, and those who routinely interact with victims and survivors may lack awareness or tools to properly identify and assist victims. [4]

The current low level of awareness about child trafficking among health care providers, the lack of provider training on identification and culturally sensitive trauma-informed care of victims, and the paucity of resources available for referral to long-term mental health and social services continue to interfere with the health care sector's ability to more effectively respond to and meet the full spectrum of health needs of commercially sexually exploited minors [11]. In essence, the inability of health care providers to either engage in victim identification through the recognition of red flags or forge trusting patient-provider relationships wherein a minor may feel comfortable disclosing their predicament without fear of being judged severely limits the role of health care. Overcoming these barriers is an essential preliminary step to improving the health sector's role in prevention and intervention. Preventing the victimization of at-risk youth, identifying victimized minors, and responding appropriately to an identification require the formal education and training of health care providers and should be carried out in the safest manner possible so as to minimize harm to the minor and the provider.

Retraumatization in Health Care

It should be noted that the provision of health care itself can be inadvertently retraumatizing to commercially sexually exploited youth. For example, the tightening of the blood pressure cuff around the arm or the insertion of the stethoscope down the shirt without warning may trigger memories or flashbacks of an abusive or violent event and may provoke an intense visceral reaction setting into motion the "fight-or-flight" response and leading to angry outbursts, dramatic emotional displays, complete disengagement, or dissociation. In addition, due to the stigma, complex trauma, and polyvictimization experienced at the hands of adults, minors who have been commercially sexually exploited may have difficulty trusting authority figures and may display their distrust and contempt for authority in the health care setting. In turn, clinical providers and auxiliary support staff may not always possess the skill or the time to respond to the adolescent's seemingly irrational behavior in a constructive manner and may unfortunately revert to emotionally driven reactions and disparaging labels such as "difficult," "disturbed," "non-compliant," "painful," or other pejoratives.

To compound the stigma they encounter in other aspects of society, some sex-trafficked minors also report experiencing judgmental and punitive attitudes from health care providers [11]. The experience of being negatively judged and mistreated may indeed be due to health care providers' premature assessments of a minor's moral character but may also be exacerbated by the minor's own shame, guilt, and lack of self-worth.

One way to encourage a positive and constructive response to victims of polyvictimization, regardless of profession, is to always see them through a lens that attempts to understand how their past and current experiences have influenced their attitudes and behaviors. Constant mental reminders of the horrific trauma they have endured, including at the hands of adults on whom they relied for love and protection, will help inspire compassion, patience, and respect even in the face of a "defiant" or "disrespectful" minor.

Culturally Sensitive Trauma-Informed Care and Provider Education

Lack of access to treatment and follow-up care may prevent victims from seeking support. However, when they do present to the health care setting, victim identification and delivery of care can be difficult due to the complex nature of the exploitation. Excessive exposure to traumatic events may heighten vulnerabilities in children who may subsequently experience a range of reactive processes alongside the PTSD symptoms. As a result, these children may carry several diagnoses and end up in multiple child-serving systems, including the education, juvenile justice, child welfare, and health care systems. In addition, professionals in each system may use different frameworks to assess and treat this population and may have varying degrees of understanding of their symptoms. In order to avoid retraumatization by well-meaning providers, it is important to adopt a common comprehensive framework that will improve the communication between the different providers and take into consideration the vulnerabilities of complex trauma survivors.

An approach that takes into account the impact of adverse childhood experiences while considering cultural differences in customs and beliefs is crucial in creating a validating, safe environment and increasing the effectiveness of care delivery to victims and survivors of trauma. The trauma-informed approach to service delivery recognizes the pervasiveness of trauma and emphasizes the physical, emotional, and psychological safety of survivors. Trauma-informed care is a strength-based approach to care delivery that focuses on empowerment, while minimizing stigma and fostering healing and recovery [50]. As an example, when addressing the minor, the term survivor—more so than victim—may have therapeutic value and help strengthen resiliency.

For many trafficked minors, shame is one of the most salient barriers to seeking services. Provider education and training concerning trust building, culturally sensitive services, and co-occurring behavioral, mental, and health problems may positively affect the quality of care [51]. In order to provide culturally sensitive care, providers should make an effort to learn and understand the victim's culture, beliefs, practices, assumptions, and level of acculturation. When working with victims of

CSE and sex trafficking, it is important to create a safe environment, where they would not feel judged or blamed.

Multidisciplinary Response

Responding to the needs of commercially sexually exploited youth, particularly those with limited support systems prior to being exploited, requires a multidisciplinary approach to care. Providers should assess immediate needs and provide referrals to appropriate services. In the health care setting, a multidisciplinary response may entail not only physical and mental health treatment but also consultation of other pertinent professionals such as addiction specialists, child abuse specialists, forensic examiners, social workers, and other pertinent disciplines. In addition, since most trafficked minors have been isolated from their families and friends, a multidisciplinary approach may entail referral to family therapy if and when the situation and timing are appropriate. It is important to ensure that comprehensive wraparound services are put into place in order to create a safety net of providers working simultaneously and collaboratively to minimize a minor's risk of re-victimization. Lastly, case management to assist in the coordination of care between different providers and across systems is crucial to the success of treatment.

Currently, one of the scarcest resources is age-appropriate safe housing for exploited and trafficked minors. Providers should work with the Department of Children and Families and local anti-trafficking organizations to determine the best options for emergency shelter, short-term housing, and long-term housing through which minors can begin to heal and reconstruct their lives. A practical and accessible resource for providers is the National Human Trafficking Resource Center (NHTRC). By calling the NHTRC 24-h hotline (1-888-373-7888), providers can obtain information about service providers and other resources available in their local area.

Since CSE and sex trafficking are a form of child abuse, child welfare agencies responsible for investigating reports of suspected child maltreatment should be equipped to receive reports of commercially sexually exploited minors, to coordinate an effective response, and to protect these minors. Furthermore, having a separate category (distinct from other forms of child maltreatment) may facilitate the collection of data needed to support the implementation of service programs specific for this population. A successful model of such a program is the Massachusetts Suffolk County Department of Children and Families (DCF) and its close collaboration with the District Attorney (DA) and the Support to End Exploitation Now (SEEN) Coalition. When a report of child maltreatment is identified as involving a commercially sexually exploited or sex-trafficked minor, DCF notifies local law enforcement and makes a discretionary referral to the DA office and the SEEN case coordinator. The SEEN Coalition promptly strategizes with cross-sector partners to mobilize multidisciplinary teams and resources to provide wraparound services for the child in question [52]. Replication of Suffolk County's child welfare response model would require proper training of child welfare agency staff, mechanisms for cross-sector communication, partnerships with local service providers, improved awareness among mandated reporters, and guidelines for recognizing and responding to the needs of at-risk and exploited minors.

Conclusion

Although there has been increased general awareness and understanding of the problem of commercial sexual exploitation and sex trafficking of minors in the United States, there are still critical gaps in prevention, identification, treatment, and response that merit attention. The increasing use of terms such as *commercially sexually exploited* and *sex-trafficked minors* to replace terms such as *child* or *juvenile prostitutes* and *sexual deviants* suggests a slow, yet critical paradigm shift to one that recognizes the abusive and manipulative nature of this crime. Importantly, this terminology is essential in advancing our understanding of these complex criminal practices as acts of abuse and violence committed *against* minors, rather than crimes committed by minors deserving of juvenile detention and correction. With this perspective, the development and implementation of evidence-based age-appropriate primary prevention strategies are more likely to be pursued and funded at the state and local levels.

One major challenge that society faces in the fight against commercial sexual exploitation and sex trafficking of minors is the limited ability to identify victimized youth. Indeed, in the health care sector, the commercial sexual exploitation and sex trafficking of minors are infrequently identified and often underreported. In fact, as previously mentioned, sex trafficking of minors has been cited as the most underreported and undertreated form of child abuse [49]. Reasons for this may include *victim-related barriers* to disclosure (e.g., insecure attachment, fear of retribution, fear of deportation, fear of being placed back into an abusive home, distrust of authority, feelings of shame and complicity), lack of awareness among providers who routinely interact with this population, and *provider-related barriers* to reporting (e.g., fear of causing more harm than good, fear of actuating deportation, fear of betraying the minor's trust, poor understanding of mandatory reporting guidelines). While there is a paucity of educational opportunities on this topic that are specifically designed for health care providers, formal curricula and training for students, residents in training, and practicing physicians may improve the health sector's ability to identify and treat victims [28, 53–55].

There is an abundance of evidence to support a trauma-informed approach in the treatment of complex trauma and polyvictimization. The trauma-informed framework offers guidance for providing services to trauma survivors in an empowering manner that will promote healing and minimize inadvertent retraumatization. In the health care setting, trauma-informed care is based on an understanding that trauma is ubiquitous and may impact an individual's behaviors, feelings, thoughts, personality, and interactions with health care providers. It is important to recognize that even individuals who stand resilient in the face of adversity may suffer the emotional, physiological, and developmental sequelae of traumatic events. This may depend on the victim age, gender, support system, beliefs, and cultural background. Understanding the additional influence of culture and the vulnerabilities related to the trauma (such as trauma reminders) may reduce retraumatization in the health care setting and increase genuine participation in treatment.

Finally, health care providers should understand that no one provider alone can respond to the broad range of needs of commercially sexually exploited or sex-trafficked minors. Whenever resources allow, a multidisciplinary team approach to assisting exploited and trafficked minors will lead to a more comprehensive and effective health sector response. Ensuring that the immediate and long-term needs of these patients are met is an important first step to recovering these minors and minimizing their risk for re-exploitation. Warm referrals to services within and outside of the health care system are frequently indicated. By securing wraparound services, health care providers can play a prominent role in fostering healing and recovery.

Future work in this field could focus on the development of a national centralized systems-integrated database to facilitate collecting and tracking data on victims of trafficking across systems and across states. Such a database may also enhance real-time cross-sector communication of vital information to and from first responders identifying and assisting victims of trafficking. Furthermore, efforts to increase public awareness of the problem provide specialized education and training for health care providers who routinely interact with minors and elucidate more effective prevention strategies, screening tools, and treatment protocols that may help reduce vulnerability and stigma and support victims as they grow and progress from surviving to thriving.

Commercially sexually exploited and trafficked minors are all around us. They are the hidden and forgotten children of our generation and the many generations before us. The commercial sexual exploitation and trafficking of minors is a violation of children's rights—their right to live a life free from neglect, exploitation, and abuse. While lawmakers have now passed trafficking legislation in all 50 states, there is still much work to be done in its prevention and eradication. Despite progress in raising awareness and understanding commercial sexual exploitation and trafficking as abhorrent crimes committed against minors, we continue to fall short in moving the public mindset and attitude to reflect that same understanding. The stigma attached to commercially sexually exploited and trafficked individuals, particularly once they age out of adolescence into adulthood, is a heavy psychological and emotional burden for these once innocent ordinary children. Any significant reduction in the vulnerability of minors or the stigma they bear once victimized will require a more nuanced understanding and acceptance of the ways in which society repeatedly fails to protect and assist these minors early in life. Health care providers have the unique opportunity to lead and role model a different attitude and approach to these children—one of compassion, understanding, validation, and empowerment.

Disclosures The authors have no conflicts of interest to disclose.

References

1. International Labor Organization (ILO). ILO global estimate of forced labour: results and methodology. Geneva: ILO; 2012. http://www.ilo.org/wcmsp5/groups/public/@ed_norm/@declaration/documents/publication/wcms_182004.pdf.
2. ECPAT. International. Commercial sexual exploitation of children. http://resources.ecpat.net/EI/Csec_definition.asp.
3. Office of Juvenile Justice and Delinquency Prevention (OJJDP). Commercial sexual exploitation of children/sex trafficking. http://www.ojjdp.gov/mpg/litreviews/CSECSexTrafficking.pdf.
4. Institute of Medicine (IOM) and National Research Council (NRC). Confronting commercial sexual exploitation and sex trafficking of minors in the united states. Washington, DC: IOM-NRC; 2013.
5. Victims of Trafficking and Violence Protection Act of 2000, Public Law 106–386. Washington, DC: 106th United States Congress; 2000. http://www.state.gov/documents/organization/10492.pdf.
6. United States Department of State. U.S. laws on trafficking in persons. http://www.state.gov/j/tip/laws/.
7. International Programme on the Elimination of Child Labour (IPEC)/International Labour Organization (ILO). Commercial sexual exploitation of children and adolescents: the ILO's response. Geneva: IPEC/ILO; 2008. http://www.ilo.org/ipecinfo/product/download.do?type=document&id=9150.
8. Estes RJ, Weiner NA. The commercial sexual exploitation of children in the U.S., Canada, and Mexico. Philadelphia: University of Pennsylvania, School of Social Work, Center for the Study of Youth Policy; 2002.
9. Smith L, Vardaman S, Snow M. The national report on domestic minor sex trafficking. Arlington: Shared Hope International; 2009. http://sharedhope.org/wp-content/uploads/2012/09/SHI_National_Report_on_DMST_2009.pdf.
10. Centers for Disease Control and Prevention. The social-ecological model: a framework for prevention. http://www.cdc.gov/ViolencePrevention/overview/social-ecologicalmodel.html.
11. Macias Konstantopoulos W, Ahn R, Alpert EJ, McGahan A, William TP, Castor JP, et al. An international comparative public health analysis of sex trafficking of women and girls in eight cities: achieving a more effective health sector response. J Urban Health. 2013;90(6):1194–204.
12. Hom KA, Woods SJ. Trauma and its aftermath for commercially sexually exploited women as told by front-line service providers. Issues Ment Health Nurs. 2013;34:75–81.
13. Wilson H, Widom C. The role of youth problem behaviors in the path from child abuse and neglect to prostitution: a prospective examination. J Res Adolesc. 2010;20(1):210–36.
14. Widom C, Kuhns J. Childhood victimization and subsequent risk for promiscuity, prostitution and teenage pregnancy: a prospective study. Am J Public Health. 1996;86(11):1607–12.
15. Williamson C, Prior M. Domestic minor sex trafficking: a network of underground players in the Midwest. J Child Adol Trauma. 2009;2:1–16.
16. Kruger A, Harper E, Harris P, Sanders D, Levin K, Meyers J. Sexualized and dangerous relationships: listening to the voices of low-income African American girls placed at risk for sexual exploitation. West J Emerg Med. 2013;14(4):370–6.
17. Van Brunschot EG, Brannigan A. Childhood maltreatment and subsequent conduct disorders: the case of female street prostitution. Int J Law Psychiatry. 2002;25:219–34.
18. Reid JA. An exploratory model of girl's vulnerability to commercial sexual exploitation in prostitution. Child Maltreat. 2011;16(2):146–57.

19. Congressional Testimony of Ernie Allen, President and CEO of National Center for Missing & Exploited Children for the Subcommittee on Crime, Terrorism and Homeland Security, Committee on the Judiciary. "Domestic minor sex trafficking." Washington, DC: United States House of Representatives; 2010. http://judiciary.house.gov/_files/hearings/pdf/allen100915.pdf.

20. Durso LE, Gates GJ. Serving our youth: findings from a national survey of service providers working with lesbian, gay, bisexual, and transgender youth who are homeless or at risk of becoming homeless. Los Angeles: The Williams Institute with True Colors Fund and The Palette Fund; 2012.

21. Cochran BN, Stewart AJ, Ginzler JA, Cauce AM. Challenges faced by homeless sexual minorities: comparison of gay, lesbian, bisexual, and transgender homeless adolescents with their heterosexual counterparts. Am J Public Health. 2002;92(5):773–7.

22. Whitbeck L, Xiaojin C, Tyler K, Johnson K. Mental disorder, subsistence strategies, and victimization among gay, lesbian, and bisexual homeless and runaway adolescents. J Sex Res. 2004;41(4):329–42.

23. United States Department of Health and Human Services Administration for Children, Youth and Families (ACYF). Guidance to states and services on addressing human trafficking of children and youth in the United States. Washington, DC: ACF; 2013. https://www.acf.hhs.gov/sites/default/files/cb/acyf_human_trafficking_guidance.pdf.

24. Lillywhite R, Skidmore P. Boys are not sexually exploited? A challenge to practitioners. Child Abuse Rev. 2006;15(5):351–61. doi:10.1002/car.952.

25. Ijadi-Maghsoodi R, Todd EJ, Bath EPJ. Commercial sexual exploitation of children and the role of the child psychiatrist. J Am Acad Child Adolesc Psych. 2014;53(8):825–9.

26. American Psychological Association (APA). Report of the APA task force on the sexualization of Girls. Washington, DC: APA; 2010. http://www.apa.org/pi/women/programs/girls/report-full.pdf.

27. Greenbaum VJ. Commercial sexual exploitation and sex trafficking of children in the United States. Curr Probl Pediatr Adolesc Health Care. 2014;44:245–69.

28. Alpert EJ, Ahn R, Albright E, Purcell G, Burke TF, Macias-Konstantopoulos WL. Human trafficking: guidebook on identification, assessment, and response in the health care setting. Boston: MGH Human Trafficking Initiative, Division of Global Health and Human Rights, Department of Emergency Medicine, Massachusetts General Hospital, and Committee on Violence Intervention and Prevention, Massachusetts Medical Society; 2014. http://www.massmed.org/humantrafficking.

29. Zimmerman C, Hossain M, Yun K, Gajdadziev V, Guzun N, Tchomarova M, et al. The health of trafficked women: a survey of women entering posttrafficking services in Europe. Am J Public Health. 2008;98(1):55–9.

30. Zimmerman C. Stolen smiles: a summary report on the physical and psychological consequences of women and adolescents trafficked in Europe. London: London School of Hygiene and Tropical Medicine; 2006.

31. Oram S, Stöckl H, Busza J, Howard LM, Zimmerman C. Prevalence and risk of violence and the physical, mental, and sexual health problems associated with human trafficking: systematic review. PLoS Med. 2012;9(5):e1001224. doi:10.1371/journal.pmed.1001224.

32. Clawson HJ, Goldblatt-Grace L. Finding a path to recovery: residential facilities for minor victims of domestic sex trafficking. Washington, DC: Office of the Assistant Secretary for Planning and Evaluation, U.S. Department of Health and Human Services; 2007.

33. Williamson E, Dutch N, Clawson H. Medical treatment of victims of sexual assault and domestic violence and its applicability to victims of human trafficking. Washington, DC: Office of the Assistant Secretary for Planning and Evaluation, U.S. Department of Health and Human Services; 2010.

34. Drocton P, Sach C, Chu L, Wheeler M. Validation set correlates of anogenital injury after sexual assault. Acad Emerg Med. 2008;15(3):231–8.

35. Suglia SF, Enlow MB, Kullowatz A, Wright RJ. Maternal intimate partner violence and increased asthma incidence in children: buffering effects of supportive caregivers. Arch Pediatr Adolesc Med. 2009;163(3):244–50.

36. Breiding MJ, Ziembroski JS. The relationship between intimate partner violence and children's asthma in 10 US states/territories. Pediatr Allergy Immunol. 2011;22:e95–100.
37. Hossain M, Zimmerman C, Abas M, Light M, Watts C. The relationship of trauma to mental disorders among trafficked and sexually exploited girls and women. Am J Public Health. 2010;100(12):2442–9.
38. Choi H, Klein C, Shin MS, Lee HJ. Posttraumatic stress disorder (PTSD) and disorders of extreme stress (DESNOS) symptoms following prostitution and child abuse. Vio Against Women. 2009;15(8):933–51.
39. Yates GL, Mackenzie RG, Pennbridge J, Swofford A. A risk profile comparison of homeless youth involved in prostitution and homeless youth not involved. J Adolesc Health. 1991;12(7):545–8.
40. Kilpatrick DG, Saunders BE, Smith DW. Youth victimization: prevalence and implications. Washington, DC: U.S. Department of Justice, Office of Justice Programs; 2003.
41. Deykin EY, Buka SL. Prevalence and risk factors for posttraumatic stress disorder among chemically dependent adolescents. Am J Psychiatry. 1997;154(6):752–7.
42. Finkelor D, Turner H, Hamby S, Ormrod R. Polyvictimization: children's exposure to multiple types of violence, crime, and abuse. Juvenile justice bulletin, national survey of children's exposure to violence. Washington, DC: Office of Juvenile Justice and Delinquency Prevention; 2011.
43. Courtois CA, Ford JD, editors. Treating complex traumatic stress disorders: an evidence-based guide. New York: The Guilford Press; 2009.
44. Cook A, Spinazzola J, Ford J, Lanktree C, Blaustein M, Cloitre M, et al. Complex trauma in children and adolescents. Psychiat Ann. 2005;35(5):390–8.
45. Dennis J. Women are victims, men make choices: the invisibility of men and boys in the global sex trade. Gend Issues. 2008;25(1):11–25.
46. Family Violence Prevention Fund. Turning pain into power: trafficking survivors' perspectives on early intervention strategies. San Francisco: Futures Without Violence; 2005.
47. Baldwin SB, Eisenman DP, Sayles JN, Ryan G, Chuang KS. Identification of human trafficking victims in the health care settings. Health Hum Rights. 2011;13(1):1–12.
48. Lederer LJ, Wetzel CA. The health consequences of sex trafficking and their implications for identifying victims in healthcare facilities. Ann Health Law. 2014;23(1):61–91.
49. Estes RJ, Weiner NA. The commercial sexual exploitation of children in the United States. In: Cooper SW, Estes RJ, Giardino AP, Kellogg ND, Vieth VI, editors. Medical, legal and social science aspects of child sexual exploitation: a comprehensive review of pornography, prostitution and internet crimes. St. Louis: GW Medical; 2005.
50. Elliott DE, Bjelajac P, Fallot RD, Markoff LS, Reed BG. Trauma-informed or trauma-denied: principles and implementation of trauma-informed services for women. J Commun Psych. 2005;33(4):461–77.
51. Tucker CM, Marsiske M, Rice KG, Jones JD, Herman KC. Patient-centered culturally sensitive health care: model testing and refinement. Health Psychol. 2011;30(3):342–50.
52. Piening S, Cross T. From "The Life" to my life: sexually exploited children reclaiming their futures. Suffolk county Massachusetts' response to Commercial Sexual Exploitation of Children (CSEC). Boston: Children's Advocacy Center of Suffolk County; 2012.
53. Ahn R, Alpert EJ, Purcell G, Konstantopoulos WM, McGahan A, Cafferty E, Eckardt M, Conn KL, Cappetta K, Burke TF. Human trafficking: review of educational resources for health professionals. Am J Prev Med. 2013;44(4):283–9.
54. Chisolm-Straker M, Richardson LD, Cossio T. Combating slavery in the 21st century: the role of emergency medicine. J Health Care Poor Underserved. 2012;23(3):980–7.
55. Grace A, Ahn R, Macias KW. Integrating curricula on human trafficking into medical education and residency training. JAMA Pediatr. 2014;168(9):793–4.

Chapter 12
Stigma and Health Services Use Among Veterans and Military Personnel

Lauren K. Richards, Elizabeth M. Goetter, Magdalena Wojtowicz, and Naomi M. Simon

Veterans represent one of the country's most underserved populations. Among the nation's 22 million veterans, and over two million current active duty service members who return from deployments with varying physical and mental health concerns, access to needed healthcare services is a pressing matter [1]. In the realm of physical healthcare needs, common concerns requiring timely access to healthcare treatment include physical injuries, chronic pain, and traumatic brain injury [2, 3]. In addition, the unmet mental healthcare needs of veterans remain a persistent and serious issue, as despite high rates of psychological difficulties [4], veterans have disproportionately low rates of mental health service utilization [4, 5]. The mismatch between healthcare need and use among veterans increases the long-term costs associated with illness chronicity. Therefore, a top priority in recent years has been to identify and eliminate barriers to healthcare among veterans and military personnel, who experience exposures that place them at increased risk for the development of injuries, PTSD, depression, anxiety, and substance use disorders among other concerns [2, 4, 6, 7].

As mental health clinicians, our particular expertise allows for an in-depth discussion of how stigma impacts access to and experience of mental healthcare among veterans. It is from this perspective that we expand this discussion to explore stigma as it relates to general healthcare access for common health concerns among veterans. Stigma is a major contributing factor to service underutilization among veterans [8–10]. Given the debilitating consequences of unmet healthcare needs, an examination and synthesis of the extant research regarding the impact of stigma on

L.K. Richards, PhD (✉) • E.M. Goetter, PhD
M. Wojtowicz, PhD • N.M. Simon, MD, MSc
Department of Psychiatry, Harvard Medical School,
Red Sox Foundation and Massachusetts General Hospital
Home Base Program, Boston, MA, USA
e-mail: lrichards3@mgh.harvard.edu

© Springer International Publishing Switzerland 2016
R. Parekh, Ed W. Childs (eds.), *Stigma and Prejudice: Touchstones in Understanding Diversity in Healthcare*, Current Clinical Psychiatry,
DOI 10.1007/978-3-319-27580-2_12

service use is crucial in order to inform the development of novel interventions. This chapter reviews the various barriers to healthcare utilization faced by today's veterans, and given our area of expertise, we expand upon stigma as a primary barrier to mental health service use. We explore the different sources and types of stigma that are unique to veterans and military personnel and the impact of stigmatization on healthcare utilization. Finally, a review of the current state of healthcare for veterans as well as the effectiveness of existing anti-stigma interventions informs our recommendations for future directions. The development and implementation of innovative approaches to eliminating stigma-based treatment barriers is vital to improving treatment engagement and health outcomes, thus alleviating the disproportionate burden of physical and mental illness among veterans.

Barriers to Healthcare Service Use Among Veterans

The majority of studies investigating barriers to healthcare utilization among veterans and service members have identified barriers within three categories of healthcare use determinants: need variables (medical and psychiatric symptoms), enabling variables (environmental access-related factors), and predisposing variables (sociodemographic and personal characteristics) [11]. Across studies, the presence and severity of medical and psychiatric symptoms have been consistently associated with increased healthcare use among veterans [12–14]. In a large-scale, nationally representative sample of US veterans, Elhai and colleagues [13] examined the extent to which medical and mental health symptoms predicted medical and mental healthcare service utilization and found that both physical and mental health impairments were the strongest predictors of both VA and non-VA outpatient medical and mental healthcare utilization. However, several studies have identified healthcare environmental characteristics such as long waiting times, difficulty navigating the healthcare system, extensive paperwork, difficulty communicating with providers, and difficulty scheduling appointments as major impediments to utilization among veterans [13, 15–17]. Additional oft-cited barriers include affordability, transportation, childcare responsibilities, geographical constraints, and interference with employment [15, 16]. Further, evidence suggests that perceived barriers are common even in patients who have already engaged in care [16, 18] and that vulnerable veteran populations, including those with mental health problems, physical disabilities, and racial/ethnic minority status, perceive higher levels of healthcare barriers [16].

Predisposing variables including sociodemographic characteristics such as male gender, older age, combat exposure, lack of private insurance, and service-connected disability status have been associated with increased healthcare use in VA settings [13, 15–17]. Female gender, unemployment, and higher level of education have been linked to non-VA medical healthcare utilization [13]. In addition to sociodemographic variables, personal beliefs and attitudes regarding illness and healthcare demonstrate strong associations with utilization [18]. For example, in a national sample of women veterans, 19 % of participants reported delaying or failing to initiate needed medical healthcare at a VA hospital, and this delayed or uninitiated care was associated with less positive perceptions about care and less knowledge regarding the availability of services there [15]. Another study demonstrated that stigma-related barriers, such as having concerns about the social consequences of seeking treatment, were more powerful barriers than institutional factors in the VA system [5].

The stigma faced by veterans in the healthcare system impacts both medical and mental healthcare experiences. Veterans return from deployments with significant physical and mental health needs, requiring care at several levels of the system. In the following sections, we discuss how healthcare-related stigma may impact treatment seeking and quality of care among veterans. We begin with a discussion of the impact of stigma as it pertains to common medical problems experienced among veterans and then emphasize the particular relevance of stigma in the arena of mental health service use. Stigmatizing beliefs regarding mental illness and treatment have been established as powerful deterrents to seeking mental health treatment in the civilian population [19], and stigma may be an even more powerful barrier among veterans [18, 20].

Healthcare-Related Stigma Among Veterans

Physical Health Concerns

Physical injuries, chronic pain, and traumatic brain injuries are common among veterans returning from theater. The traumatic loss of limbs due to combat exposure is one of the most severe injuries experienced by veterans of all eras [21]. Traumatic loss of limbs has a profound effect on quality of life, presenting physical and emotional challenges [21], which appear to be largely centered around adjusting to limb amputation. Poorer adjustment is associated with psychological symptoms such as depression and anxiety, poorer self-reported physical health, and social stigma (see Horgan et al. for a review) [22]. Chronic pain is also a common complaint among veterans [23], and particularly among OEF/OIF veterans, as this cohort experiences multiple deployments that include intense combat and increased risk for physical injury [2]. Data suggest that the majority of veterans returning from the conflicts in Iraq and Afghanistan experience chronic pain [24]. Therefore, treatment of chronic pain has been identified as a priority area, and recommendations for optimal pain management emphasize a multidisciplinary and integrated approach. Stigma among those with chronic pain encompasses both patient and clinician beliefs about the condition and its treatment. For example, in the civilian literature, internalized stigma experience among sufferers of chronic pain includes feelings of alienation, experiences of discrimination, and the perception that others question the legitimacy of their sometimes invisible illness [25]. There has been little research conducted to illuminate the impact of stigma among chronic pain sufferers in the veteran population, but extant findings suggest that both internalized stigma and clinician attitudes toward chronic pain may shape the illness experience. A recent qualitative study of chronic pain among OEF/OIF veterans revealed several common stigmatizing beliefs among veterans related to their pain including the belief that others will not understand their pain, the belief that their pain is a weakness, and a belief that it would not be perceived as legitimate given its invisibility [26]. These stigmatizing beliefs discouraged them from discussing their pain with others, thus limiting opportunities for often needed social support [26]. The public's knowledge of outcomes and sequelae following TBI has been found to be limited and misinformed. This includes inaccurate ideas about the duration and extent of recovery and the specific difficulties associated with TBI [27–31]. Similar misperceptions have been endorsed by nonexpert health professionals (i.e., health providers who do not have specialist knowledge about TBI) [28]. There is also evidence suggesting that community-dwelling individuals and university students hold some negative attitudes toward civilians with TBI, including viewing these individuals as having less desirable personal characteristics, such as being less friendly, mature, responsible, and intelligent[32, 33]. Negative perceptions of individuals with TBI may have a significant impact on outcomes following injury by increasing stress, reducing social support, and affecting employment opportunities [34, 35]. In fact, these variables, along with injury severity, have been found to affect successful return to employment, quality of life, and social reintegration following TBI [35, 36].

Mental Health

Several studies have demonstrated that mental health stigma is prevalent among military personnel [4, 10, 37]. Broadly, mental health-related stigma encompasses a range of perceptions related to (1) the extent to which one will be evaluated or devalued by others, including the general public (formally defined in the literature as anticipated, enacted, or public stigma), and family members and friends (formally defined as personal stigma) for experiencing a mental health problem and/or seeking treatment, and (2) internalized negative beliefs about mental illness and treatment (formally defined as self-stigma or endorsed stigma) [10, 20, 38, 39].

There are several theorized reasons that stigma may be a particularly concerning issue among veterans that are substantiated with accumulating empirical support. First, several researchers posit that the worth placed on competence, emotional toughness, and stoicism and the devaluation of weakness in military culture contribute to increased stigmatizing beliefs about mental illness and treatment among veterans [40, 41]. Indeed, in our experience, beliefs related to self-reliance are commonly reported among both Vietnam era and Operation Enduring Freedom (OEF) and Operation Iraqi Freedom (OIF) veterans, including concerns about being perceived as weak by others for having a mental illness, the perception that therapy is a sign of weakness, and the belief that one should handle one's own mental health problem [18, 42–44]. A recent qualitative study of treatment-seeking OEF/OIF combat veterans illustrated a distinct belief regarding personal responsibility in this group. Participants reported the perception that the public blames them for their problems because they volunteered for service and "knowingly put themselves at risk" [42]. Additional stigmatizing concerns include feelings of embarrassment, fear of being labeled with a mental illness, and being perceived as "dangerous" and "crazy" [42–44].

Second, while sources of personal stigma in civilian populations are typically circumscribed to family members and friends, for veterans this network extends to fellow service members and leaders, suggesting that veterans and service members may contend with concern about stigmatizing attitudes and behaviors from multiple sources [39]. Concern that having a mental illness or seeking mental health treatment would weaken peer confidence among unit members is a commonly cited belief among service members [4, 42], as is the fear that leadership would treat one differently or even blame one for one's psychological problem [4]. One study demonstrated that veterans with mental health concerns perceived angry reactions or distancing not only by relatives and friends but by fellow service members as well [45]. Another study of OEF/OIF veterans found that veterans' negative beliefs about unit support were significant predictors of mental health stigma [43]. Two recent studies have explicitly investigated the role of unit organization and leadership on mental health stigma among veterans. Britt and colleagues [45] found that soldiers' perceptions of their direct supervisors' negative leadership behaviors predicted their own stigmatizing beliefs about mental illness, whereas Kelley and colleagues [46] found that feeling supported by unit members was associated with reduced mental health-related stigma. Supporting these findings, Blais and Renshaw [47] found that combat veterans reported more concerns about stigma from military personnel than family members or friends, suggesting that stigma from military sources may be a more powerful deterrent to treatment seeking than stigma from other sources.

Third, while beliefs related to the negative career consequences of having a mental health problem and seeking mental health treatment are also experienced by civilians, there are additional concerns – primarily related to privacy – that may be unique to military personnel, particularly among active duty service members. Concerns regarding negative perceptions and evaluations by coworkers and superiors have been consistently reported in the veteran literature and are similar to concerns reported by civilians [20, 42, 44, 45]. For example, a recent study reported that one third of OEF/OIF veterans endorsed concerns about stigma in the workplace, citing beliefs that coworkers would think they are not capable of doing their jobs and that career options would be narrowed [20]. However, while civilian mental health records are typically inaccessible to colleagues or supervisors, among those who are still active duty service members, health records may be viewed by commanding officers and can influence military career-related decisions, including discharge status [10, 48]. Within military populations, there are indications that active duty personnel perceive greater mental health-related stigma than non-active members [49]. Given that active duty personnel are more likely to experience combat-related psychopathology [50], these findings suggest that career-related stigma may be particularly salient among these individuals and interfere with seeking and engaging in needed treatment.

Fourth, stigma is more prevalent among individuals with mental health concerns than those without, and research indicates that veterans often experience higher rates of mental disorders – including PTSD, depression, and substance use – and associated impairment than the general population [51, 52]. Epidemiological studies document that up to 43 % of veterans returning from the recent conflicts in the Middle East meet diagnostic criteria for a mental health disorder [4, 53], and several studies suggest that veterans with psychological illness perceive greater stigma than those without [4, 43]. A striking example is the finding that recently returning troops who screened positively for a mental health problem were twice as likely to report fear of stigmatization than those who did not [4]. A more recent study found that individuals with probable diagnoses of depression and PTSD reported being more concerned about stigma from loved ones and in the workplace than those without these conditions [20]. Overall, in our professional experience with this population at high risk for mental illness, stigma tends to be more prevalent among those who are most in need of psychological treatment.

In addition to the aforementioned unique types and sources of stigma among veterans regarding the consequences of having a mental illness and seeking treatment, other stigmatizing beliefs specifically reflecting concerns about psychological treatment itself have been frequently endorsed, including the perception that therapy is not effective, concerns about taking medications, and fears about the side effects of psychotropic drugs [9, 20, 43, 54]. Stigmatizing beliefs regarding treatment providers specifically have also been cited. In one study of both Vietnam and Iraq/Afghanistan veterans, participants endorsed the belief that mental health providers would not understand their problems [18]. Others have reported that a significant percentage of OEF/OIF soldiers are mistrustful of mental health providers [49] and feel they cannot be understood by individuals who have not been deployed [9].

Special Considerations: Female Veterans, Veterans with Military Sexual Trauma, and Racial/Ethnic Minorities

Female veterans, veterans who have experienced military sexual trauma (MST), as well as sexual orientation and racial/ethnic minorities, represent veteran subpopulations that may have distinct stigma-related concerns and merit a brief but separate discussion. For women, these unique stigmatizing concerns appear to center around seeking treatment at VA settings. Women represent a growing proportion of today's military service members and are diagnosed with mental health conditions at higher rates than men [55]. However, research examining medical and psychological treatment utilization among women veterans has predominantly been conducted in VA settings, which historically accommodated a male-only population. In these reports, female veterans have expressed specific concerns about fitting in, the lack of availability of specialized services, and provider's lack of sensitivity and/or skill regarding unique healthcare needs of women [5, 15, 17, 56, 57] which are distinct from general treatment-seeking stigmatizing beliefs among male veterans discussed above. With respect to the latter concern, few studies have examined the role of provider attitudes in shaping women veterans' healthcare experiences. Research in this area suggests that gender awareness – encompassing providers' use of negative stereotypes, sensitivity to women's healthcare needs, and knowledge about caring for female patients (see Vogt et al. 2001 [58] for a detailed illustration) – impacts the treatment experience among female veterans [56, 58]. In a rare study examining gender awareness among VA hospital providers, Vogt and colleagues [58] reported that healthcare workers lacked sensitivity to female patients' particular privacy needs and the constraints of their caregiving responsibilities. These concerns appear to impact women veteran's treatment-seeking behaviors for medical [17] and mental healthcare [57]. In one study examining treatment-seeking behaviors among women with PTSD in the VA, the availability of specialized mental health treatment programs was the most important determinant of treatment access among women veterans [57]. Not surprisingly, women's level of comfort with VA mental health services was positively associated with treatment engagement [57]. Still, women veterans are more likely to access treatment outside of the VA [54], which may be at least in part attributable to negative beliefs about receiving treatment in the VA environment.

Stigma may also be a particular concern among veterans seeking MST-related care. The estimated prevalence of military sexual trauma among service members ranges from 25 to 40 % [59, 60], and veterans who have experienced MST are more likely to have physical and mental health comorbidities [59, 61] and higher associated need for treatment. However, low rates of reporting MST and seeking treatment for these concerns are consistently reported [62]. Even in nonveteran populations, stigma associated with sexual violence/trauma, including self-blame, embarrassment, and fear of not being believed, is commonly reported [63, 64]. Unfortunately, fewer data exist regarding stigmatizing beliefs among veterans with MST. Two recent qualitative analyses offer preliminary explorations of the particular stigma faced by both female and male veterans with MST. Burns and colleagues [62] provide an in-depth examination of servicewomen's experiences with MST and identified stigma-related concerns regarding fears about the reactions from others, confidentiality, negative career impact, and unit cohesion as barriers to reporting and seeking treatment. In addition, confusion regarding what constituted sexual assault was a distinct reason for not seeking MST-related care [62]. In a second qualitative analysis of barriers to care among 20 male veterans with MST who had engaged in care at a VA, stigma-related barriers were endorsed by all participants. Further, the authors indicated that most of these were directly related to the sexual nature of the trauma and were distinct from more general stigma-related concerns about seeking psychological treatment. These included embarrassment and shame, privacy concerns, self-blame, and sensitivity to reactions of providers [65]. While the literature regarding stigma specific to MST among veterans is nascent, these qualitative data suggest that military personnel seeking care for MST may have additional stigmatizing concerns beyond those endorsed when seeking treatment for non-MST-related concerns.

Other minority groups, including sexual orientation and racial/ethnic minority veterans, may also experience particular stigma that impacts service utilization. With respect to LGBT individuals, the civilian literature suggests that worry regarding the consequence of disclosing one's sexual minority status is associated with healthcare underutilization in this group [66, 67]. Researchers suggest that LGBT veterans may experience more fear about disclosing their orientation than civilians, as LGB sexual orientation has historically led to dismissal from the military, and transgender identity still can lead to discharge [68]. There are very little published data regarding healthcare use stigma among LGBT veterans; however, researchers investigating VA hospital use suggest that LGBT veterans may view care at VA hospitals as an extension of their service and that fears about disclosure are common for this reason [68]. Recent preliminary studies consistently indicate that LGBT veterans endorse stigmatizing concerns regarding the attitudes and behaviors of medical staff [69, 70]. Endorsed concerns included fear of nonacceptance by providers, being treated differently, losing benefits, and being seen as less competent [70]. These stigmatizing beliefs have been linked to service underutilization. Over one quarter of veterans in an online survey reported avoiding using at least one service at a VA because of fear of stigma [69]. Overall, it appears that sexual minority individuals face substantial stigma that deters them from seeking care and that increasing provider awareness, sensitivity, and incorporation of LGBT issues into treatment would enhance needed care among these individuals.

Finally, it is worth noting that research in both veteran and nonveteran populations has demonstrated racial/ethnic disparities in treatment access, healthcare experiences, and health outcomes [71–74]. The broader, nonveteran literature demonstrates that racial/ethnic minority individuals who have experienced discrimination or racism have poorer physical and mental health [75, 76] and that racial/ethnic minorities with mental illness may face "double stigma" related to both their racial minority status and psychiatric status, which may deter them more than nonminorities from seeking needed services [77]. Attitudes toward mental health system and providers, including mistrust of treatment practices and lack of cultural competence of providers, have also been posited to contribute to reduced access among racial/ethnic minorities [77]. However, there are virtually no data regarding particular stigmatizing experiences related to healthcare among racial/ethnic minority veterans. We briefly discuss related findings that may help to better conceptualize racial minority veterans' healthcare experiences and provide a framework for future research. Overall, research suggests that particular experiences with racism and discrimination during military service are associated with mental health outcomes [78], suggesting a greater need for healthcare services relative to Caucasian service members. For example, several studies suggest that racial/ethnic minorities are at higher risk for PTSD (e.g., [78, 79]). Research regarding mental health treatment among racial/ethnic minority veterans suggests that provider sensitivity to race and ethnicity is associated with better self-reported ratings of mental health [72]. In addition, the provision of mental health services from a race-matched clinician was associated with increased disclosure of mental health problems and length of treatment [80], suggesting that increasing cultural sensitivity, as well as the availability of racial/ethnic minority providers could enhance outcomes. However, as mentioned above, there is a dearth of research that builds on these preliminary findings. Further research is needed to identify particular ethnic or culturally based stigmatizing beliefs and experiences, as well as to investigate how such stigma is associated with healthcare utilization among racial/ethnic minority veterans.

Stigma and Healthcare Utilization Among Veterans

Physical Health

Traumatic limb loss, chronic pain, and traumatic brain injuries often require ongoing comprehensive medical care, and elimination of barriers to care access for these concerns is an ongoing goal to meet healthcare needs. Rehabilitation for traumatic limb loss is a comprehensive process involving multiple components of the healthcare system, and access to such treatment is imperative to reduce the acute and long-term consequences of limb loss among veterans. The VA hospital has pointed to several challenges to providing care for these individuals including the complexity of injuries and associated medical procedures and the difficulty of providing a continuum of care to individuals who present at various stages of their injuries [81]. In addition, it seems likely that the various barriers to healthcare detailed above (including geographic constraints, comorbid medical and psychological conditions) may be amplified among veterans with limb amputations, thus creating further barriers to accessing needed healthcare.

Stigma and healthcare access for chronic pain appears to highlight clinician attitudes toward chronic pain patients. Among civilian physicians, lack of knowledge and training in pain management and negative perceptions of patients with chronic pain (including the perception of chronic pain patients as frustrating and the perception that treating pain is time consuming) have been identified as sources of stigma and have been shown to negatively impact pain treatment [82, 83]. Among veterans, Dobscha and colleagues reported on VA primary care clinicians' attitudes and treatment of chronic pain among veterans and found that while providers identified pain management as a high priority, they felt they often could not provide optimal pain treatment [84]. Stigmatizing beliefs that impacted their provision of care include the perception of patients as "frustrating," and concerns that their use of prescription opioids to manage pain may contribute to physical dependence among their veteran patients [84].

To date, there is limited research investigating stigma and healthcare use in veterans with TBI. One study found that approximately half of caregivers of OEF/OIF veterans with TBI reported that they perceived they had stigmatizing views toward the veterans [85]. This included frequent perceptions that the veteran was treated with less courtesy and respect than other people and that others were afraid of the veteran [85]. Furthermore, the perceived discrimination against the veteran with

TBI was associated with greater caregiver stress and social isolation [85]. Additional research is needed to gain a better understanding of potential biases perceived by veterans with TBI and the impact of these perceptions on recovery and psychosocial functioning.

Mental Health

As mentioned above, mental health stigma is a prevalent concern among veterans that seemingly has negative implications for mental health treatment utilization. In a large study of treatment engagement among VA patients with PTSD of all eras, Spoont and colleagues [86] found that less than 40 % of veterans received psychotherapy within 6–12 months of their diagnosis. Further, research suggests that recently returning veterans who have served in Afghanistan and Iraq, who face more recent combat-related and readjustment concerns, are less likely to access care than older veteran cohorts [87]. In a large national survey of OEF/OIF veterans who screened positive for PTSD or depression, nearly half reported that they had not received any mental healthcare in the previous year [88]. Another study found that up to 70 % of Iraq and Afghanistan veterans who met criteria for a psychological disorder were not interested in treatment [4]. Active duty personnel may be even less likely to access mental health treatment, despite higher rates of combat-related psychopathology [50]. Data suggest that only one quarter of active duty troops with psychiatric diagnoses actually receive treatment [4, 44].

Research suggests that stigma is a primary barrier to seeking needed psychological treatment among veterans, with studies generally demonstrating that greater perceived stigma is associated with lower intentions to seek care [47] or more negative attitudes toward seeking care [39]. More precisely, findings suggest that self-stigma, compared to public stigma, is a stronger predictor of treatment-seeking attitudes [8, 39, 47]. For example, in a sample of active duty and retired service members, Held and Owens [39] found that self-stigma mediated the relationship between public stigma and negative treatment-seeking attitudes. Blais and Renshaw [8] echoed these findings in a study of National Guard reservists, demonstrating that the association between public stigma and intentions to seek mental healthcare was fully mediated by self-stigma. These findings suggest that internalized negative personal beliefs about treatment are the most potent deterrent to treatment utilization and have important implications for the development of targeted anti-stigma interventions.

While the studies described above have assessed how various stigmatizing beliefs impact intentions and attitudes toward seeking care, fewer studies have examined the role of stigma on actual healthcare utilization. This is an important distinction, as stigmatizing beliefs that are reported as a perceived barrier to care may be different from what predicts use of services [89]. Indeed, findings linking public and self-stigma to healthcare use have been mixed. Several studies demonstrate that stigma is associated with reduced mental healthcare utilization [12, 20, 43], while others indicate that stigma is not associated with prospective use [90] and, in some cases, is associated with increased likelihood of use [53, 91, 92]. In a study of OEF/OIF veterans and active duty service members, Pietrzak and colleagues [43] found that stigmatizing beliefs regarding mental health treatment were negatively associated with receiving mental health counseling or medication services in the previous 6 months. A more recent study provided an in-depth examination of the impact of self-stigma on mental health service use in a sample of OEF/OIF veterans [20]. The authors found that personal beliefs about mental illness and treatment seeking, but not public stigma from others, were related to decreased mental health and substance abuse service use in the previous 6 months. Notably, only self-stigma was associated with actual service use, although the majority of participants reported concerns about public stigma [20]. On the other hand, in a study of Vietnam era and OEF/OIF veterans, Rosen and colleagues [92] found that stigma was not prospectively associated with initiating psychotherapy, despite the fact that one third of participants endorsed public and self-stigma. Similarly, while stigma-related barriers were the most commonly endorsed among a range of possible barriers in a sample of Iraq and Afghanistan veterans, stigma was not associated with mental healthcare use [90]. Moreover, findings from two studies indicate that greater perceived stigma was associated with greater mental health treatment engagement, with perceived stigma being positively correlated to number of treatment sessions in two veteran samples [53, 92].

In sum, accessing needed healthcare services for chronic physical conditions and mental health difficulties is impeded by various types of stigma. Public and self-stigma are very commonly reported among service members and veterans and are consistently associated with negative attitudes toward treatment seeking across studies. Further, self-stigma seems to be more strongly associated with treatment-seeking intentions than public stigma. Stigma does not appear to reliably predict actual treatment-seeking behaviors, as research examining the role of stigmatizing beliefs on actual utilization is mixed [12, 53]. These discrepant findings may best be explained by sample characteristics, such that the studies described above that did not find that stigma was related to service use were conducted in hospital or mental health clinic settings among veterans with mental health diagnoses [53, 90, 92], versus veterans in the community who have not yet initiated any kind of services [12, 20]. The relative lack of prospective studies renders it difficult to fully understand this relationship, and more studies utilizing prospective designs are needed to better elucidate the way in which stigma influences treatment-seeking behavior. Finally, the relationship between need (i.e., presence and severity of mental illness), stigma, and service use is also highlighted in these studies and is synthesized here. Overall, it appears that individuals with more severe psychiatric symptoms appear to be more likely to both endorse stigma and to seek treatment [20]. These findings provide several important insights into the types of stigma to be addressed in the development of interventions, and to whom they should be targeted, which are discussed in greater detail in the last section of this chapter.

Increasing Access to Healthcare Among Veterans: Amputation System of Care, Integrated Primary Care, Women's Clinics, and Telemedicine

Long-term medical care for veterans with war-related medical illnesses and injuries has largely been undertaken by the DOD and VA healthcare systems [93]. Rehabilitation of veterans to their highest level of functioning has been challenging, particularly among veterans with the most severe injuries, such as traumatic limb loss. The priority placed on increasing access to evidence-based, comprehensive, and high-quality services has led to a "paradigm shift" within the VA healthcare system [81]. This shift has placed an emphasis on person-centered care, where the patient plays an active role in guiding his or her care. A stunning example of such reform is best exemplified by the VA hospital's "Amputation System of Care," which emphasizes a balance between access to care and expertise, calling for a multidisciplinary approach to treating veterans closer to their homes while also providing the most advanced technologies and expert knowledge regarding limb amputation and rehabilitation (see Sigford et al. for a comprehensive explication) [81]. Advances in such healthcare reform have been crucial steps in ensuring that all veterans obtain access to a full palate of services, while also receiving specialized care for their particular concerns.

There is a strong evidence base for a variety of psychological and pharmacological approaches to mental health problems frequently encountered by military service members and veterans (e.g., prolonged exposure therapy for PTSD, antidepressants, and cognitive behavioral therapy for depression), and several recent treatment innovations have led to increased avenues by which veteran service members access to mental healthcare. Two developments specifically within the VA system – integrated primary care and specialized women's services – as well as the use of telemedicine have helped increase treatment access among veterans in this setting.

Research indicates that primary care settings are associated with less mental health-related stigma than specialty mental health clinics [4] and that veterans with mental health concerns are more likely to present to primary care [94]. In response, a mandated model of integrated primary care was developed to increase access to mental health screening and initial care in VA hospitals [95]. The VA-wide policy initiative for the development of primary care mental health clinics (PMHCs) has since become a widely used model for integrated care, offering mental health assessment, treatment, and appropriate referral in a less stigmatizing healthcare setting (see Pomerantz et al. [96] for a review). An emerging body of research regarding the effectiveness of this model on increasing access to care suggests generally positive results. Specifically, initial mental healthcare treatment in a primary care setting is associated with greater subsequent treatment engagement in specialty mental health clinics [97–99]. A recent study examined the effect of a three-session brief trauma treatment (BTT) delivered in a VA PMHC and found that more than 60 % of patients later engaged in specialized mental health services [97]. This represents an increase from previously reported specialty care treatment engagement rates ranging from 1 to 13 % [100, 101]. Similarly, another study examined mental health treatment outcome in a longitudinal cohort who screened positive in primary care for a mental health concern and found that following a positive screen for depression or PTSD, over half of the sample received high-quality care that was consistent with treatment guidelines [100]. Rather than initiating services in a separate, specialty mental healthcare clinic, these integrative methods appear to make mental health treatment more approachable and less stigmatizing for veterans.

Treatment adaptations addressing the unique stigma-related barriers to care faced by female veterans have also been implemented within the VA. As previously discussed, the availability of specialized, gender-specific mental health services for women is a primary determinant of treatment access [57]. To address these concerns, the VA has focused on increasing the provision of gender sensitive mental health services. The development of the Women's Stress Disorder Treatment Team (WSDTT) has provided specialized mental health services for women by clinicians with expertise regarding the unique clinical needs of women veterans and returning service members. These developments include ensuring a gender-matched provider and providing group and individual CBT for trauma-related disorders among women. Studies evaluating these clinics indicate success in reducing stigma-based concerns and discomforts among women associated with seeking care at a VA [57]. Overall, the integration of services and the development of women-specific services appear to reduce mental health-related stigma and enhance treatment engagement through providing high-quality screening, treatment, and care coordination.

Finally, the use of telemedicine has become increasingly available in a variety of treatment settings and has expanded the reach of health treatment among veterans. In general, telemedicine includes, but is not limited to, the use of face-to-face video teleconferencing, Internet, smartphones, and tablets to deliver mental healthcare, and research demonstrates its efficacy in reducing both practical (i.e., geography, transportation) and stigma-related (i.e., confidentiality concerns, negative beliefs about seeking traditional face-to-face psychological treatment) barriers to accessing mental healthcare [102]. Telemedicine has become a crucial component to care for medical as well as mental health concerns. While we did not identify any studies that explicitly examined the effect of telemedicine versus face-to-face therapy on reducing stigma, one study demonstrated that female OEF/OIF veterans felt that a web-based mental health screening program increased their comfort with seeking mental healthcare [103]. Further, participants reported being "more truthful" in their answers to mental health screening questions via the Internet compared to in person [103]. Overall, these data confirm the efficacy of telemedicine as a viable and cost-effective treatment modality and provide early indications that it may effectively reduce self-stigma and increase access to needed mental healthcare.

Anti-stigma Interventions for Mental Health Treatment in Particular

While, as evidenced above, stigma can affect nearly every stage of general health-care experience among veterans, it is our opinion that stigma is the most salient barrier to mental health treatment, and we devote the remainder of this chapter to discussing current progress in reducing stigma as well as outlining recommendations for future directions for increasing access to care for mental health concerns exclusively. Despite compelling empirical evidence that stigma is a salient barrier to accessing mental healthcare among veterans, there appears to be very little research examining stigma reduction interventions in veteran and military populations. Some authors have proposed conceptual models of anti-stigma intervention strategies for veterans and service members drawing from the empirical anti-stigma literature in the civilian population [38, 104, 105]. In a recent review, Dickstein and colleagues [38] thoughtfully proposed relevant targets for anti-stigma efforts specific to military populations. These included reducing inaccurate perceptions and stereotypes about mental illness and treatment, reducing self-blame, and resolving uncertainty about symptoms and treatment [38]. Current proposals for anti-stigma approaches to address these targets appear to emphasize the potential effectiveness of an educational component, stressing the provision of accurate information to challenge misguided perceptions regarding mental illness and treatment [104, 105]. In military populations, this may include providing targeted psychoeducation about mental health symptoms (e.g., post-traumatic stress disorder, depression), their course, and treatment options [38, 104, 105]. Another proposed intervention includes promoting contact with individuals with a mental illness and/or TBI to reduce negative attitudes and stereotypes about these concerns. One school-based intervention focused on reducing stigmatization of individuals with brain injuries found that contact with a person with an acquired brain injury was more effective in promoting positive attitudes than education alone [106]. In the military context, contact interventions consist of exposure to well-respected and/or high ranking soldiers who have struggled with mental illness and received treatment to facilitate discussions of these potentially stigmatizing experiences in a supportive context [104, 105]. Other ideas for anti-stigma interventions have been proposed, including cognitive reappraisal techniques, values-based work, and empowerment (see Dickstein et al. [38] for a review). Despite these theoretical advances, empirical support for anti-stigma approaches in military populations is lacking. We identified two studies that examined the impact of psychoeducational programs on attitudes toward mental illness and treatment, and both report promising results [103, 107]. Gould and colleagues [107] evaluated the effectiveness of a PTSD psychoeducational program among service members of the UK Armed Forces and found that the provision of education regarding stress and PTSD significantly improved attitudes toward mental illness and treatment seeking. More recently, Sadler and colleagues [103] found that 31 % of female OEF/OIF veterans who received an individualized web-based psychoeducation program reported increased comfort with seeking mental health services, and over two thirds indicated their intention to follow up with recommendations to seek treatment.

Overall it appears that while there are promising theoretical frameworks for directly targeting and reducing treatment-deterring stigma among veterans and military personnel, the literature on this topic is emerging, and stigma still remains a potent barrier to care. Additionally, it is not clear that an anti-stigma intervention would not be susceptible to the same stigma-related barriers as mental health treatment itself. Therefore, we provide further recommendations for the development of targeted anti-stigma campaigns in the next section.

Future Directions

Recommendations for Anti-stigma Interventions for Mental Health

Our review of the literature regarding stigma among veterans and service members revealed a number of promising avenues for the development of targeted and effective anti-stigma interventions. First, as discussed above, the literature suggests that self-stigma is perhaps the most salient form of stigma and is more strongly associated with treatment-seeking attitudes and behaviors than public or personal stigma (e.g., [8]). Several authors have recommended that anti-stigma strategies be targeted toward altering negative internalized beliefs regarding mental illness and treatment rather than at changing the perception of the public [8, 20]. Examples of beliefs reflective of self-stigma such as seeking treatment is a sign of weakness or that one should handle one's own problems would be suitable targets for psychoeducation interventions. Furthermore, studies should pay particular attention to how interventions impact self-stigma, rather than stigma more broadly. Information that normalizes help seeking may serve to correct misperceptions and mitigate the negative impact on treatment-seeking attitudes and behaviors. In addition, information regarding how to recognize early signs and symptoms of trauma and adjustment-related difficulties may be particularly helpful in military service members who may have combat exposure. For example, Vogt and colleagues [20] found that the majority of OEF/OIF veterans reported intentions to seek treatment only when symptoms are severe and suggest that an educational component that bolsters recognition of the benefit of seeking treatment early may prevent a chronic course of debilitating symptoms. It has been our clinical experience that veterans often think they did not have it "as bad" as other veterans or that by seeking care for their problems, they invalidate the struggles of those who may have "had it worse." Interventions might also address these beliefs and find a way to emphasize the importance of self-care in a way that does not undermine the values of self-sacrifice and teamwork that pervade military culture.

A recent and more nuanced finding suggests that veterans may be ambivalent about their treatment seeking beliefs, rather than adopting polarizing perceptions of mental health treatment. In a study utilizing a comprehensive measure of stigmatizing beliefs about mental illness and treatment, Vogt and colleagues [20] found that half of the sample of OEF/OIF veterans appeared to be undecided about their beliefs around mental illness and treatment rather than holding categorically positive or negative views. This finding highlights the possibility that many individuals may benefit from motivation-enhancing interventions [20], which may be particularly effective in resolving ambivalence, correcting misperceptions, and increasing engagement in needed mental healthcare.

Second, the literature suggests that stigma may be less of a barrier among individuals who have already initiated some form of treatment [53]. Because individuals with no prior treatment engagement appear to particularly vulnerable to the treatment deterring effects of stigmatizing beliefs [49], anti-stigma interventions might target this group specifically to be optimally effective. In these cases, the use of telemedicine may be the most effective way to provide psychoeducational material to these individuals, given their initial reluctance to physically present for care. Results from a preliminary study of the effectiveness of a web-based psychoeducational program are promising and suggest that continued program development and evaluation research in this area might promote treatment initiation among treatment-naive service members [103]. An additional potentially helpful avenue to provide needed stigma-reducing education is through family members and/or friends of veterans. The provision of treatment encouraging information from a trusted source may more strongly influence treatment-seeking attitudes and behaviors. Future research could examine the effect of an intervention model that includes delivering treatment encouraging messages indirectly to veterans through the provision of psychoeducation to family members and friends.

Third, we recommend implementing targeted efforts within military systems, as this represents a crucial juncture at which anti-stigma interventions could promote treatment utilization. Perceptions of unit cohesion and leadership behaviors appear to be linked to stigmatizing beliefs about mental illness and treatment [45], and a positive unit climate is correlated with reduced stigma associated with seeking treatment for PTSD [46]. Therefore, providing education to unit leaders about the benefit of a supportive environment, along with specific training about how to talk about mental illness and encourage care seeking in a supportive manner, may help to create a climate of reduced stigma wherein soldiers may feel more comfortable addressing mental health concerns. Related recommendations include increasing contact with fellow soldiers or veterans who have struggled with mental illness and sought treatment [104, 105] given that messages encouraging treatment seeking may be better received if delivered by veterans with similar experiences themselves. Given that veterans have reported mistrust of clinicians who have not been deployed [9], this may be a particularly effective avenue to increase treatment engagement. While these contact-promoting recommendations have mostly focused on their application to military contexts [105], contact with veterans or fellow service members in clinical settings may promote a more immediate initiation of needed services, particularly among veterans who express ambivalence, and for whom acting upon transitory motivation is crucial. Preliminary findings suggest that having veteran service members on staff in an outpatient clinic setting may increase willingness to initiate needed mental health services among prospective patients [108]. While further research is needed to explore if and how this model explicitly influences stigmatizing beliefs, the inclusion of veterans as part of mental health clinics appears to be an effective way to facilitate the difficult process of connecting with care.

Finally, larger-scale reforms regarding the normalization of mental illness in the military may substantially reduce stigmatizing beliefs about mental illness and treatment. To normalize mental illness, educational efforts aimed at reconceptualizing mental illness as equivalent in severity and treatment worthiness to other physical injuries incurred during war could help to reduce mental illness-related stigma and increase treatment seeking. Efforts within a military context include promoting psychiatric and physical injury equivalence through officially recognizing and honoring individuals with "invisible" psychiatric wounds of war as is done to those with physical wounds. While this remains a controversial topic in the United States, some nations have expanded their Purple Heart honor (a decoration awarded to soldiers physically wounded or killed) to include PTSD in an effort to destigmatize mental illness and promote access to needed treatment.

Conclusions

We have found that stigma among military veterans and service members is a significant deterrent to seeking needed treatment for medical problems and contributes to access-related mental health disparities. In particular, individuals with traumatic limb loss, chronic pain, and traumatic brain injuries face several stigma-related obstacles to accessing needed healthcare services including personal beliefs and interpretations of their illness, medical provider bias, and social stigma. In the realm of mental health, personal beliefs regarding mental illness and psychological treatment represent the most potent forms of stigma and therefore suitable targets for interventions. Our findings identify the following avenues for future work that would further our understanding of stigma and treatment seeking, as well as reduce stigma to improve treatment engagement and health outcomes among veterans: (1) additional research employing prospective designs to better understand the ways in which stigma exerts its influence on actual treatment-seeking behaviors; (2) a focus on addressing particular stigmatizing beliefs among vulnerable veteran populations including individuals with limb loss and chronic pain and gender, sexual, and ethnic minorities; (3) the development of novel anti-stigma interventions that target those most in need (i.e., treatment-naïve veterans with mental illness), that utilize novel modalities to reach them (i.e., telemedicine), and that incorporate influential sources (i.e., fellow service members, family, and friends); and (4) continued advocacy for the recognition of and sensitivity to mental illness within military settings. While large-scale extensive change will not be immediate, we hope that progress informed by continued efforts at any level will contribute to significant reductions in stigma and increased access to treatment for needed care among our historically marginalized veterans.

References

1. Veterans Health Administration. Analysis of VA health care utilization among Operation Enduring Freedom (OEF), Operation Iraqi Freedom (OIF), and Operation New Dawn (OND) Veterans. 2013:1–13. Available from: http://www.publichealth.va.gov/epidemiology/reports/oefoifond/health-care-utilization/index.asp.
2. Outcalt SD, Ang DC, Wu J, Sargent C, Yu Z, Bair MJ. Pain experience of Iraq and Afghanistan Veterans with comorbid chronic pain and posttraumatic stress. J Rehabil Res Dev. 2014;51(4): 559–70.
3. Owens BD, Kragh JF, Wenke JC, Macaitis J, Wade CE, Holcomb JB. Combat wounds in operation Iraqi freedom and operation enduring freedom. J Trauma [Internet]. 2008 [cited 8 Apr 2015];64(2):295–9. Available from: http://www.ncbi.nlm.nih.gov/pubmed/18301189.
4. Hoge CW, Castro CA, Messer SC, McGurk D, Cotting DI, Koffman RL. Combat duty in Iraq and Afghanistan, mental health problems and barriers to care. US Army Med Dep J [Internet]. [cited 1 Feb 2015];7–17. Available from: http://www.ncbi.nlm.nih.gov/pubmed/20088060.
5. Ouimette P, Vogt D, Wade M, Tirone V, Greenbaum MA, Kimerling R, et al. Perceived barriers to care among veterans health administration patients with posttraumatic stress disorder. Psychol Serv [Internet]. 2011 [cited 4 Feb 2015];8(3):212–23. Available from: http://www.researchgate.net/publication/232567638_Perceived_barriers_to_care_among_veterans_health_administration_patients_with_posttraumatic_stress_disorder.
6. Kang HK, Hyams KC. Mental health care needs among recent war veterans. N Engl J Med [Internet]. 2005 [cited 4 Feb 2015];352(13):1289. Available from: http://www.ncbi.nlm.nih.gov/pubmed/15800224.
7. Seal KH, Metzler TJ, Gima KS, Bertenthal D, Maguen S, Marmar CR. Trends and risk factors for mental health diagnoses among Iraq and Afghanistan veterans using department of veterans affairs health care, 2002–2008. Am J Public Health [Internet]. 2009 [cited 28 Jan 2015];99(9):1651–8. Available from: http://www.pubmedcentral.nih.gov/articlerender.fcgi?artid=2724454&tool=pmcentrez&rendertype=abstract.
8. Blais RK, Renshaw KD. Self-stigma fully mediates the association of anticipated enacted stigma and help-seeking intentions in national guard service members. 2014;26(2):114–9.
9. Stecker T, Shiner B, Watts B V, Jones M, Conner KR. Treatment-seeking barriers for veterans of the Iraq and Afghanistan conflicts who screen positive for PTSD. Psychiatr Serv [Internet]. 2013;64(3):280–3. Available from: http://www.ncbi.nlm.nih.gov/pubmed/23450385.
10. Vogt D, Di Leone B a L, Wang JM, Sayer N a, Pineles SL, Litz BT. Endorsed and Anticipated Stigma Inventory (EASI): a tool for assessing beliefs about mental illness and mental health treatment among military personnel and veterans. Psychol Serv [Internet]. 2013;11(1):105–13. Available from: http://www.ncbi.nlm.nih.gov/pubmed/24274110.
11. Andersen RM. Revisiting the behavioral model and access to medical care: does it matter? J Health Soc Behav [Internet]. 1995 [cited 27 Jan 2015];36(1):1–10. Available from: http://www.ncbi.nlm.nih.gov/pubmed/7738325.
12. Blais RK, Hoerster KD, Malte C, Hunt S, Jakupcak M. Unique PTSD clusters predict intention to seek mental health care and subsequent utilization in US veterans with PTSD symptoms. J Trauma Stress [Internet]. 2014 [cited 4 Feb 2015];27(2):168–74. Available from: http://www.ncbi.nlm.nih.gov/pubmed/24634206.
13. Elhai JD, Grubaugh AL, Richardson JD, Egede LE, Creamer M. Outpatient medical and mental healthcare utilization models among military veterans: results from the 2001 National survey of veterans. J Psychiatr Res [Internet]. 2008 [cited 4 Feb 2015];42(10):858–67. Available from: http://www.ncbi.nlm.nih.gov/pubmed/18005993.
14. Schnurr PP, Friedman MJ, Sengupta A, Jankowski MK, Holmes T. PTSD and utilization of medical treatment services among male Vietnam veterans. J Nerv Ment Dis [Internet]. 2000 [cited 4 Feb 2015];188(8):496–504. Available from: http://www.ncbi.nlm.nih.gov/pubmed/10972568.

15. Washington DL, Bean-Mayberry B, Riopelle D, Yano EM. Access to care for women veterans: delayed healthcare and unmet need. J Gen Intern Med [Internet]. 2011 [cited 4 Feb 2015];26 Suppl 2:655–61. Available from: http://www.pubmedcentral.nih.gov/articlerender.fcgi?artid=3191223&tool=pmcentrez&rendertype=abstract.

16. Bauer MS, Williford WO, McBride L, McBride K, Shea NM. Perceived barriers to health care access in a treated population. Int J Psychiatry Med [Internet]. 2005 [cited 4 Feb 2015];35(1):13–26. Available from: http://www.ncbi.nlm.nih.gov/pubmed/15977942.

17. Vogt D, Bergeron A, Salgado D, Daley J, Ouimette P, Wolfe J. Barriers to veterans health administration care in a nationally representative sample of women veterans. J Gen Intern Med. 2006;21:19–25.

18. Sayer NA, Friedemann-Sanchez G, Spoont M, Murdoch M, Parker LE, Chiros C, et al. A qualitative study of determinants of PTSD treatment initiation in veterans. Psychiatry [Internet]. 2009 [cited 4 Feb 2015];72(3):238–55. Available from: http://www.ncbi.nlm.nih.gov/pubmed/19821647.

19. Corrigan P. How stigma interferes with mental health care. Am Psychol [Internet]. 2004 [cited 16 Jul 2014];59(7):614–25. Available from: http://www.ncbi.nlm.nih.gov/pubmed/15491256.

20. Vogt D, Fox AB, Di Leone BAL. Mental health beliefs and their relationship with treatment seeking among U.S. OEF/OIF veterans. J Trauma Stress [Internet]. 2014 [cited 4 Feb 2015];27(3):307–13. Available from: http://www.ncbi.nlm.nih.gov/pubmed/24839077.

21. Dougherty PJ. Long-term follow-up study of bilateral above-the-knee amputees from the Vietnam war. J Bone Joint Surg Am [Internet]. 1999 [cited 1 Jul 2015];81(10):1384–90. Available from: http://www.ncbi.nlm.nih.gov/pubmed/10535588.

22. Horgan O, MacLachlan M. Psychosocial adjustment to lower-limb amputation: a review. Disabil Rehabil [Internet]. [cited 1 Jul 2015];26(14–15):837–50. Available from: http://www.ncbi.nlm.nih.gov/pubmed/15497913.

23. Kazis LE, Miller DR, Clark J, Skinner K, Lee A, Rogers W, et al. Health-related quality of life in patients served by the Department of Veterans Affairs: results from the Veterans Health Study. Arch Intern Med [Internet]. 1998 [cited 23 Apr 2015];158(6):626–32. Available from: http://www.ncbi.nlm.nih.gov/pubmed/9521227.

24. Lew HL, Otis JD, Tun C, Kerns RD, Clark ME, Cifu DX. Prevalence of chronic pain, posttraumatic stress disorder, and persistent postconcussive symptoms in OIF/OEF veterans: polytrauma clinical triad. J Rehabil Res Dev [Internet]. 2009 [cited 23 Apr 2015];46(6):697–702. Available from: http://www.ncbi.nlm.nih.gov/pubmed/20104399.

25. Waugh OC, Byrne DG, Nicholas MK. Internalized stigma in people living with chronic pain. J Pain. 2014;15(5):550.e1–10. Elsevier Ltd.

26. Matthias MS, Miech EJ, Myers LJ, Sargent C, Bair MJ. A qualitative study of chronic pain in operation enduring freedom/operation Iraqi freedom veterans: "A burden on my soul". Mil Med [Internet]. 2014;179(1):26–30. Available from: http://www.ncbi.nlm.nih.gov/pubmed/24402981.

27. Hux K, Schram CD, Goeken T. Misconceptions about brain injury: a survey replication study. Brain Inj. 2006;20(5):547–53.

28. Guilmette TJ, Paglia MF. The public's misconception about traumatic brain injury: a follow up survey. Arch Clin Neuropsychol. 2004;19(2):183–9.

29. Swift TL, Wilson SL. Misconceptions about brain injury among the general public and non-expert health professionals: an exploratory study. Brain Inj. 2001;15(2):149–65.

30. Benedict RHB, Cookfair D, Gavett R, Gunther M, Munschauer F, Garg N, et al. Validity of the Minimal Assessment of Cognitive Function in Multiple Sclerosis (MACFIMS). J Int Neuropsychol Soc. 2006;12(4):549–58.

31. Ralph A, Derbyshire C. Survivors of brain injury through the eyes of the public: a systematic review. Brain Inj. 2013;27(13–14):1475–91.

32. McLellan T, Bishop A, McKinlay A. Community attitudes toward individuals with traumatic brain injury. J Int Neuropsychol Soc. 2010;16(4):705–10.

33. Linden MA, Crothers IR. Violent, caring, unpredictable: public views on survivors of brain injury. Arch Clin Neuropsychol. 2006;21(8):763–70.
34. Link BG, Phelan JC. Stigma and its public health implications. Lancet. 2006;367(9509): 528–9.
35. Resch JA, Villarreal V, Johnson CL, Elliott TR, Kwok O-M, Berry JW, et al. Trajectories of life satisfaction in the first 5 years following traumatic brain injury. Rehabil Psychol. 2009;54(1):51–9.
36. Doig E, Fleming J, Tooth L. Patterns of community integration 2–5 years post-discharge from brain injury rehabilitation. Brain Inj. 2001;15(9):747–62.
37. Stecker T, Fortney J, Hamilton F, Sherbourne CD, Ajzen I. Engagement in mental health treatment among veterans returning from Iraq. Patient prefer adherence [Internet]. 2010 [cited 4 Feb 2015];4:45–9. Available from: http://www.pubmedcentral.nih.gov/articlerender.fcgi?artid =2853904&tool=pmcentrez&rendertype=abstract.
38. Dickstein BD, Vogt DS, Handa S, Litz BT. Targeting self-stigma in returning military personnel and veterans: a review of intervention strategies. Mil Psychol. 2010;22:224–36.
39. Held P, Owens GP. Stigmas and attitudes toward seeking mental health treatment in a sample of veterans and active duty service members. Traumatology (Tallahass Fla). 2012;(X).
40. Lorber W, Garcia HA. Not supposed to feel this: traditional masculinity in psychotherapy with male veterans returning from Afghanistan and Iraq. Psychotherapy (Chic) [Internet]. 2010 [cited 4 Feb 2015];47(3):296–305. Available from: http://www.ncbi.nlm.nih.gov/pubmed/ 22402087.
41. Nash WP, Silva C, Litz B. The historic origins of military and veteran mental health stigma and the stress injury model as a means to reduce it. Psychiatr Ann [Internet]. 2009 [cited 4 Feb 2015];39(8):789–94. Available from: http://www.researchgate.net/publication/247914594_ The_Historic_Origins_of_Military_and_Veteran_Mental_Health_Stigma_and_the_Stress_ Injury_Model_as_a_Means_to_Reduce_It.
42. Mittal D, Drummond KL, Blevins D, Curran G, Corrigan P, Sullivan G. Stigma associated with PTSD: perceptions of treatment seeking combat veterans. Psychiatr Rehabil J [Internet]. 2013;36(2):86–92. Available from: http://www.ncbi.nlm.nih.gov/pubmed/23750758.
43. Pietrzak RH, Johnson DC, Goldstein MB, Malley JC, Southwick SM. Perceived stigma and barriers to mental health care utilization among OEF-OIF veterans. Psychiatr Serv. 2009;60(8):1118–22.
44. Stecker T, Fortney JC, Hamilton F, Ajzen I. An assessment of beliefs about mental health care among veterans who served in Iraq. Psychiatr Serv [Internet]. 2007 [cited 4 Feb 2015];58(10):1358–61. Available from: http://www.ncbi.nlm.nih.gov/pubmed/17914017.
45. Britt TW, Wright KM, Moore D. Leadership as a predictor of stigma and practical barriers toward receiving mental health treatment: a multilevel approach. Psychol Serv. 2012;9(1): 26–37.
46. Kelley CL, Britt TW, Adler AB, Bliese PD. Perceived organizational support, posttraumatic stress disorder symptoms, and stigma in soldiers returning from combat. Psychol Serv [Internet]. 2014;11(2):229–34. Available from: http://www.ncbi.nlm.nih.gov/pubmed/ 24364593.
47. Blais RK, Renshaw KD. Stigma and demographic correlates of help-seeking intentions in returning service members. J Trauma Stress [Internet]. 2013 [cited 3 Jan 2015];26(1):77–85. Available from: http://www.ncbi.nlm.nih.gov/pubmed/23335155
48. Porter TL, Johnson WB. Psychiatric stigma in the military. Mil Med [Internet]. 1994 [cited 4 Feb 2015];159(9):602–5. Available from: http://www.ncbi.nlm.nih.gov/pubmed/7800175.
49. Kim PY, Thomas JL, Wilk JE, Castro CA, Hoge CW. Stigma, barriers to care, and use of mental health services among active duty and national guard soldiers after combat. Psychiatr Serv. 2010;61(6):582–8.
50. Vogt DS, Samper RE, King DW, King LA, Martin JA. Deployment stressors and posttraumatic stress symptomatology: comparing active duty and national guard/reserve personnel from Gulf war I. J Trauma Stress [Internet]. 2008 [cited 4 Feb 2015];21(1):66–74. Available from: http:// www.ncbi.nlm.nih.gov/pubmed/18302185.

51. Levy BS, Sidel VW. Health effects of combat: a life-course perspective. Annu Rev Public Health [Internet]. 2009 [cited 4 Feb 2015];30:123–36. Available from: http://www.ncbi.nlm.nih.gov/pubmed/18925871.
52. O'Toole BI, Catts SV, Outram S, Pierse KR, Cockburn J. The physical and mental health of Australian Vietnam veterans 3 decades after the war and its relation to military service, combat, and post-traumatic stress disorder. Am J Epidemiol. 2009;170(3):318–30.
53. Harpaz-Rotem I, Rosenheck R, Pietrzak R, Mph P, Southwick S. Determinants of prospective engagement in mental health treatment among symptomatic Iraq/Afghanistan veterans. J Nerv Ment Dis [Internet]. 2014;202(2):97–104. Available from: http://ovidsp.ovid.com/ovidweb.cgi ?T=JS&PAGE=reference&D=yrovfto&NEWS=N&AN=00005053-201402000-00004.
54. Elbogen EB, Wagner HR, Johnson SC, Kinneer P, Kang H, Vasterling JJ, et al. Are Iraq and Afghanistan veterans using mental health services? new data from a national random-sample survey. Psychiatr Serv [Internet]. 2013 [cited 4 Feb 2015];64(2):134–41. Available from: http://www.pubmedcentral.nih.gov/articlerender.fcgi?artid=3622866&tool=pmcentrez&rend ertype=abstract.
55. Maguen S, Cohen B, Cohen G, Madden E, Bertenthal D, Seal K. Gender differences in health service utilization among Iraq and Afghanistan veterans with posttraumatic stress disorder. J Womens Health (Larchmt) [Internet]. 2012 [cited 4 Feb 2015];21(6):666–73. Available from: http://www.pubmedcentral.nih.gov/articlerender.fcgi?artid=3366102&tool=pmcentrez&rend ertype=abstract.
56. Salgado DM, Vogt DS, King LA, King DW. Gender awareness inventory-VA: a measure of ideology, sensitivity, and knowledge related to women veterans' health care. Sex Roles [Internet]. Kluwer Academic Publishers-Plenum Publishers; [cited 4 Feb 2015];46(7–8): 247–62. Available from: http://link.springer.com/article/10.1023/A%3A1020171416038.
57. Fontana A, Rosenheck R. Treatment of female veterans with posttraumatic stress disorder: the role of comfort in a predominantly male environment. Psychiatr Q [Internet]. 2006 [cited 4 Feb 2015];77(1):55–67. Available from: http://www.ncbi.nlm.nih.gov/pubmed/16397755.
58. Vogt DS, Stone ER, Salgado DM, King LA, King DW, Savarese VW. Gender awareness among veterans administration health-care workers: existing strengths and areas for improvement. Women health [Internet]. 2001 [cited 4 Feb 2015];34(4):65–83. Available from: http://www.ncbi.nlm.nih.gov/pubmed/11785858.
59. Allard CB, Nunnink S, Gregory AM, Klest B, Platt M. Military sexual trauma research: a proposed agenda. J Trauma Dissociation [Internet]. 2011 [cited 4 Feb 2015];12(3):324–45. Available from: http://www.ncbi.nlm.nih.gov/pubmed/21534099.
60. Suris A, Lind L. Military sexual trauma: a review of prevalence and associated health consequences in veterans. Trauma violence abuse [Internet]. 2008 [cited 4 Feb 2015];9(4):250–69. Available from: http://www.ncbi.nlm.nih.gov/pubmed/18936282.
61. Katz LS, Cojucar G, Beheshti S, Nakamura E, Murray M. Military sexual trauma during deployment to Iraq and Afghanistan: prevalence, readjustment, and gender differences. Violence Vict [Internet]. 2012 [cited 4 Feb 2015];27(4):487–99. Available from: http://www.ncbi.nlm.nih.gov/pubmed/22978070.
62. Burns B, Grindlay K, Holt K, Manski R, Grossman D. Military sexual trauma among US servicewomen during deployment: a qualitative study. Am J Public Health. 2014;104(2): 345–9.
63. Ahrens CE. Being silenced: the impact of negative social reactions on the disclosure of rape. Am J Community Psychol [Internet]. 2006 [cited 28 Jan 2015];38(3–4):263–74. Available from: http://www.pubmedcentral.nih.gov/articlerender.fcgi?artid=1705531&tool=pmcentrez &rendertype=abstract.
64. Gibson LE, Leitenberg H. The impact of child sexual abuse and stigma on methods of coping with sexual assault among undergraduate women. Child Abuse Negl [Internet]. 2001 [cited 4 Feb 2015];25(10):1343–61. Available from: http://www.ncbi.nlm.nih.gov/pubmed/11720383.
65. Turchik JA, McLean C, Rafie S, Hoyt T, Rosen CS, Kimerling R. Perceived barriers to care and provider gender preferences among veteran men Who have experienced military sexual trauma: a qualitative analysis. Psychol Serv. 2012;10(2):213–22.

66. Barbara AM, Quandt SA, Anderson RT. Experiences of lesbians in the health care environment. women health [Internet]. 2008 [cited 4 Feb 2015];34(1):45–62. Available from: http://www.researchgate.net/publication/254379423_Experiences_of_Lesbians_in_the_Health_Care_Environment.

67. Shipherd JC, Green KE, Abramovitz S. Transgender clients: identifying and minimizing barriers to mental health treatment. J Gay Lesbian Ment Health [Internet]. 2010 [cited 4 Feb 2015];14(2):94–108. Available from: http://www.researchgate.net/publication/233448568_Transgender_Clients_Identifying_and_Minimizing_Barriers_to_Mental_Health_Treatment.

68. Sherman MD, Kauth MR, Shipherd JC, Street RL. Communication between VA providers and sexual and gender minority veterans : a pilot study. Psychol Serv. 2014;11(2):235–42.

69. Simpson TL, Balsam KF, Cochran BN, Lehavot K, Gold SD. Veterans administration health care utilization among sexual minority veterans. Psychol Serv [Internet]. 2013 [cited 26 Jan 2015];10(2):223–32. Available from: http://www.ncbi.nlm.nih.gov/pubmed/23730965.

70. Shipherd JC, Mizock L, Maguen S, Green KE. Male-to-female transgender veterans and VA health care utilization. Int J Sex Heal [Internet]. Taylor & Francis Group; 2012 [cited 5 Feb 2015];24(1):78–87. Available from: http://www.tandfonline.com/doi/abs/10.1080/19317611.2011.639440?journalCode=wijs20#preview.

71. Chow JC-C, Jaffee K, Snowden L. Racial/ethnic disparities in the use of mental health services in poverty areas. Am J Public Health [Internet]. 2003 [cited 4 Feb 2015];93(5):792–7. Available from: http://www.pubmedcentral.nih.gov/articlerender.fcgi?artid=1447841&tool=pmcentrez&rendertype=abstract.

72. Hausmann LR, Gao S, Mor MK, Schaefer Jr JH, Fine MJ. Understanding racial and ethnic differences in patient experiences with outpatient health care in Veterans Affairs Medical Centers. Med Care [Internet]. 2013;51(6):532–9. Available from: http://journals.lww.com/lww-medicalcare/Abstract/2013/06000/Understanding_Racial_and_Ethnic_Differences_in.9.aspx.

73. Merrill RM, Allen EW. Racial and ethnic disparities in satisfaction with doctors and health providers in the United States. Ethn Dis [Internet]. 2003 [cited 4 Feb 2015];13(4):492–8. Available from: http://www.ncbi.nlm.nih.gov/pubmed/14632269.

74. Smedley BD, Stith AY, Nelson A, editors. Unequal treatment: Confronting racial and ethnic disparities in health care. Washington, DC: The National Academies; 2003.

75. Harrell JP, Hall S, Taliaferro J. Physiological responses to racism and discrimination: an assessment of the evidence. Am J Public Health [Internet]. 2003 [cited 4 Feb 2015];93(2):243–8. Available from: http://www.pubmedcentral.nih.gov/articlerender.fcgi?artid=1447724&tool=pmcentrez&rendertype=abstract.

76. Williams DR, Neighbors HW, Jackson JS. Racial/ethnic discrimination and health: findings from community studies. Am J Public Health [Internet]. 2003 [cited 4 Feb 2015];93(2):200–8. Available from: http://www.pubmedcentral.nih.gov/articlerender.fcgi?artid=1447717&tool=pmcentrez&rendertype=abstract.

77. Gary FA. Stigma: barrier to mental health care among ethnic minorities. Issues Ment Health Nurs. 2005;26:979–99.

78. Loo CM, Fairbank JA, Chemtob CM. Adverse race-related events as a risk factor for posttraumatic stress disorder in Asian American Vietnam veterans. J Nerv Ment Dis [Internet]. 2005 [cited 4 Feb 2015];193(7):455–63. Available from: http://www.ncbi.nlm.nih.gov/pubmed/15985840.

79. Beals J, Manson SM, Shore JH, Friedman M, Ashcraft M, Fairbank JA, et al. The prevalence of posttraumatic stress disorder among American Indian Vietnam veterans: disparities and context. J Trauma Stress [Internet]. 2002 [cited 4 Feb 2015];15(2):89–97. Available from: http://www.ncbi.nlm.nih.gov/pubmed/12013069.

80. Rosenheck R, Fontana A, Cottrol C. Effect of clinician-veteran racial pairing in the treatment of posttraumatic stress disorder. Am J Psychiatry [Internet]. 1995 [cited 4 Feb 2015];152(4):555–63. Available from: http://www.ncbi.nlm.nih.gov/pubmed/7694904.

81. Sigford BJ. Paradigm shift for VA amputation care. J Rehabil Res Dev [Internet]. 2010 [cited 1 Jul 2015];47(4):xv–xix. Available from: http://www.ncbi.nlm.nih.gov/pubmed/20803396.

·82. Ponte CD, Johnson-Tribino J. Attitudes and knowledge about pain: an assessment of West Virginia family physicians. Fam Med [Internet]. [cited 23 Apr 2015];37(7):477–80. Available from: http://www.ncbi.nlm.nih.gov/pubmed/15988631.

83. Green CR, Wheeler JR, Marchant B, LaPorte F, Guerrero E. Analysis of the physician variable in pain management. Pain Med [Internet]. 2001 [cited 23 Apr 2015];2(4):317–27. Available from: http://www.ncbi.nlm.nih.gov/pubmed/15102236.

84. Dobscha SK, Corson K, Flores JA, Tansill EC, Gerrity MS. Veterans affairs primary care clinicians' attitudes toward chronic pain and correlates of opioid prescribing rates. Pain Med. 2008;9(5):564–71.

85. Phelan SM, Griffin JM, Hellerstedt WL, Sayer NA, Jensen AC, Burgess DJ, et al. Perceived stigma, strain, and mental health among caregivers of veterans with traumatic brain injury. Disabil Health J. 2011;4(3):177–84. Elsevier Inc.

86. Spoont MR, Murdoch M, Hodges J, Nugent S. Treatment receipt by veterans after a PTSD diagnosis in PTSD, mental health, or general medical clinics. Psychiatr Serv [Internet]. 2010 [cited 4 Feb 2015];61(1):58–63. Available from: http://www.ncbi.nlm.nih.gov/pubmed/20044419.

87. Harpaz-Rotem I, Rosenheck RA. Serving those who served: retention of newly returning veterans from Iraq and Afghanistan in mental health treatment. Psychiatr Serv [Internet]. 2011 [cited 5 Feb 2015];62(1):22–7. Available from: http://www.ncbi.nlm.nih.gov/pubmed/21209295.

88. Schell TL, Marshall GN. Survey of individuals previously deployed for OEF/OIF. In: Tanielian T, Jaycox LH, editors. Invisible wounds of war: psychological and cognitive injuries, their consequences, and servcies to assist recovery. Santa Monica: RAND Center for Military Health Policy Research; 2008. p. 81–115.

89. Vogt D. Mental health-related beliefs as a barrier to service use for military personnel and veterans: a review. Psychiatr Serv. 2011;62(2):135–42.

90. Hoerster KD. Association of perceived barriers with prospective use of VA mental health care among Iraq and Afghanistan veterans. Psychiatr Serv. 2012;63(4):380.

91. Kehle SM, Polusny MA, Murdoch M, Erbes CR, Arbisi PA, Thuras P, et al. Early mental health treatment-seeking among U.S. national guard soldiers deployed to Iraq. J Trauma Stress [Internet]. 2010 [cited 4 Feb 2015];23(1):33–40. Available from: http://www.ncbi.nlm.nih.gov/pubmed/20104591.

92. Rosen CS, Greenbaum MA, Fitt JE, Laffaye C, Norris VA, Kimerling R. Stigma, help-seeking attitudes, and use of psychotherapy in veterans with diagnoses of posttraumatic stress disorder. J Nerv Ment Dis. 2011;199(11):879–85.

93. Gross ML. Why treat the wounded? Warrior care, military salvage, and national health. Am J Bioeth [Internet]. 2008 [cited 1 Jul 2015];8(2):3–12. Available from: http://www.ncbi.nlm.nih.gov/pubmed/18570066.

94. Magruder KM, Frueh BC, Knapp RG, Davis L, Hamner MB, Martin RH, et al. Prevalence of posttraumatic stress disorder in veterans affairs primary care clinics. Gen Hosp Psychiatry. 2005;27:169–79.

95. Kirchner JE, Ritchie MJ, Pitcock JA, Parker LE, Curran GM, Fortney JC. Outcomes of a partnered facilitation strategy to implement primary care-mental health. J Gen Intern Med [Internet]. 2014 [cited 4 Feb 2015];29 Suppl 4:904–12. Available from: http://www.ncbi.nlm.nih.gov/pubmed/25355087.

96. Pomerantz AS, Kearney LK, Wray LO, Post EP, Mccarthy JF. Mental health services in the medical home in the Department of Veterans Affairs : factors for successful integration. Psychol Serv. 2014;11(3):243–53.

97. Harmon AL, Goldstein ESR, Shiner B, Watts B V. Preliminary findings for a brief posttraumatic stress intervention in primary mental health care. Psychol Serv [Internet]. 2014 [cited 4 Feb 2015];11(3):295–9. Available from: http://www.ncbi.nlm.nih.gov/pubmed/24588106.

98. Szymanski BR, Bohnert KM, Zivin K, McCarthy JF. Integrated care: treatment initiation following positive depression screens. J Gen Intern Med [Internet]. 2013 [cited 23 Feb 2015];28(3):346–52. Available from: http://www.pubmedcentral.nih.gov/articlerender.fcgi?artid=3579958&tool=pmcentrez&rendertype=abstract.

99. Wray LO, Szymanski BR, Kearney LK, McCarthy JF. Implementation of primary care-mental health integration services in the veterans health administration: program activity and associations with engagement in specialty mental health services. J Clin Psychol Med Settings [Internet]. 2012 [cited 8 Feb 2015];19(1):105–16. Available from: http://www.ncbi.nlm.nih.gov/pubmed/22383016.

100. Shiner B, Tang C, Trapp AC, Konrad R, Bar-On I, Watts B V. The provision of mental health treatment after screening: exploring the relationship between treatment setting and treatment intensity. Gen Hosp Psychiatry [Internet]. [cited 4 Feb 2015];36(6):581–8. Available from: http://www.ncbi.nlm.nih.gov/pubmed/25138536.

101. Watts B V, Shiner B, Zubkoff L, Carpenter-Song E, Ronconi JM, Coldwell CM. Implementation of evidence-based psychotherapies for posttraumatic stress disorder in VA specialty clinics. Psychiatr Serv [Internet]. 2014 [cited 23 Feb 2015];65(5):648–53. Available from: http://www.ncbi.nlm.nih.gov/pubmed/24430622.

102. Morland LA, Raab M, Mackintosh M-A, Rosen CS, Dismuke CE, Greene CJ, et al. Telemedicine: a cost-reducing means of delivering psychotherapy to rural combat veterans with PTSD. Telemed J E Health [Internet]. 2013 [cited 4 Feb 2015];19(10):754–9. Available from: http://www.pubmedcentral.nih.gov/articlerender.fcgi?artid=3787338&tool=pmcentrez&rendertype=abstract.

103. Sadler AG, Mengeling MA, Torner JC, Smith JL, Franciscus CL, Erschens HJ, et al. Feasibility and desirability of web-based mental health screening and individualized education for female OEF/OIF reserve and national guard war veterans. J Trauma Stress [Internet]. 2013 [cited 4 Feb 2015];26(3):401–4. Available from: http://www.ncbi.nlm.nih.gov/pubmed/23696367.

104. Ben-Zeev D, Corrigan PW, Britt TW, Langford L. Stigma of mental illness and service use in the military. J Ment Health [Internet]. 2012 [cited 15 Jan 2015];21(3):264–73. Available from: http://www.ncbi.nlm.nih.gov/pubmed/22250849.

105. Greene-Shortridge TM, Britt TW, Castro CA. The stigma of mental health problems in the military. Mil Med. 2007;172(2):157–61.

106. Irwin LG, Fortune DG. Schools-based interventions for reducing stigmatization of acquired brain injury: the role of interpersonal contact and visible impairment. Arch Clin Neuropsychol. 2014;29(2):194–205.

107. Gould M, Greenberg N, Hetherton J. Stigma and the military: evaluation of a PTSD psychoeducational program. J Trauma Stress [Internet]. 2007 [cited 4 Feb 2015];20(4):505–15. Available from: http://www.ncbi.nlm.nih.gov/pubmed/17721966.

108. Patient Satisfaction Survey Data. Unpubl Data, Red Sox Found Massachusetts Gen Hosp Home Base Progr. 2014.

Chapter 13
I Pity the Poor Immigrant: Stigma and Immigration

Schuyler W. Henderson

Introduction: Global Movement, Local Interventions

In 2013, the United Nations Population Division reported a mid-year International Migrant Stock of 231, 522, 215 people [1]. The percentage of immigrants in any country ranged from about 85 % of the population, in the United Arab Emirates, to fractions of a per cent [1]. Multiple factors influence who immigrates and why, including global socioeconomic determinants, safety, politics, work opportunities, health-care needs, and family reunification. In 2013, the majority of immigrants (nearly 59 %) lived in developed countries—North America, Europe, Australia/ New Zealand, and Japan [2]. Of the immigrants in developed countries, 60 % came from developing countries; the large majority of immigrants (86 %) in developing countries came from other developing countries [2].

Immigration may be a global phenomenon, but its demographics arc local. For example, in 2013, the United States was about 14 % immigrant, but 37 % of the population of New York City is foreign born, including nearly 50 % of Queens residents; foreign-born mothers account for 51 % of births in the city [3]. Where are the immigrants coming from? In the United States overall, Mexicans account for approximately 30 % of the immigrants, followed by people from China, India, the Philippines, El Salvador, Vietnam, Cuba, Korea, the Dominican Republic, and Guatemala. In New York City, however, Dominicans are the largest group, but account "for only 12 % of the foreign born. Six countries on the nation's top 10 list—Philippines, El Salvador, Korea, Vietnam, Cuba, and Guatemala—were not

S.W. Henderson
Child and Adolescent Psychiatry, Bellevue Hospital, New York, NY, USA

Department of Child and Adolescent Psychiatry, New York University,
One Park Avenue, 7th Floor, New York, NY 10016, USA
e-mail: schuyler.henderson@nyumc.org

© Springer International Publishing Switzerland 2016
R. Parekh, Ed W. Childs (eds.), *Stigma and Prejudice: Touchstones in Understanding Diversity in Healthcare*, Current Clinical Psychiatry,
DOI 10.1007/978-3-319-27580-2_13

among the city's top ten groups, and the last 3 not even among the city's top 20 groups" [4].

These trends support the notion that, broadly speaking, immigrants make choices about where they will live based on larger socioeconomic factors like work opportunities, health-care availability, and family reunification but these choices are also influenced by their place of origin. For example, 143,770 Bosnians were resettled in the United States between 1993 and 2006, the majority in Chicago and St. Louis, but there were class and religious differences in the Chicago and St. Louis populations that reflected socioeconomic and cultural factors from when they were in Bosnia [5].

The vastly diverse migrant population includes physicians and other health-care workers, as well as those who will come into health-care systems needing care. In health-care systems, among the plethora of policies typical of the modern medical world ranging from hand hygiene to not talking about patients in elevators are ones that reflect medical encounters with immigrants. One increasingly common policy is that if somebody's first or preferred language is not English (not uncommon in a place like New York City with between 200 and 800 languages spoken [3, 6]), a medical interpreter needs to be present for an interview, not the patient's child or uncle, not a passing dietician who speaks a similar language, not the physician's butchered efforts to shout a few words remembered from a college class—a medical interpreter, in person or on the phone.

The policy is in place for a clear medical reason: optimal patient care requires an accurate and nuanced history. Deaf, hard-of-hearing, and non-English speaking patients—the latter group typically comprised of migrants, first-generation citizens, refugees and tourists, and less often second-generation children of immigrants—all deserve optimal care. In the United States, the policy is also a political intervention. It runs counter to a nativist approach that insists, "You're here, you should be speaking English."

Another hospital policy, more controversial on a national scale but adopted by a number of large hospital systems in New York City, is that nobody is turned away on account of immigration status. In an era of widespread and popular anti-immigrant sentiment, policies of this nature are not universally observed, beyond national mandates to provide emergency and obstetric care; in fact, some hospitals have shown themselves to be willing to deport patients who are undocumented [7].

Interpreter services and providing care regardless of immigration status result in better public health: preventing people from getting the medical care they need will not make any population healthier. But these policies also directly resist *stigma*, both in the health-care setting itself and in larger society by setting an example.

Goffman famously defined stigma as a "deeply discrediting" attribute that reduces the bearer "from a whole and usual person to a tainted, discounted one" [8]. These hospital policies oppose stigma precisely because they do not accept that a language or a type of documentation taints somebody as meriting insufficient medical care, nor do they acquiesce to the diminution of a person. Your language or place or birth does not mean you have a less privileged place in the (usually) highly valued doctor-patient relationship.

Why should it matter if hospital systems have interventions that can reduce stigma? What is so bad about stigma, other than its general unpleasantness? Stigma has significant and immediate public health consequences for immigrant communities—and therefore for the communities in which immigrants live. These include frank barriers in access to care, as happens when clinics are expected to check documentation, dissuading people from seeking services, and perceived barriers (e.g., reticence to come to services because of concerns about how you will be perceived in a clinical milieu); there are also barriers in the provision of care, such as decreased services for vulnerable populations (consider pregnant migrants put into detention centers or asthmatic child migrants who are not brought to a primary care physician); and subsequent public health hazards (populations who are suspicious of public health surveillance may be less willing to get treatment for reportable and contagious illnesses).

The ramifications of stigma for already vulnerable populations are pervasive throughout health care. Stigma exacerbates vulnerability. Rarely is stigma applied to the powerful, and inequalities that are pervasive in society disproportionately fall upon those who are more stigmatized; and then social inequalities bleed into worse health-care disparities. This in turn feeds a downward cycle, where, for those already burdened with worse access to health care, stigmatization prevents access, while stigma itself may affect both structural-level and community-level and individual constructions of the self, resulting in less healthy lives [9].

This chapter examines the relationship between anti-immigrant sentiment and stigma in the health-care field, beginning with an examination of the tight parallels between anti-immigrant sentiment and stigma, and how both are often characterized as a "natural" phenomenon. This is followed by a closer examination of three domains where stigma and anti-immigrant sentiment intersect prominently with health, often to the disadvantage of immigrants: in epidemiology, in health-care politics, and in the notion that immigrants harbor more stigma toward medicine (particularly mental health). Given the prominence and power of stigma as rhetoric [10], it is imperative to look at how stigma infiltrates discourses in and around the practice of health care, to reveal the operations of stigma and point to the strategies required to counter its pernicious efficacy. This is followed by a section reviewing ways of countering stigma in relation to immigrants in health care. The chapter ends with concluding thoughts about what, ultimately, an investigation of stigma and anti-immigrant sentiment demands of us. The purpose is to not so much to show that stigma has negative health consequences, which has been adequately and comprehensively demonstrated, but to see *how* this happens in immigrant populations and, ultimately, how stigma is a way of avoiding important questions raised by immigration.

Migration and Stigma

Both stigma and anti-immigrant sentiment can appear to be natural ways of thinking, partly because they are so ubiquitous and partly because, like everything else, they can be given evolutionary explanations: for example, fear of contamination or encroachment into one's own ecological niche and competition for finite resources, respectively. But although they are prevalent and powerful, they are not necessarily natural or instinctive.

The movement of creatures across the Earth is an enduring feature of life itself. From the migration of blue whales across oceans and of monarch butterflies across continents to frogs hopping from pond to pond, creatures move. Geographical movement is an ecological process responsive to fluctuations in temperatures, changes in competition, and the flourishing of edibles, and it is a driving force for evolution, speciation, and diversity; it is why we are not still single cells bubbling in a thermal vent deep under the ocean.

Throughout human history, people have migrated. They have done so for ecological reasons and also with an innate human curiosity about new frontiers. Two million years ago, *Homo erectus* left Africa; approximately 140,000 years ago, *Homo sapiens* spread out across Eurasia and, 12,500 years ago, crossed Beringia into the Americas—these time frames remain a matter of debate, but then controversies are never far from the topic of migration [11, 12].

As humans migrated, they established societies and civilizations, mapping a social geography of families, kinship systems, communities, villages, towns, principalities, sovereign states, countries, and nations, each nurturing languages and customs, over the physical topography of the Earth. Migration became more than a geographical movement; it became a movement across social boundaries into new cultural landscapes, where one might find churches instead of mosques, baklava instead of chocolate sundaes. These differences in the cultural landscapes have provoked shock as well as fascination, fear as well as respect, and disgust as well as desire.

With such strongly evoked emotions, it is not surprising that the history of migration has often been marked by aggressive encounters between peoples: migration has been colonial and exploitative, associated with war, domination, and genocide. Indeed, human history is a long narrative of conquest, atrocities, and violence, in which migrants have been victims, perpetrators, and both.

There is another history of migration, also based on how people experience the emotional and psychological shock of cultural difference. This is the history of migrations that have been peaceful, convivial, and beneficial for both the migrants and those that they arrive among, spurring curiosity, friendships, new ideas, cuisines, and the sharing of expertise and customs. Pleasant though this is, the contentious debates that have always swirled around migration are sometimes more revealing about what is at stake in migration than rose-tinted views of camaraderie, chop suey, and chicken vindaloo. Migration challenges core concepts of who we are: migration challenges the atavistic idea that we belong to or own a particular patch of land or a certain part of our shared Earth, the extent to which we are defined by where we come from and how much of who we are is constituted by our nation, our origins, our race, and our ancestry. Underneath the insults about who is civilized and who is not (in which we are typically more civilized than they are) are difficult questions about the nature of civility itself: what do we owe each other as hosts and guests? What respect do we afford differences within this host-guest relationship?

Stigma is a way of avoiding these questions; it creates a discourse in which these questions are precisely not asked. Stigma takes the problems we face in our encounter with another person (e.g., who are we to make claims about ourselves and our place on Earth, and what do we owe to those who have come to our doorstep?) and insists that the problems belong to them. This is one of the ways, along with intimidation and passion, in which stigma effectively modulates a discourse: it denaturalizes a natural set of problems into another's error or sin, it places the burden of problematization onto the Other, and in doing so, it reifies superiority.

To hear this dynamic in anti-immigrant sentiment, and how close it so often comes to issues of health and hygiene, consider the words of Michael Savage, the radio talk show host: "We're getting refugees now who have never used a telephone, a toothbrush, or toilet paper. You're telling me they're going to assimilate? They will never assimilate. They come here and they bring their destitute ways to this country, and they never assimilate" [13]. The way Savage explains it, the problem is in them. There is no concession that the problem at hand is shared and involves dialogue and blending—how we welcome migrants and how we employ them and protect them and invite them in with the promise of a dream with statues in harbors: these issues are solved by transposing the problem onto their intransigence and their failure to stop being who they are. And they remain marked and lesser; they are, according to Savage, neither competent in the basic modes of civilized conversation and hygiene nor willing to become so.

In this manner, the immigrant is stigmatized as naturally uncivil by those whose ability to detect the natural incivility elevates them into a position of perspicuous civility, a process that simultaneously erases the immigrant's civility and the incivility of the prejudiced. There is no necessarily natural or instinctive basis for anti-immigrant sentiment, but the rhetoric insists that there is and simultaneously justifies the prejudice.

Anti-immigrant sentiment and stigma are natural companions, which is why they so often encounter one another in the biomedical world. Social cognitive models of stigma define the visibilities and assumed relationships as attributions and stereotypes, which then result in prejudice and discrimination (see, e.g., Corrigan [16]). Link and Phelan, ever attentive to the social pragmatics of conceptual models, strive to include these pragmatics within the definitions of the models themselves; they insist that to understand stigma, one has to also account for the role of power. As they say, "it takes power to stigmatize" ([17], pg. 375).

Stigma and anti-immigrant sentiment are rooted in fundamental (and easily manipulated) fears of strangers, of the unknown figure knocking at the door, bearing sickness and contagion; in both, primal, genetic, atavistic sentiments about the dangerousness of the unknown Other are immersed in legendary stories of tribal victory and defeat, danger, toxicity, and undetectable murderousness and then justified by contemporary anecdote, the filters of experience, and the missampling inherent in stories (*crazy person pushes man into subway, immigrant from West Africa taken to hospital with flu*); and in both, links are formed between what is invisible (fears, threats, hidden dangers) and what is visible (the attribute that becomes "deeply discrediting"), in which a relationship is assumed between an invisible underlying danger and the phenotypes. As an example, consider how "bearded" became metonymic with religious terrorism in the years after 9/11 [14, 15].

What is less remarked upon, but worth observing, is how both stigma and anti-immigrant sentiment intimate a secret: a hidden motive, a sneaky propensity toward violence and murder, and a smuggled pathology. In a twist typical of discriminatory practices, the act of stigmatization provides ostensibly self-evident justifications to exert power: the fact that they are exposing their secret with the mark of stigma without divulging it makes them dishonest, spies, and inherently untrustworthy, and they therefore must be excluded.

For this reason, both stigma and anti-immigrant sentiment are associated with physical and psychological pathology and contagion. The bearers of a dangerous secret may be bearers of a dangerous disease, and vice versa, the one being a metaphor for the other. And where there are metaphors of health, there will be real consequences in health-care systems. We now turn to look at how these notions of secrecy and danger infiltrate paradigms for understanding migrants—in other words, how stigma influences medical practices.

Dangerous Secrets: Stigma and Epidemiologies of Immigration

A historical, epidemiologic reality underlies a fear of the transmission of disease through migration, in so far as the movements of people have long been associated with the movements of disease, whether it is the exchange of smallpox and syphilis between the Old World and the New or the spreading of epidemics such as the *Ebola* virus or severe acute respiratory syndrome. But as reflected in Savage's claims, there is also a significant and lengthy history of associating immigration with sickness and morbidity beyond conventional epidemiology, representing a frank, or subtle, belief in the dirtiness and dangerousness of the foreigner: the soiled, the unwashed, the lice-ridden, the shaggy and dissolute bearers of worms, transporting disease and madness from afar. This becomes a way of insisting that there is a natural rationale for anti-immigrant sentiment, which can then shift political stigmatization into the ostensibly neutral realm of public health. And the natural sciences become implicated.

In the *Washington Times*, Stephen Dinan begins a report about a detention facility by saying, "Communicable diseases continue to be a problem at the New Mexico facility built to house illegal immigrant families surging across the U.S.-Mexico border, and the immigrants themselves aren't taking their own health care very seriously, according to an audit released Monday" [18]. What on the surface appears to be a plain opening sentence is profoundly political: the use of the militaristic "surge," not only echoing strategies for the "surge" in Iraq but also, in this case, evoking an invasion: the euphemism of "house" as a verb, when the facility is not so much housing people as preventing them from creating a new house in the United States. Layered over this is the ersatz blandness of public health's passive voice, where communicable diseases "continue to be a problem" (for whom? How?) and the glib, casual slur that immigrants aren't taking their health care very seriously, suggesting some combination of idiocy, ignorance, and savagery. The author of the report, General John Roth, echoes Michael Savage, adding that, "Family unit illnesses and unfamiliarity with bathroom facilities continued to result in unsanitary conditions."

Blame is placed on the immigrants. How an unhealthy situation created by the New Mexico facility is *causing* these problems, rather than the immigrants themselves, is glossed over. Dinan does report that one "hiccup the investigators did find is that some CBP [Customs and Border Protection] officers at one facility weren't trained in how to segregate immigrant children with communicable diseases." This is an impressive act of elision: a single problem was indeed found (so the facility is not perfect!) and yet the problem is not the segregation of these families into a facility, but how to further segregate them. If you recall the notion that stigma involves a dangerous secret, notice how the children themselves are problematized, where the secret, hard-to-detect pathology is located in them; and, in a stunning rhetorical flourish, this problem is a mere hiccup: *they* have disgusting diseases that require quarantine; *we* occasionally get the hiccups—mild, transient, more amusing than worrying, and very public. That is the difference between stigmatizing them and our bemused self-deprecation.

The easy adoption of the empirical tones of public health for perpetuating stigma does not mean that public health is necessarily stigmatizing, but nor can it be ignored how epidemiologies, however neutral they may try to be and however benign their intent, can replicate or reify associations between migration and pathology. The search itself as well as any correlations uncovered suggests that the foreign bear the contagion of the mysterious world from which they've come, carry the parasites, and smuggle in disease and mental disorder.

The principles and work of epidemiological research in immigrant health can be involved closely in policing borders and defining immigrants in such a way that the immigrants will be stigmatized (see, e.g., Davidovitch and Zalashik [19]), but they may also be benevolent, sincere, and efficacious: for example, by identifying health needs (including unfamiliar diseases, or by noting that migration may increase the risk of psychosis [e.g., Cantor-Grae and Selton [20]] or elevated prevalence of PTSD and depression in refugee populations [e.g., Zimbrean [21]]), justifying interventions, determining outcomes, providing focused services, and ensuring that physicians check for etiologies that may not be common in native-born populations.

Nevertheless, recalling that stereotype plus power results in discrimination, the assumption of a foreigner's propensity to disease, whether communicable or not, is put to use to argue for segregation and for imposing rules that control the movement of people. The historical use of real or imagined correlations between migration, illness, and mental illness to create unsatisfactory policy around immigration or to perpetuate myths that then validate prejudice and bigotry requires that we reflect on how epidemiology can be complicit in stigma (for an example from Australia, see Bashford [22]; for a fascinating historical overview of how different locales construct and use epidemiological correlations, see Markel and Stern [23]).

A difference between epidemiological inquiry and the generation of stigma is not just a matter of intent. If epidemiology is bound to the rules of its science, stigma is not so easily contained. One of the pragmatic dangers of stigma is that its boundaries blur so that it can easily adopt the empirical language of epidemiology (for a parallel example, consider how self-interested arguments clamoring for "sound science" usurp very real uncertainties and humilities of scientific inquiry to undermine a political response to the findings of climate science). Scientific ambiguities and imprecisions (e.g., the *risk* of increased psychosis; the ongoing questions as to *why* there is a risk) can bleed into general bigotries, just as studies of populations can be translated into stereotypes. A visceral response to stigma, even when associated with a calmer, more sensitive epidemiology, can generalize into racism and xenophobia, providing a rationale for disenfranchisement.

Such blurring, in epidemiology, is a problem, but the science of epidemiology is designed to restrict the blurring and to relegate it to accident, or chance, using statistical models, as best it can. The blurring associated with stigmatization is not an accident. It is an active process. The rhetoric of stigma blurs boundaries between confidence and speculation, mimicking but undermining the dynamic between confidence and speculation in scientific discourses.

We see this in how the contours of anti-immigrant rhetoric are sharply defined, while the insinuations are simultaneously precise and imprecise, certain but speculative (in much the same way as a stereotype can be simultaneously precise and imprecise, certain but speculative). For example, when a school board did not renew the contract of a principal who reportedly mandated an English-only policy in school, there was an unsurprisingly critical response by commentators in the media, including Laura Ingraham who said,

> You're not helping these kids, right, by giving these kids a sense that they don't have to speak English to get ahead. You do have to speak English to get ahead. You do have to speak English to assimilate. Now a lot of these kids are probably illegal aliens in this school, I would imagine. Right? Maybe some of them have parents who are illegal aliens, and so they have that kind of situation they're dealing with [24].

Speaking Spanish (the appreciable marker) is easily and comfortably associated with criminality ("illegal"). Indeed, speaking Spanish is an indicator itself of a criminal person; it is a smoking gun, a snapshot of someone at the scene of a crime. But the rhetoric is one of cool scrutiny with just enough hedging ("probably," "I would imagine," "maybe") to suggest thoughtfulness. The confidence and hidden uncertainty of stigmatization move from opinion to fact.

Evil Intent: Stigma and the Stealing of Health Care

Ideally, epidemiology seeks to uncover the hidden prevalence of disease in a population; stigma seeks to expose a population to discrimination on account of a hidden danger, a secret that is not being revealed. The hidden danger is typically evil, aggressive intent: often, random murder in the case of the madman, a desire to infect in the case of the sick person, and stealing in the case of the immigrant. The epidemiological discourse around immigration and health can inform the stereotypes of stigma. The health policy discourse around immigration and health care is already heavily informed by stigma—in this case, by cultivating a sense of the immigrants' dangerousness not only through disease but in accusations of theft and exploitation.

Many public, televised debates around health-care policy are infused with the rhetoric of stigma. Immigrants, so essential to the economy, so hard-working, heeding promises made by societies that require immigration so that they have laborers and paying more into the economies and health-care systems than they are taking out of it (see, e.g., Zallman et al. [25]) are treated as though they are thieves, stealing health care. They are implicated in a moral crime that is no crime (wanting decent health care) and told that their movement is somehow intrinsically sneaky (as though nobody else ever sought work for health benefits) and that the health-care system is suffering from their pernicious robberies.

These debates have infused the writing of legislation. The Personal Responsibility and Work Opportunity Reconciliation Act states worriedly that the availability of public benefits would "constitute an incentive for immigration to the United States" [26]. Kullgren observes that there is no evidence that public benefits "lure undocumented immigrants to the United States" [27]. But even if it is true, blaming immigrants for wanting public benefits is a perverse mechanism for making their very ambition (a purportedly celebrated virtue of the immigrant) into a sin. Public infrastructure is a logical and meaningful incentive for migration and indeed is folded into the attractive possibilities of the American Dream.

In the PRWORA, however, and in much of the rhetoric around immigration and US health care, the United States is cast as a victim: they are coming here to steal services we've paid for; they come here to make use of our medical care and to exploit our system. The implication is that the immigrant is no longer the go-getting newcomer drawn to citizenship but rather the thief in the night, the conniving outsider. The shared fear at the heart of stigma and anti-immigrant prejudice is revealed: they are trying to make victims of us.

The PRWORA, however, still allows for "emergency medical care" and "immunizations with respect to immunizable diseases and for testing and treatment of symptoms of communicable diseases whether or not such symptoms are caused by a communicable disease." These have significant pragmatic ramifications for the delivery of barebones public health provisions and recognize a fundamental moral need to provide the most basic and immediate medical care. Kullgren, however, identifies multiple public health problems associated with this approach (including, e.g., a lack of preventative care that would *prevent* people from showing up with a chronic but untreated illness for emergency care) [27]. The medicolegal act also frames "aliens" as people with sly, selfish goals, as leeches on the body politic, and then imagines them as bloody, damaged beings (careless enough to require emergency services) who probably have dangerous diseases (need immunizations) and are trying to have children here (dropping their anchor babies on American soil).

Even as PRWORA construes health-care systems as the victim and diminishes immigrants, there is an ethical halo: a Good Samaritan beneficence in the provision of emergency care and a worldly Public Health perspective in providing immunizations (even if the public health effects of this act are counterproductive), giving the enactment an imprimatur of *our* ethics, community orientation, and science against *their* sneaky, insidious thievery. It should be understood that health-care systems or practitioners that limit the care they are willing to provide to groups of people to emergency and prenatal care are not operating essential medical services; they are providing moral cover for their failure to do so while promoting stigmatizing perceptions of those populations.

Health-Care Stigma Within Immigrant Communities

But what about stigma and health *within* immigrant communities themselves? Stigmatizing others can exist within stigmatized populations: indeed, stigma is no barrier to stigma. It has been suggested that stigma around physical and mental health is more prevalent in immigrant populations [28–30] and that this subsequently results in suboptimal care (e.g., Wynaden et al. [31], and Interian et al. [32]). There are three notes of caution to inject here.

First, it is worth questioning whether the concept of stigma is being used to explain unfamiliarity with a new system (which may manifest in reticence, awkwardness, discomfort, and embarrassment, not dissimilar to the shame so often associated with stigma). Returning to the *Washington Times* article, notice how the delivery of services is characterized:

> Part of the issue is the immigrants themselves, some of whom have never seen a doctor before, don't follow up afterward, either for themselves or their children.
> "If detainees do not attend sick call or stand in line to receive daily medications, they remain sick and their illnesses tend to get worse," the inspector general said.

In this overcrowded facility, who among the inmates knows how to attend "sick call," and when to stand in line, and what for? Would a journalist or inspector general know the procedures and regulations and organization of health care should they suddenly show up in a detention facility in a foreign country? Would they know how to "follow up," either for themselves or their children? Explanations for why people do not seek services require an inside-out approach, not an overarching explanation of "stigma" [32] or, as in the Dinan article, the intimation of ignorance or callousness.

Second, it has been argued that stigma may be related to how people present to services and, in particular, that somatic complaints replace psychological ones because the stigma associated with what is perceived as psychological illness is greater than with what is perceived as physiological illness. For example, colleagues treating children in an emergency room argued that children in one population came in with headaches and neurological symptoms because those symptoms were less stigmatized than underlying anxiety, which was more often the etiology of these symptoms. This somatization hypothesis has been challenged, for example, in a study by Montesinos et al. [34] in female Turkish migrants. The somatization hypothesis also reflects a bias: somatic symptoms are very much part of psychopathology [34] and may be understood as such in native-born populations but then perceived as excuses, or a response to stigma, in non-native-born population. To put it another way, the assumption that we recognize somatic symptoms but they do not is infused with the stigma associated with foreignness: they are doing something devious with their somatic symptoms, masking the reality of the disorder, while they are also more bodily, less conscious of their minds.

Stigma toward people with physical and mental disorders will be present in migrant communities, but cannot be seen as a sole, or even predominant, explanatory for how migrants access health-care services or communicate within those services. Stigma is produced within cultures, and as cultures are diverse, when it does appear, it will appear differently in different populations [29, 36]. In one study that looked at stigma and depression in immigrant and native-born women, Nadeem et al. [37] showed ethnic differences in stigma (measured by three questions about what might keep people from services: "being embarrassed to talk about personal matters with others," "being afraid of what others might think," and "family members might not approve") and found that in immigrant women in general, elevated perceptions of stigma was correlated with less help seeking. But Nadeem et al. also show how perceptions of stigma may be less powerful than expected: the very same research found that immigrant Latinas were most likely to want mental health care and were among the most likely to report stigma [37].

Any assumption that immigrants attach more stigma to health is itself problematic. In fact, what happens is that migrants' presumed treatment of a stigmatized population (the mentally ill, epileptics, etc.) becomes stigmatizing. For example, migrants are stigmatized as people who do not understand the reality of psychiatric or medical illness, in part because of their presumed cruelty to people who have these illnesses. The discourse around stigma may reproduce the stigma, exoticism, and stereotyping, cultivating the view that the migrant is more primitive and therefore more likely to have lurid, theological, unenlightened views of mental illness.

Finally, when examining stigma within migrant communities, there may be a parallel cultural gamesmanship at work, where health services are imagined as operating in cultural opposition to "traditional" services (despite findings that, e.g., in Cambodian refugees in the United States, use of alternative and complementary medicine was positively associated with an increased use of "Western" providers [38].

Countering Stigma Around Immigration Within Health Care

So how do we address stigma? How do we address stigma toward, and within, vulnerable populations? A primary way of addressing stigma is through education and public relations campaigns: advertisements in newspapers and billboards on subway walls. Interventions of this type assume that stigma or prejudice is a natural state, albeit an ignorant one, that can be counteracted with more information. This, unfortunately, is just scratching the surface. Anti-stigma campaigns that address the symptoms of stigma—isolation, internalization, and misunderstandings—through peer support may be more effective (see, e.g., Yang et al. [39]), but many campaigns involve spending money at ad agencies and in glossy magazines without much evidence of efficacy.

Within a health-care setting, in order to address stigma against migrant populations, an individual approach of respect for migration can be adopted. When working with immigrant populations, health-care workers can begin by not treating migration as a single event, but a process, typically divided up into pre-migration, migration, and post-migration, all of which can be useful for a clinical history but also for understanding the person (see Table 13.1).

Clinical attentiveness to immigrants in the individual encounter can be cultivated in health-care systems. A more politically active approach can be more effective at reducing stigma. Identifying and fighting stigma through policy and legislation against discrimination have been effective against stigma around certain illnesses in certain places and times (consider the partial success in reducing stigma around HIV in some, but not all, parts of the world). This tends to be more effective around physical illness and less effective with mental illness and with immigration (even in racist societies, frank racism is less acceptable than anti-immigrant rhetoric). Why is this the case? There are certainly compounding effects (e.g., class and race,

Table 13.1 Using a tripartite model to explore migration

Pre-migration	Tell me about the reasons why you left your home country. What are the things that compelled you to leave? What are the things that attracted you to coming here? What happened prior to departure?
Migration	Tell me about your journey here and any challenges you might have had along the way. How did you get to where you are now? Did your whole family come at the same time, or were you separated for a while? How was that separation for you?
Post-migration	Tell me about the family and friends you left behind. How do you keep in touch with them? Do they plan to come join you? Describe any concerns about your life right now. What are you most happy about? What are your plans looking ahead? What do you hope to achieve? Where are you going to find support here?

Adapted from Henderson SW, Sung D, and Baily C [citation from immigration chapter in cultural diversity book]

socioeconomic drift, and legal problems) that compound stigma around immigration and the relative concealability of the stigmatized features [40].

Another reason why stigma is so hard to dissociate from immigration and mental illness is that the categories of foreignness and madness are so heterogeneous and so mutable that stigma itself helps us understand what they are, in a way that is not necessarily true of, say, racial stigma, sexual stigma, or stigma around physical disability. Stigma around madness helps us define mental illness; stigma around immigration helps us identify the targets of anti-immigrant policy. Stigma is not an ideal way of making sense of immigration and mental illness, to say the least, but recognizing its role here is necessary to avoid two pitfalls: romanticism and fungibility.

Romanticism, in this case, is when mental illness and immigration fall prey to an anti-stigmatic correction where the stigma is flipped on its head. In this case, the madness or anti-immigrant sentiment no longer provokes disgust; it provokes desire; the secret is now purportedly enviable, rather than dangerous. The process is similar to when supposedly positive stereotypes are used to replace negative ones, purportedly countering stigma. We see this when the immigrant is not seen as hiding a dangerous secret, but where the secret is a delicious mystery (usually exotic or erotic) or when the madman whose secret is not a desire to attack but a connection with the otherworldly or creativity itself. Romanticism may be more pleasant than stigma in its mood, but it is not a counter to stigma; it replicates the workings of stigma, only it is excited about the secret, instead of fearing it.

The other pitfall is fungibility: this is when there is an attempt to change stigmatized language in order to replace the stigmatized concept, but the stigma merely follows along. A long-standing example is the trail of the words used to describe what it is currently called intellectual disability. As *moron*, *imbecile*, and *idiot* gave way to *mental subnormality* and *mental handicap*, through to *mentally retarded*, the theoretically unstigmatized terms became markers of stigma [41]. Stigma is fungible: it can move unchanged into whatever is thought to replace it.

Education and polite advocacy risk more than just a romanticism or fungibility; they risk tepid success or frank failure. Given the widespread use of madness as pejorative (*crazy* or *lunatic* is ubiquitous in political debates), how prisons are repositories for many with mental illness, and the marginalization of mental health in the health-care system, and the widespread proliferation of anti-immigrant sentiment, the casual imprisonment of immigrants at borders, and the ease with which medical care can be refused immigrants, it is clear that the efforts of many in these arenas have been marginally successful at best. If the underlying mechanisms of stigma are not addressed, the stigma will confound the sentimental efforts of romanticizing and the attempt to change attitudes only through a change in language. So how can stigma be addressed?

A broader approach to defeating stigma is to foster the principle of welcome (see, e.g., Lobo [43]). Instead of putting up barriers to protect hospitals from migrants, hospitals can welcome migrants, with policies like those described at the beginning of the chapter—having medical interpreter services and not checking migration status. Stigma traffics in insinuation, suspicion, and implication to drive people away; principles of welcome bring people in by opening up communication to confront or dispel insinuation and implication, and contact can bring about a leap into trust that no dangerous secret is being harbored. Religious traditions are full of examples of moments when instead of driving somebody away, arms are flung open in welcome, a celebration of shared humanity: popes hugging people with diseases, priests caring for the contagious, and churches becoming sanctuaries to prevent immigrants from being deported [44]. This can be a model for medicine as well.

There are limits to an attitude of welcome as a cure to stigma. The leper may appreciate the papal touch and still may not want to be reduced to a symbol of the Godliness and compassion in another. Cosmopolitanism [45], welcome, and miscegenation appropriate difference from the grips of stigma and make those differences interesting. But people don't necessarily want to be interesting; people do not want to be specimens explaining themselves. Patients may want culturally competent doctors, nurses, social workers, and other care providers, but they may not want their culture of origin to excite the physician. This is the thorny area where curiosity meets microaggression, with prickly questions like "But where are you from?" or "Where is your family from?"

Nevertheless, patronizing, pitying, or curious breaches of difference may be better conversations to be having than stigmatizing cries for quarantine or murder, and they are conversations where common grounds can be found, misunderstandings negotiated, and core values not only espoused but interrogated (see, e.g., Derrida [46]).

These principles become more powerful when they become enforced. Responses can begin in individual, local, policy-based interventions in health-care systems, as noted at the outset of this chapter with hospital policies that guarantee medical interpreters and that refuse to make their services dependent upon citizenship documentation. Comprehensive policies can guarantee that immigration status is not a barrier to services while addressing real concerns, like language and paperwork.

In the fields of health, this means:

1. Identifying the bigotry and prejudice in rhetoric that uses, or abuses, the tools and concepts of epidemiology, medicine, and psychiatry to isolate and stigmatize immigrants, such as political practices acting as though they are public health ventures: prison camps for immigrants are not places where people are "housed"; the public health problems associated with the prison camps are not because the imprisoned families are immigrants.
2. The next step is recognizing how effective these rhetorics are at cultivating and naturalizing stigma toward immigrant populations when they become legitimized. Policies and laws based in stigma must be opposed, even if they appear to have a Good Samaritan halo, such as the presumed beneficence of the PRWORA.
3. Partner with powerful institutions to delegitimize how they or their representatives participate in the social sanctioning of stigma against immigrants (an example of this process is when the American Psychiatric Association formally rejected the association of homosexuality with mental illness in 1973, followed by the American Psychological Association [42]). The same organizations can wholeheartedly refuse to participate in practices that stigmatize immigrants, including, for example, taking stands against those that require their practitioners refuse services to some or any migrant populations.

4. Contextualize the stigma. *The stigma is operating effectively for a reason.* Addressing stigma requires understanding and addressing the political power of stigma and therefore the structures that benefit from the stigma. To see how these operate in action, immigrants are stigmatized as sickly people who are coming to steal for a health-care system they did not pay for. In one respect at least, incorporating stigma into debates about health care is distraction. The notion that the world's hordes are begging to get health care in the United States is a comforting one, but illusory, based in patriotism and exceptionalism that serves a dual purpose: if the system is so great, we do not need to pay more for it (while its deficits are not a function of funding, but of exploitation by immigrants); and stigma in health-care debates pulls the eye away from the extent to which public health care has atrophied and how health-care dollars are siphoned into private insurance and investors.

   It is also part of a larger attack on public institutions: we need private health care, so that we can ensure that "illegals" don't get what they don't deserve. Let us be clear: the stigma about immigration and public health-care funding benefits those who would use the contagions of stigma to poison public institutions. Addressing this stigma needs to address these larger issues: empowering and financing public institutions not from a position of the phony Good Samaritan (as we see in PRWORA) but as essential, cost-effective, cost-reducing, disparity-reducing public health investments.

5. Understand the role of those generating the stigma and make them accountable for it [41]. Stigma is an intentional misunderstanding; a misunderstanding is not nonsense, surreal, or absurd, but a mishandling of the truth, a misapprehension of the real. Stigma falls into the category of misunderstandings that are not susceptible to simple correction and are reinforced not just by selective sampling of facts but by the benefits that accrue to stigmatizing. A misunderstanding of the Krebs cycle could be corrected. The misunderstanding fomented by stigma is protected from correction through cognitive strategies (particularly the metaphorical grain of truth; latching onto that grain of truth as synecdochal for a whole truth), emotional bluster, and its own vindictive logic: the problem is not in the attributions of stigma, but in the stigmatized, where if there is "misunderstanding," then the "mis" belongs to the stigmatized. Anti-stigma campaigns should therefore be addressed to those who are stigmatizing and they should address not only the stereotypes and the discrimination, but the benefits the stigmatizing are accruing from the stigma.

Conclusion

Migration is fundamental to human nature. This has produced great adventures and great changes in cultures and societies but has also posed, and continues to pose, great challenges, particularly in how we see ourselves and others. For health-care providers and researchers, these challenges cannot be ignored. The close parallels between stigma and anti-immigrant sentiment become visible in the encounter between migrants and health-care systems, influencing epidemiology and health policy and affecting the delivery of care for individual migrants. To address the problems of stigma and anti-immigrant sentiment, it is important to discern how stigma influences interventions that do not appear to be directly influenced by stigma and to move beyond education campaigns to address root causes.

Future Directions

All too often, stigma is a general explanation for diffuse if powerful experiences of exclusion, encompassing many different experiences, social pressures, and expectations. Research can be conducted into more precise dissection of stigma and the actual mechanisms through which stigma prevents people from getting care (see, e.g., the work of Paterson et al. [47] on how stigma has been researched in populations with hepatitis C). Given the extent to which anti-stigma initiatives are informed by the research, more granularity and specificity in understanding stigma will improve interventions and prevent naïve or stigmatizing perpetuations of stigma.

At the same time, returning stigma to broader social contexts will guide comprehensive principles for anti-stigma initiatives. Immigration, sickness, and madness generate the types of fear produced by difference—unfamiliar looks, tongues, attitudes, and customs and practices—indicating that the Other is not quite human: an animal, a predator, a monster (see, e.g., Santa Ana [48]; Casanavo [49]). Stigma is a way of acting on this difference to turn the fear into a social practice.

In research and anti-stigma initiatives, stigma is seen as a bad thing, understandably so. But another question needs to be asked: why does stigma attach itself to a particular difference at a particular point in time? In this chapter, the discussion has revolved around connections—metaphorical, real, and stigmatized—between sickness, madness, and foreignness. These connections do not adequately or wholly elucidate an affinity or correlation between illness and foreignness, but rather describe a common pathway in how difference is understood and then stigmatized. *Why* is stigma operating so effectively here and mapping itself over this connection between illness and foreignness? One could argue that stigma is itself fundamentally, if metaphorically, a confused, sick, foreign response to difference, or, alternatively, that concepts of sickness and madness necessarily imply the kinds of difference that can be exploited and magnified in stigma. To put it another way, stigma *adequately* describes a confused, foreign response to difference that constitutes the categories of immigration, sickness, and madness.

Migration challenges core concepts of who we are. Madness and sickness also challenge core concepts of who we are: our identities, our moods, our rationality, our bodies, our mortality. Where these entwine with the five components of stigma identified by Link and Phelan [50]—a socially salient difference, stereotyping, differentiation into "us" and "them," active discrimination, and the exercise of power—the questions are lost and displaced onto another, who is defined, derided, and disempowered.

Confronting stigma against migrant populations, then, is not simply a matter of education or protest. It entails a willingness to ask those questions about oneself, one's own ownership of selfhood and of a place (in geography, in society), as well as one's indebtedness to and trust in others, without foreclosing the answer. Defeating stigma against migrant populations means being able to address hard questions in oneself, not in others.

References

1. United Nations. Global migration database. 2014. Available at: http://www.un.org/en/development/desa/population/migration/data/empirical2/index.shtml. Accessed 18 June 2015.
2. United Nations. International migration report 2013. 2013. Available at: http://www.un.org/en/development/desa/population/publications/pdf/migration/migrationreport2013/Full_Document_final.pdf#zoom=100.
3. Department of City Planning. Population facts. 2015. Available at: http://www.nyc.gov/html/dcp/html/census/pop_facts.shtml. Accessed 25 June 2015.
4. Department of City Planning. The newest New Yorkers (2013 ed.). 2013. Available at: http://www.nyc.gov/html/dcp/pdf/census/nny2013/nny_2013.pdf. Accessed 25 June 2015.
5. Palmer JR. Patterns of settlement following forced migration: the case of Bosnians in the United States. 2014. Available at: http://johnrbpalmer.com/BosnianMigrants.pdf. Accessed 25 June 2015.
6. Turin M. New York, a graveyard for languages. BBC News Magazine. 2012. Available at: www.bbc.co.uk/news/magazine-20716344. Accessed 25 June 2015.
7. Monga P, Keller A, Venters H. Prevention and punishment: barriers to accessing health services for undocumented immigrants in the United States. Laws. 2014;3(1):50–60.
8. Goffman E. Stigma: notes on the management of spoiled identity. Englewood Cliffs: Prentice-Hall; 1963.
9. Viruell-Fuentes EA, Miranda PY, Abdulrahim S. More than culture: structural racism, intersectionality theory, and immigrant health. Soc Sci Med. 2012;75(12):2099–106.
10. Soderlund M. Role of news media in shaping and transforming the public perception of Mexican immigration and the laws involved. Law Psychol Rev. 2007;31:167.
11. Pearson OM. Africa: the cradle of modern people. In: The origins of modern humans: biology reconsidered. Hoboken: Wiley; 2013. p. 1–43.
12. Waters MR, Wier Stafford T. The first Americans: a review of the evidence for the late-pleistocene peopling of the Americas. In: Paleoamerican odyssey. College Station: Center for the Study of the First Americans; 2013. p. 541–60.
13. Aronow Z. Media matters. Posted on 25 June 2008. Available at: http://mediamatters.org/video/2008/06/25/savage-were-getting-refugees-now-who-have-never/143856. Accessed 18 Mar 2015.
14. Horry R, Wright DB. Anxiety and terrorism: automatic stereotypes affect visual attention and recognition memory for White and Middle Eastern faces. Appl Cogn Psychol. 2009;23(3):345–57.
15. Kapitan L. Imagine the other: drawing on art therapy to reduce hate and violence. Art Ther. 2012;29(3):102–3.
16. Corrigan PW. Mental health stigma as social attribution: implications for research methods and attitude change. Clin Psychol Sci Pract. 2000;7(1):48–67.
17. Link BG, Phelan JC. Conceptualizing stigma. Annu Rev Sociol. 2001;27:363–85.

18. Dinan S. Disease plagues illegal immigrants; lack of medications, basic hygiene blamed. Washington Times. 6 Oct 2014. Available at: http://www.washingtontimes.com/news/2014/oct/6/diseases-still-problem-illegal-immigrant-families/#ixzz3W5jRP600. Accessed 17 Apr 2015.
19. Davidovitch N, Zalashik R. Medical borders: historical, political, and cultural analyses. Sci Context. 2006;19(03):309–16.
20. Cantor-Graae E, Selten JP. Schizophrenia and migration: a meta-analysis and review. Am J Psychiatr. 2005;162(1):12–24.
21. Zimbrean P. Risk factors and prevalence of mental illness in refugees. In: Refugee health care. New York: Springer; 2014. p. 149–62.
22. Bashford A. At the border contagion, immigration, nation. Aust Hist Stud. 2002;33(120): 344–58.
23. Markel H, Stern AM. Which face? Whose nation? Immigration, public health, and the construction of disease at America's ports and borders, 1891–1928. Am Behav Sci. 1999;42(9): 1314–31.
24. Uwimana S. Media matters. Posted on 20 Mar 2014. http://mediamatters.org/research/2014/03/20/right-wing-media-seize-on-principals-spanish-sp/198556. Accessed 17 Apr 2015.
25. Zallman L, Woolhandler S, Himmelstein D, Bor D, McCormick D. Immigrants contributed an estimated $115.2 billion more to the Medicare trust fund than they took out in 2002–09. Health Aff. 2013;32(6):1153–60.
26. Personal Responsibility and Work Opportunity Reconciliation Act (PRWORA). Pub L No. 104–193, 110 Stat 2260.
27. Kullgren JT. Restrictions on undocumented immigrants' access to health services: the public health implications of welfare reform. Am J Public Health. 2003;93(10):1630–3.
28. Perlick DA. Special section on stigma as a barrier to recovery: introduction. Psychiatr Serv. 2001;52:1613–4.
29. Chung K, Ivey SL, Guo W, Chung K, Nguyen C, Nguyen C, Chung C, Tseng W. Knowledge, attitudes, and practice toward epilepsy (KAPE): a survey of Chinese and Vietnamese adults in the United States. Epilepsy Behav. 2010;17(2):221–7.
30. Cook TM, Wang J. Descriptive epidemiology of stigma against depression in a general population sample in Alberta. BMC Psychiatry. 2010;10(1):29.
31. Wynaden D, Chapman R, Orb A, McGowan S, Zeeman Z, Yeak S. Factors that influence Asian communities' access to mental health care. Int J Ment Health Nurs. 2005;14(2):88–95.
32. Interian A, Martinez IE, Guarnaccia PJ, Vega WA, Escobar JI. A qualitative analysis of the perception of stigma among Latinos receiving antidepressants. Psychiatr Serv. 2007;58(12): 1591–4.
33. Castro A, Farmer P. Understanding and addressing AIDS-related stigma: from anthropological theory to clinical practice in Haiti. Am J Public Health. 2005;95(1):53–9.
34. Montesinos AH, Rapp MA, Temur-Erman S, Heinz A, Hegerl U, Schouler-Ocak M. The influence of stigma on depression, overall psychological distress, and somatization among female Turkish migrants. Eur Psychiatry. 2012;27:S22–6.
35. Ritsner M, Ponizovsky A, Kurs R, Modai I. Somatization in an immigrant population in Israel: a community survey of prevalence, risk factors, and help-seeking behavior. Am J Psychiatry. 2000;157(3):385–92.
36. Weiss MG, Jadhav S, Raguram R, et al. Psychiatric stigma across cultures: local validation in Bangalore and London. Anthropol Med. 2001;8:71–87.
37. Nadeem E, Lange JM, Edge D, Fongwa M, Belin T, Miranda J. Does stigma keep poor young immigrant and US-born black and Latina women from seeking mental health care? Psychiatr Serv. 2007;58(12):1547–54.
38. Berthold SM, Wong E, Schell T, Marshall G, Elliott M, Takeuchi D, Hambarsoomians K. US Cambodian refugees' use of complementary and alternative medicine for mental health problems. Psychiatr Serv. 2007;58(9):1212–8.

39. Yang LH, Lai GY, Tu M, Luo M, Wonpat-Borja A, Jackson VW, Lewis-Fernández R, Dixon L. A brief anti-stigma intervention for Chinese immigrant caregivers of individuals with psychosis: adaptation and initial findings. Transcult Psychiatry. 2014;51(2):139–57.
40. Chaudoir SR, Earnshaw VA, Andel S. "Discredited" versus "discreditable": understanding how shared and unique stigma mechanisms affect psychological and physical health disparities. Basic Appl Soc Psychol. 2013;35(1):75–87.
41. Cheshire JR, William P. Dignifying intellectual disability. Ethics Med. 2014;30(2):71.
42. Herek GM. Sexual stigma and sexual prejudice in the United States: a conceptual framework. In: Contemporary perspectives on lesbian, gay, and bisexual identities. New York: Springer; 2009. p. 65–111.
43. Lobo M. Gestures of judgement and welcome in public spaces: hypervisible migrant newcomers in Darwin, Australia. J Cult Geogr. 2015;32(1):54–67.
44. Dinan S. Church network offers sanctuary to illegal immigrants to avoid deportation. Washington Times. 14 Sept 2014. Available at: http://www.washingtontimes.com/news/2014/sep/24/sanctuary-2014-church-network-helping-illegal-immi/. Accessed on 24 June 2015.
45. Hannerz U. Cosmopolitanism. In: A companion to the anthropology of politics. Malden: Blackwell; 2004. p. 69–85.
46. Derrida J. On cosmopolitanism and forgiveness, translated by Mark Dooley and Michael Hughes with a preface by Simon Critchley and Richard Kearney. London/New York: Routledge; 2001.
47. Paterson BL, Backmund M, Hirsch G, Yim C. The depiction of stigmatization in research about hepatitis C. Int J Drug Policy. 2007;18(5):364–73.
48. Santa Ana O. Like an animal I was treated: anti-immigrant metaphor in US public discourse. Discourse Soc. 1999;10(2):191–224.
49. Casanova H. Commentary: undocumented immigrants being dehumanized. 2007. Available at: http://archives.gcah.org/xmlui/bitstream/handle/10516/4250/article45.aspx.htm?sequence=2. Accessed 10 Apr 2015.
50. Link BG, Phelan JC. Stigma and its public health implications. Lancet. 2006;367(9509):528–9.

Part II
Innovative Ways to Bridge Differences

Chapter 14
Limited English-Proficient (LEP) Patients: The Importance of Working with Trained Medical Interpreters to Promote Equitable Healthcare

Katia M. Canenguez and Anabela M. Nunes

Introduction

Approximately 60 million people in the United States speak a language other than English at home. Half of these individuals report that they speak English less than "very well." These individuals are considered to have limited English proficiency (LEP). Linguistic barriers can lead to patient misunderstanding of treatment, misdiagnosis, significant delays in treatment, patient's poor decision-making, ethical compromises (e.g., difficulty obtaining informed consent, medical errors, and patients not being given all available options of care), and rise in the cost of medical care. Overall, linguistic barriers have been associated with lower healthcare access and poorer physical and mental health. Providing medical interpreter services is vital to promoting equitable healthcare and in overcoming the stigma and prejudice that can be associated with being a patient with LEP.

Effective communication is achieved not only by addressing linguistic barriers but also by better understanding the various cultural beliefs patients hold in relation to healthcare. When learning about a patient's culture, healthcare providers can become aware of their patient's (as well as their own) prejudices and biases. This awareness can help healthcare providers think about ways of providing culturally sensitive services.

K.M. Canenguez, PhD, EdM (✉)
Department of Child and Adolescent Psychiatry,
Massachusetts General Hospital, Yawkey Center for Outpatient
Care 55 Fruit Street, Boston, MA 02114, USA
e-mail: kcanenguez@mgh.harvard.edu

A.M. Nunes, MBA
Interpreter Services, Massachusetts General Hospital, Boston, MA USA

© Springer International Publishing Switzerland 2016
R. Parekh, Ed W. Childs (eds.), *Stigma and Prejudice: Touchstones in Understanding Diversity in Healthcare*, Current Clinical Psychiatry,
DOI 10.1007/978-3-319-27580-2_14

Providing culturally appropriate services can improve communication, access to healthcare, and eventually health outcomes. In the following chapter, the authors will discuss the role of the medical interpreter, the importance of effective communication, the benefits of partnering with medical interpreters in meeting hospital-wide quality and safety requirements, how partnering with medical interpreters helps to reduce the overall cost of delivering healthcare, and how healthcare providers can partner with medical interpreters to improve the quality of care and health outcomes in LEP patients. Medical interpreters are instrumental in bridging the communication gap when there are language and cultural differences. The goal of this chapter is to make the reader aware of both the established and innovative ways in which working with medical interpreters can help in overcoming the stigma and prejudice that can be associated with being a patient with LEP.

The authors would like make note that in this book chapter, the term "healthcare provider" refers to clinicians, researchers, and healthcare educators. Patient cases will be presented to help illustrate several of the topics discussed. Some of these cases are well known in the medical literature, and others will be blended cases shared by colleagues from various institutions.

Who Is the Medical Interpreter?

Gricelda Zamora, a 13-year-old daughter of Spanish-speaking parents, often served as the interpreter whenever the parents needed to communicate with English-speaking persons. When Gricelda herself got sick with severe abdominal pain and was rushed to the hospital, no interpreter was provided for the parents. After a pregnancy test, she was discharged with a diagnosis of gastritis. The parents were told to bring her back if symptoms worsened, otherwise to follow up with a doctor in 3 days [1]. Without a medical interpreter, what the parents understood was to follow up with a doctor in 3 days. After 2 days however, Gricelda got sicker and the parents brought her back. By then it was too late and Gricelda died from a ruptured appendix.

There is no question that effective communication is essential to deliver quality and safe care, contributing to overall good outcomes; that it is critical to ensure that patients are able to follow instructions and adhere to treatment plans; and that this can be accomplished by partnering with professional medical interpreters.

Medical interpreters are professionals who are fluent in at least two languages, one of which is English, who are trained and proficient in the skills and ethics of medical interpretation and have extensive knowledge in medical terminology and concepts in both languages to be able to facilitate accurate, complete, and impartial medical interpretation between a healthcare provider and a non-English or limited English-proficient (LEP) patient or family. The work of the professional medical interpreter is to foster the therapeutic relationship between patient and healthcare

Table 14.1 The roles of the professional medical interpreter

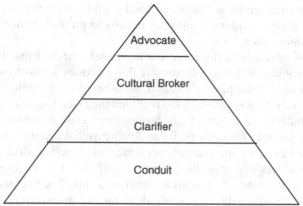

provider by facilitating direct and effective communication. The authors would like to point out that research has not been consistent, and several papers have used the term *bilingual* (i.e., speaks two languages) to refer to interpreters who speak more than two languages. For the sake of this chapter, the authors will use the term bilingual, taking into consideration that there are medical interpreters who speak more than two languages.

Medical interpreters have different roles within the medical encounter, and they move between these roles seamlessly as necessary to ensure good communication and understanding. The roles of the medical interpreter are conduit, clarifier, cultural broker, and advocate [2]. Often, these roles are depicted as a pyramid to show the more predominant role at the base of the pyramid; and the roles less often assumed as the pyramid reaches its apex (Table 14.1). As a conduit the medical interpreter renders a message from one language into another, without adding or omitting information and without changing the message. Medical interpreters are skilled in managing the flow of communication, they have participants speak in turns and allow for each speaker to finish, including the medical interpreter, before speaking. This is by far the role which medical interpreters assume most of the time.

As message clarifiers, medical interpreters pay close attention to terminology or concepts that may be difficult to understand by the patient, by the healthcare provider, and by the medical interpreter. In order for medical interpreters to be effective conduits, they must first fully understand the original message. If the message and the intended meaning are not clear, then medical interpreters will ask the healthcare provider or the patient to explain terminology or concepts.

Medical interpreters at times must also provide cultural context while interpreting when they feel that there may be confusion due to cultural misunderstandings. Cultural values vary greatly among individuals. Each person experiences culture based on a variety of factors, such as socioeconomic status, education, and life experiences. In an encounter you may have various cultures at play, and cultures play a part in how you interpret information. In a medical encounter, you have the healthcare provider's culture, the patient's culture, the medical interpreter's culture, and the Western healthcare culture. Although the medical interpreters are by no means cultural experts, they can offer healthcare providers and patients cultural context as needed to promote understanding and effective communication.

The role of advocate is the more controversial role and one that medical interpreters may choose to take on only if those actions support better clinical outcomes and only if the patient's health, well-being, and dignity are compromised; and no other interventions have resolved the issue [3]. The reason is that one of the fundamental tenets of the professional code of ethics for medical interpreters is the need for impartiality and professional distance. Being impartial ensures that the communication is accurate and objective. Both patients and healthcare providers can trust the objectivity of the interpretation when the medical interpreter is not seen as taking anyone's side. The professional medical interpreter could easily be perceived as having greater power within an encounter due to the understanding of both languages. Therefore, medical interpreters must skillfully navigate the role of advocate in order to ensure objective, quality interpretation.

When Should You Request a Medical Interpreter?

The United States is becoming increasingly more diverse, and the number of LEP individuals continues to grow. According to the US Census data, the Hispanic population grew by 43 % between 2000 and 2010 [4]. Additionally, according to the 2011 American Community Survey Report, approximately 21 % of the US population speaks a language other than English at home. That's approximately 60 million people. And of those about 25 million have self-identified as speaking English less than very well [4]. Furthermore, it is anticipated that the Affordable Care Act will allow more diverse populations to enter the healthcare system. In a report published by the Kaiser Family Foundation, of the 24 million projected new enrollees of private health insurance, about 23 % will speak a language other than English at home [5]. Providing medical interpreter services is critical to effective communication between healthcare providers and patients. Healthcare institutions and staff should gather information on the patients' preferred language to communicate healthcare information with healthcare professionals. Given the changing demographics and the need to provide culturally sensitive care, it is necessary to partner with professional medical interpreters.

Having an organization that reflects the diverse population it serves is also necessary to improve interactions and create a more culturally and linguistically sensitive organization. This will increase access by minorities, promote research in new areas, and enable leadership to address the needs of the diverse groups. However, workforce diversity has not kept pace with the changing demographics. This requires creating pipelines to increase enrollment in schools that feed these professions, a process that will take time [6].

How Healthcare Providers Can Contribute in Supporting Effective Communication

Providing professional medical interpreters when caring for patients who are LEP is a matter of quality and safety. Language barriers have been shown to be the cause of medical errors in LEP patients. Evidence shows that LEP patients are more likely to suffer from adverse events in hospitals resulting in harm or death, as compared to their English counterparts [7]. There is also evidence that working with untrained ad hoc interpreters results in a significantly higher number of errors with clinical consequences [8]. Ad hoc interpreters are untrained individuals who are bilingual and who are asked to interpret. These can include family members, staff members, bystanders, or anyone else who volunteers or is asked to provide interpretation and has not been trained as a professional medical interpreter.

In a study conducted in 2003 by Glen Flores, M.D., transcripts of interpreted pediatric encounters were analyzed. The study compared the errors in interpretation between encounters that were facilitated by medical interpreters and encounters facilitated by untrained or ad hoc interpreters. Ad hoc interpreters included bilingual healthcare providers and siblings of patients. It was concluded that the frequency of errors and the clinical significance of those errors were much greater when ad hoc interpreters were used [8]. Untrained bilingual individuals, whether they are family members or bilingual staff, may not know medical terminology and do not have the confidence to clarify terms unfamiliar to them. Patients may also not feel comfortable disclosing private healthcare information in front of family or individuals who may happen to live in the same communities as the patients. This can be a breach of confidentiality and privacy for the patient [9].

Asking untrained bilingual staff to serve as interpreters, in addition to risking poor communication, breach of confidentiality, and violating the law, also puts this staff in a difficult position [10–12]. Sometimes, if these individuals have support roles, or roles that report to the more senior staff asking them to do this, they do not feel empowered to admit that they don't feel comfortable doing this. They may fear for their job security. Also, they may be concerned with the perception that they don't want to be helpful and feel embarrassed to admit when they don't know certain terminology. Furthermore, calling on colleagues to interpret is taking them away from their primary job responsibilities and asking them to do something that falls outside of their scope of practice. This can result in poor job performance. It can also create resentment among other colleagues who may have to cover the responsibilities of those being pulled in to interpret.

It's important to note that different institutions have different systems in place to provide medical interpretation. Requirements may differ between a medical center and a research institution, for example. Some research institutions may have to follow strict IRB requirements pertaining to the enrollment of limited English-proficient (LEP) subjects. These requirements may dictate the need to have specific materials available in other languages, such as translated consent forms, as well as requirements for having interpreters available during the enrollment process when subjects speak another language. These requirements may vary from institution to institution. In some healthcare facilities, medical interpretation is provided by bilingual employees who have been trained as medical interpreters and are hired as dual-role employees. Others may have medical interpreters available only remotely, by telephone or by video or both.

There are also several reasons why a family member should not be asked to interpret for a patient. When allowed to interpret, English-speaking family members often end up speaking for the patients and not interpreting; they often answer healthcare provider's questions right away in English without interpreting for the patient and leaving the patient out of their healthcare discussion [13]. Family members may withhold information from healthcare providers or from the patient themselves [14]. This prevents patients from being active participants in their healthcare, healthcare discussions, and treatment plans. These types of encounters can make it difficult for the patient to feel connected to their healthcare provider. When a patient does not feel connected to their healthcare provider, they are less likely to communicate their concerns which can lead to negative treatment outcomes.

Thus, healthcare providers should encourage families to be present in the healthcare encounter, if the patient so chooses, as caregivers and supporters for the patients, but advocate for effective communication by having a medical interpreter facilitate the communication. The evidence supports that partnering with professional medical interpreters improves clinical outcomes and contributes to the decrease in healthcare disparities in LEP patients, compared to patients without language barriers [15]. One study demonstrated shorter lengths of stay and lower readmissions for LEP patients who had professional medical interpreters at admission and at discharge [16]. Another study that analyzed transcripts of appointments, some facilitated by ad hoc interpreters and others by professional medical interpreters, found that the errors committed by ad hoc interpreters were "significantly more likely to have potential clinical consequences" [8].

Some healthcare providers also have limited language skills and may attempt to conduct appointments without the help of a professional medical interpreter, even when interpreter services are readily available. Some even welcome the opportunity to "practice" their second language with patients [17]. While healthcare providers can certainly use their limited second-language skills to chat with patients, this should not happen when discussing medical care. Patients are often embarrassed to let their healthcare providers know they do not understand them. Often, patients may speak some English. In fact they may be able to check in for an appointment without an interpreter. However, medical conversations, even with English speakers, can be complex. When you add a language barrier to that encounter, it adds to the complexity and to the risk of misunderstanding and miscommunication. Many fear being stigmatized and worry about how they may be perceived due to their limited English language ability.

In many cultures, this inability to communicate for themselves in the dominant language can create a form of social disability, particularly in elders, which can have an impact on their self-esteem and their perceived authority and status within the family unit [18].

For example, a 50-year-old Vietnamese woman arrived for her appointment. At the desk she was asked for her name and date of birth, which she was able to give with her limited English. Upon checking in, the staff at the front desk said to her "you don't need an interpreter, right?" She felt embarrassed for not knowing English. She did not want to cause more work for the staff person and did not want to make someone go out of their way to provide her with a medical interpreter. The patient timidly shook her head and sat down.

Had the staff instead said "I'm going to call now for a medical interpreter for your appointment," the patient would have kindly accepted the offer knowing that she would need the help in order to effectively communicate with her healthcare provider. This case example serves as a reminder that best practice is to preemptively offer a medical interpreter to prevent this stigma.

Another example is that of a 48-year-old Haitian woman who was accompanied by her 18-year-old son to her primary care appointment. Because her son spoke English, he was asked to interpret for his mother. He did not want to appear rude or unhelpful and agreed. His mother, embarrassed to reject his help, didn't advocate for herself. During the encounter questions of sexual history were left uninterpreted and unanswered due to the embarrassment between mother and son.

Quality and Safety

Partnering with professional medical interpreters is a matter of quality and safety. There is no question that language barriers contribute to poor outcomes and adverse events. Patients who are limited English proficient are twice as likely to suffer from adverse events in the hospital, as compared to English-speaking patients. Those events experienced by LEP patients are also more likely to result in harm or even death [7]. Communication is at the heart of the patient-healthcare provider encounter. Not being able to communicate effectively creates a greater risk for medical errors and other conditions, such as infections, falls, and pressure ulcers [19].

The six aims of the Institute of Medicine's (IOM) *Crossing the Quality Chasm* that healthcare institutions must fulfill in order to deliver high-quality care strongly apply to patient populations who are LEP. According to the IOM, healthcare should be safe, effective, efficient, timely, patient centered, and equitable [20]. Providing safe care ensures that the healthcare provider can be alerted to a medication allergy.

In one case for example, a 56-year-old Filipina patient was unable to accurately convey to her healthcare provider what medications she was allergic to due to a language barrier [21]. In the emergency room, the treating healthcare provider prescribed a medication the patient was allergic to.

Effective healthcare is care that is evidence based; however, inability to understand a patient's symptoms and history renders the healthcare provider unable to provide the best effective care in that situation. Efficient care refers to removing waste and providing care that is cost effective. One can argue that if a healthcare provider isn't able to communicate with his or her LEP patient, then unnecessary tests may be ordered, resulting in higher cost of care that does not benefit the patient. If the patient who was scheduled for a colonoscopy arrives for his procedure without having prepared correctly and has to be rescheduled because the instructions given to the patient were in English instead of his native Haitian Creole, then the patient is being delayed; in other words, appropriate care is not being delivered in a timely manner.

These delays in care can be prevented by addressing the language needs proactively and having material available in the patient's language or going over the instructions with a medical interpreter. Providing care that is patient centered is one of the aims of quality healthcare. This is care that revolves around the patient and considers the patient's preferences, including cultural beliefs, and in which the patient has the authority to make informed decisions [22]. As the authors have already illustrated, LEP patients are at a disadvantage when ad hoc interpreters facilitate the communication. Untrained interpreters tend to omit information they deem irrelevant or editorialize what needs to be interpreted. Rather than empowering patients with information, patients are left on the periphery of their care. Finally, the last IOM aim is equitable care [20]. If care to LEP patients is not the same as care for an English-speaking patient, when access is different and when delays in receiving care are experienced, then care is not equitable.

Cost Considerations

The case for medical interpreters does not only impact quality and safety, it can also have an impact on cost. When LEP patients are not provided with professional medical interpreters, they experience longer lengths of stay and are at greater risk of being readmitted [16, 23]. Patients who experience language barriers may not fully understand postdischarge care and medication instructions. Therefore, they are more likely to be readmitted for the same condition. In addition, as the authors have already discussed, the inability to communicate effectively can result in getting unnecessary tests which adds to the cost of caring for that patient.

Furthermore, failure to provide competent interpreter services is a violation of Title VI of the Civil Rights Act of 1964. It is considered discrimination based on national origin. When the authors speak of competent interpreters, in addition to the spoken languages, the authors also refer to American Sign Language (ASL) interpreters. Patients who need ASL interpreters are also covered under the Americans with Disabilities Act (ADA) of 1990, which prohibits discrimination based on disabilities [11].

This federal law ensures equal access to services provided by institutions that receive federal funding, such as Medicare and Medicaid. Violations of this law are investigated and enforced by the Department of Justice and the Department of Health and Human Services and can carry hefty penalties. A study of medical malpractice cases from a carrier that covers four states in the United States found that in 2.5 % of all the cases covered through that insurance carrier, language barriers had a direct or indirect impact in the patient's outcomes. This resulted in the carrier paying approximately $5 M in damages and legal fees [21].

However, it is important to note that violation of both Title VI and ADA does not always involve malpractice, and when that happens, penalties may come out of a healthcare provider's own pocket. This was the case of a physician in New Jersey who treated a patient who was deaf for over a year, but never provided the patient with a sign language interpreter, despite the patient asking for one repeatedly. The physician argued that the cost of providing an interpreter (approximately $200/visit) far exceeded the reimbursement rate of $49 per visit. They communicated by writing back and forth and by relying on family members, including the patient's child. Although the care provided was adequate, the patient sued the physician for not providing a competent interpreter, under the ADA. The malpractice carrier did not cover the penalty since there was no allegation of malpractice. The physician had to pay $400 K out of his own pocket [24].

The Informed Patient

Healthcare organizations have unique obligations. They are expected to, in an ethical manner, meet the healthcare needs of the communities they serve while being considerate of profitability [25–27]. This expectation creates a social covenant between healthcare organizations and their communities. One tool that healthcare organizations use to fulfill their social covenants and meet their ethical obligations is patient-centered communication [22].

Patient-centered communication is communication that is respectful of and responsive to the patients' preferences, needs, and values [22]. Any communication that affects patients can be patient-centered including oral, written, and nonverbal communication between patients and healthcare providers, between patients and healthcare organizations, and between and among healthcare providers and healthcare organizations [22]. It is important to remember that on a daily basis, patients in the United States, from diverse backgrounds, who hold various beliefs about healthcare, are asked to make important decisions about their medical care. In order for a patient to be able to make important decisions about their medical care, healthcare providers must share with their patient information such as what their diagnosis is, what the medical treatment options are, and what are the risks involved with each of the presented treatment options (if there are more than one). The goal is to provide the patient all the information they will need to be able to make an informed decision about their medical care.

Individuals from Western cultures believe in the value of autonomy, and within the medical field, it is believed that the patient should be in control when making decisions about their medical care. Without patient-centered communication, patients would be taken out of the loop, leaving the healthcare providers to assume or guess the patient's needs and preferences. In such a situation, autonomy would be denied. Thus, patient-centered communication is vital for healthcare organizations to provide ethical, high-quality care.

The use of patient-centered communication can also expose areas where communication-vulnerable groups receive lower-quality care and allow healthcare providers to find ways to improve care [22]. For example, it is important to remember that although Western cultures value autonomy and individualism, other cultures value collectivism. In some cultures (and in some families in every culture), healthcare decisions are made not just by the individual but by the individual and their family. LEP patients may have cultural beliefs and traditions that can influence the medical encounter and subsequent health outcomes in subtle and often invisible ways. These include minimizing reports of pain, respecting authority, and adhering to specific gender roles, as well as class biases [19]. Healthcare providers should be aware that these differences exist and should talk to their patients about their preferences.

It is important to remember that when there are differences between the healthcare provider's decision-making beliefs and that of the patient's, the differences should be respected. To do so is not to deny patient autonomy. On the contrary, when a patient feels their values are respected, they gain more trust in their healthcare provider. This helps to further open the lines of communication allowing the patient to feel more comfortable to talk to their healthcare provider about their doubts and concerns regarding treatment without the fear of being judged or dismissed. When this happens, medical healthcare providers should actively listen to their patients. Healthcare providers should learn from their patients about their healthcare practices and should also learn about their patient's cultural and personal preferences. If healthcare providers do not have the general awareness of cultural traditions or beliefs of their patients, these cultural nuances can be easily overlooked and can impact healthcare outcomes [19, 22]. The authors remind the healthcare providers that they are ultimately responsible for ensuring safe and effective communication with their patients [9].

The Importance of Cultural Sensitivity

Culturally sensitive healthcare has been described as care in which healthcare providers offer services in a manner that is relevant to patients' needs and expectations [28]. Studies have shown that the level of cultural sensitivity in the healthcare that patients perceive experiencing positively influences their adherence to treatment and ultimately their health outcomes [29, 30]. When a healthcare provider is aware of their patient's healthcare practices, they are better able to work with their patient on identifying appropriate health and mental health interventions. When a healthcare provider is responsive to their patient's preferences and cultural needs, the patient feels heard and understood. This patient is therefore more likely to stay in treatment with this healthcare provider. However, if a patient does not feel heard by their healthcare provider and instead feels stigmatized because their practices are thought to be foolish, this patient will likely not return to treatment. As a result this patient does not receive equitable care.

Beliefs around healthcare practices vary greatly. To illustrate this point, the authors will now provide examples of diverse beliefs that can be held by individuals from China, Cambodia, Southeast Asia, Haiti, and Latin American countries. For example, some Latinos believe that a woman should not leave the house for 40 days after having a baby. This is called "quarentena." This belief is likely to be held by individuals from rural parts of various countries in Latin America (e.g., Mexico). In addition, some Latinos believe that after surgery (even if it's minor surgery), one should not get out of bed too soon and should rest for several days as one's body has been "traumatizado" (traumatized). Thus, it can be shocking for some Latino patients to hear the physical therapist tell them they need to get up and walk around a day after surgery.

In China, ginseng is widely used to help with conditions such as anemia, depression, digestion, rheumatism, and many others [31]. Other individuals believe in traditional forms of healing such as cupping, practiced in Cambodia and other Southeast Asian countries. Cupping consists of placing cups on the skin surface, usually the back, and creating a vacuum by suctioning the air from the cups, usually with heat. This is believed to cleanse the body of harmful toxins [32]. The marks left on the body from cupping can easily be interpreted as abuse. It is vital for healthcare providers to be sensitive to these practices in order to gain their patient's trust. Healthcare providers should do their best to not misunderstand their patient's cultural practices as doing so can lead to the patient feeling shamed and/or alienated.

In other countries, members from the community believe in spiritual rituals for the treatment of the sick (e.g., individuals from Cambodia or Haiti). For example, in Haiti the practice of voodoo as a way to treat and cure illness is widespread. This stems from the belief that many illness are caused by spirits or "demons" [33]. These general examples presented here are meant to provide a brief glimpse of some of the beliefs patients can hold. However, patients may not tell their healthcare providers about these remedies out of fear that their healthcare providers will not understand their practices and will negatively judge them. In some communities there is stigma associated with mental illness and as such patients may conceal their symptoms. Therefore, it is important for the healthcare provider to actively involve their patients in sharing information about their healthcare practices and their understanding of their health condition.

The various beliefs about healthcare practices around the world are infinite. The best way to start learning about them is by asking each patient, in a nonjudgmental and inquisitive fashion, what their beliefs are. This goes for individuals from the United States as well as outside the United States [19]. Healthcare providers should do their best to not make assumptions and instead to learn from each of their patients. There is so much richness in diversity, and when a healthcare provider shows cultural humility and a genuine interest in learning about their patients, they are better able to communicate with their patients and gain their trust. Healthcare providers should listen closely to the language patients use to describe their symptoms and to the ways in which they conceptualize their condition. Healthcare providers should then work with the patient, using their framework, on developing a plan for treatment. When needed, healthcare providers should also educate the patient using language that makes the information accessible to their patient. This open communication leads to trust. When a patient is able to trust their healthcare provider, they are more likely to try interventions they may have refused otherwise.

When a patient feels heard and not judged, they are more likely to listen to what their healthcare provider has to say about treatment options, which leads to the patient actually being "informed." [22] Now the patient can make decisions about treatment on their own or with the support of family, friends, or a spiritual leader. Through this patient-centered approach to managing health and mental health, healthcare providers open the lines of communication. This can lead to the patient feeling more comfortable asking honest questions about treatment options. Through this process of open communication, the healthcare provider can empower their patients to try interventions they would have otherwise refused due to fear or distrust. The goal of open communication is to improve healthcare outcomes.

Disparities and Improving Health Outcomes

Through language, healthcare providers of different disciplines and specialties are able to communicate with their patients, and through communication they are able to learn about their patient's concerns so they can then provide appropriate care. Effective communication is necessary in order for the healthcare provider to achieve an empathic connection with their patient. To communicate effectively with LEP patients, healthcare providers should make sure to ask their patients about their symptoms and ask them why they believe they are experiencing these symptoms. Once a healthcare provider has a sense of what their patient's beliefs are, they can take the time to share with the patient facts about their condition and clear up any misconceptions using clear and simple language.

Communication barriers, whether literacy related, language related, or culture related, can impact healthcare outcomes. For example, language barriers can impact patients' ability to relay information about their symptoms to physicians; importantly, this can influence treatment and overall healthcare experience. Still, there are healthcare providers who may choose to conduct an interview with LEP patients without the support of interpreter services. One possible rationale may include the perception that the encounter will take too long [34, 35]. Yes, healthcare providers have a very tight schedule, but the consequences of not having an interpreter could be dire. Other healthcare providers may choose to use their limited language skills in hopes of conducting an "adequate" medical interview [36, 37]. The risk taken by these healthcare providers is ineffective communication at best and poor health outcomes at worse. Studies have found that LEP patients experience more adverse events, such as medical errors and drug side effects, when compared to English speakers [38]. In the next section cases will be discussed where healthcare providers did not work with a trained medical interpreter and patients suffered the consequences of their decision.

It is important to recognize that when a patient is not able to effectively communicate with their healthcare provider, they are being put at a disadvantage which might result in the patient receiving a lower quality of care than those from less linguistically vulnerable groups. Language barriers have been evidenced to impact healthcare utilization, patient-physician trust, treatment adherence, satisfaction with healthcare, and screening practices [39, 40]. Studies conducted with LEP patients repeatedly reveal that patients don't fully understand what is being discussed during a given encounter and feel dissatisfied with the care they receive [37, 41, 42].

In addition, if a patient can't understand what is being said during a particular encounter, they will be less likely to adhere to treatment [15]. This can lead to a frustrating dynamic where the healthcare provider does not understand why the patient is not following their treatment. These patients are usually referred to as "noncompliant." Meanwhile, the patient may be frustrated because they don't know how to tell the healthcare provider they don't understand what is being said to them. Some patients may in fact be reluctant to say anything to their healthcare provider because they don't want to be disrespectful to them.

It is well established that language barriers contribute to health disparities for LEP patients [43]. Studies have also revealed that medical care is improved when healthcare providers work with professional medical interpreters [44]. Studies revealed that when healthcare providers partner with professional medical interpreters, interpretation errors are less likely to occur [8, 45], greater patient comprehension is achieved [46], and increased patient satisfaction with communication is reported [47]. In addition studies have found an association of higher satisfaction among patients and/or healthcare providers working with professional medical interpreters than with ad hoc interpreters [34, 48–50]. Overall, study findings suggest that medical interpreters are associated with an overall improvement of care for LEP patients.

It is likely that the improved utilization and clinical outcomes are mediated by the ability of professional medical interpreters to overcome health communication barriers [15]. Professional medical interpreters, through their experience, training, and knowledge of both medical and lay terminology, are better able to communicate patients' symptoms and questions to healthcare professionals and healthcare professionals' rationale for treatment and explanations of proper use of therapy to patients [15].

Additional Cases and Stories

The literature on adverse events and medical errors when caring for LEP patients is extensive. A few cases stand out as examples to illustrate the risks involved when steps aren't taken to ensure effective communication. Cases run the spectrum of patients not adhering to treatment plans or becoming "noncompliant" to the full out malpractice as a result of poor communication.

One of the most widely known cases of poor outcomes based on language barriers is the case of an 18-year-old Cuban young man, Willie Ramirez, who was brought to a South Florida emergency room unconscious [51]. The family was Spanish speaking but no Spanish-speaking medical interpreter was available or requested. The only word the English-speaking healthcare provider could understand was "intoxicado", which sounds much like the English word "intoxicated." The staff began treating Ramirez for a drug overdose. However, the word "intoxicado" can have a significantly different meaning, such as nauseous or becoming ill from something a person ate or drank. The patient laid in a bed for 2 days with an untreated intracerebellar hemorrhage. By the time the healthcare providers realized the error in diagnosis, it was too late.

Willie became quadriplegic, an outcome that could have been avoided had the family and the doctors been able to communicate and understand each other effectively.

This case also illustrates the stigma that patients and families feel when they face the need to request a medical interpreter. Immigrants want to be seen as making an effort to learn the dominant language and sometimes overestimate their own language skills or don't want to appear "difficult" by requesting a medical interpreter. Additionally, in many cultures it is not considered polite to question figures of perceived authority, as doctors are seen in many cultures.

In another case, the wrong surgery was performed on a patient [52]. The patient spoke Spanish and the surgeon spoke Spanish. On the day of the surgery, the surgeon and the patient communicated directly during the preoperative procedures. In this case, the lack of a medical interpreter prevented the other English-speaking healthcare providers in the room from understanding the conversation between the surgeon and the patient. Had an interpreter been present, someone could have alerted the surgeon that the wrong procedure was about to take place. While much focus is placed on medical interpreters facilitating communication between English-speaking healthcare providers and LEP patients and families, it is also important to recognize the value and need of the medical interpreter in settings where other healthcare providers may be left out of the communication when a patient or family is able to communicate with a healthcare provider directly in another language.

In yet another case, a patient suffered an allegedly avoidable leg amputation due to ineffective communication. The patient, Mr. Hernandez, was admitted to the hospital due to a workplace leg injury. Mr. Hernandez spoke both English and Spanish but was more fluent in Spanish. His wife, who was born and educated in Mexico until she was 21 years of age, understood a little bit of English and was also more comfortable communicating in Spanish. The doctor and medical assistant who treated the patient reported that they spoke Spanish "well enough" to communicate with the Spanish-speaking patients [21]. Discharge instructions were provided to Mr. Hernandez in English. He was unable to effectively understand the instructions, which led to further medical complications. This case illustrates how sometimes healthcare providers and staff overestimate their own second-language fluency and may decide to not work with a medical interpreter. It also highlights that although patients may speak some level of English, they may feel more comfortable and understand their care if the communication, both oral and written, is done in their preferred language.

The Tran case illustrates situations when children are English speaking but the parents (who must provide care, follow up with treatment plans at home, and give informed consent) are themselves limited English proficient and need professional medical interpreters to communicate effectively.

> Tran, a 9-year-old Vietnamese girl, was brought to an emergency room, accompanied by her parents and 16-year-old brother. The medical staff in the emergency room asked the patient and her brother to interpret for the parents during the encounter. The patient was diagnosed with gastroenteritis. The emergency room medical staff told the family to bring their daughter back to the ER if side effects arose. However, the side effects were not discussed and the discharge paperwork was given to the family in English. At home, the patient began suffering from an aggressive infection, low blood volume, and ultimately suffered a heart attack, resulting in her death [21].

In this case, the patient had been misdiagnosed with gastroenteritis and died from a reaction to the inappropriate medication she had been prescribed.

By not having a professional medical interpreter present, the patient's family was denied the opportunity to effectively communicate with the healthcare providers. The patient's parents were not able to understand how to care for their daughter, they were not able to provide informed consent, and they were not able to understand their daughter's medical needs. Tran's parents were not able to engage in a meaningful discussion with her healthcare providers, which resulted in a dire outcome. Having minors serve as interpreters, even when they are the patients, alienates the caregivers (the parents) from understanding their child's medical condition, not to mention relying on the minor to convey their own complex medical conditions.

> In the case of patient Chan, a 59-year-old Cantonese-speaking patient, the healthcare providers didn't clearly identify the patient's language. When checking in for his medical care, his language was sometimes documented as Vietnamese and other times as Cantonese. When it came to providing care for this patient, the healthcare providers consistently relied on the patient's son as the interpreter. In this case, the patient died from an overdose of a chemotherapy drug because the son was not able to accurately interpret the given information [21].

In a third case, Sokolov, a 78-year-old Russian-speaking woman, was unable to communicate to her healthcare providers the type and intensity of leg pain she was experiencing. She did not have a medical interpreter. Upon examining the patient's leg, her healthcare provider discovered her leg was cold and had been so for some time. This resulted in an amputation for that patient.

Unconscious Bias and How It Impacts Care of LEP Patients

The reality of unconscious bias in healthcare is not disputed. Since 2003 when the Institute of Medicine (IOM) first published Unequal Treatment: Confronting Racial and Ethnic Disparities in Health Care, this has been an area of focus for healthcare institutions and for healthcare providers committed to understanding these biases and learning how to address them in order to decrease and eliminate healthcare disparities. It is well documented, for example, that African Americans receive less cardiac catheterizations and that Hispanic Americans receive less pain medication in long bone fractures than patients who are White [53, 54].

As previously mentioned, studies have shown that patients who perceive their healthcare providers as being culturally sensitive are more likely to follow and adhere to treatment plans. They are also more likely to follow the doctor's advice if they agree with or trust their doctor. Additionally, treatment plans or interventions that are inclusive of cultural behaviors and beliefs tend to be more effective [55]. However, the challenge lies in training healthcare providers to first recognize their own biases and stereotypes and, secondly, in identifying the skills needed to not let those conscious and unconscious biases affect the way in which they provide care to that particular patient.

One important aspect of this heightened sense of cultural sensitivity is to move the focus of healthcare provider training from cultural competence to cultural humility. Cultural competence infers an end point of obtaining mastery in cultural skills. However, culture is dynamic, evolving, and hardly ever the same for two individuals. Culture depends on a variety of factors, such as socioeconomic level, education, and life experiences. Focusing instead on the notion of cultural humility implies a concept of life-long learning and self-reflection by healthcare providers and creates a patient-centered environment of care that is less authoritative and more supportive of patients' engagement and sharing of beliefs and personal perspectives on health and illness [56]. Exercising cultural humility and creating an environment that is patient centered, where patients' cultural beliefs are accepted without judgment, reduce the risk of stigmatizing patients and contribute to their full participation in their care.

Conclusions

The authors believe in cultural humility and equitable healthcare for LEP patients. Exercising cultural humility and creating an environment where patients' cultural beliefs are accepted without judgment reduces the risk of stigmatizing LEP patients.

Likewise, exercising cultural humility allows the healthcare provider to identify potential areas of prejudice that can negatively impact LEP patient care. Developing partnerships with medical interpreters helps promote equitable healthcare as medical interpreters are instrumental in bridging the communication gap when there are language and cultural differences.

Healthcare providers are responsible for delivering respectful and effective healthcare to the increasingly diverse population of the United States. By being proactive in providing medical interpreter services, healthcare providers can help LEP patients feel more comfortable accepting/asking for language interpretation without the fear of being criticized for needing this support. This simple action can help in overcoming the stigma and prejudice that can be associated with being a patient with LEP. This action is important today and will become even more important given the change in the cultural demographics and the increased access to healthcare that these groups now have as a result of the Affordable Care Act.

Through language, healthcare providers are able to communicate with their LEP patients, and through communication, healthcare providers are able to learn about their LEP patient's concerns so they may be able to effectively care for them. Language barriers can impact LEP patients' ability to relay information about their symptoms to healthcare providers; importantly, this can influence treatment and overall healthcare experience. An entire encounter, and LEP patient's treatment, may suffer when a healthcare provider and a patient with LEP do not communicate effectively. The goal of medical interpretation is to facilitate effective communication between patient or family and a healthcare provider. When a healthcare provider partners with a medical interpreter, they can work together in providing appropriate care by promoting effective communication, maintaining confidentiality, and reducing bias in the transfer of information between parties. Working with professional medical interpreters bridges the gap in health inequities and helps to reduce healthcare disparities.

Healthcare providers need to recognize that language barriers place LEP patients at a disadvantage that can lead to healthcare inequality. Thus, working with professional medical interpreters is an essential step in ensuring quality of care to every patient regardless of their language proficiency. Better quality care leads to better outcomes which results in lowered healthcare costs. Consistently, studies have demonstrated that working with professional medical interpreters is associated with an overall improvement of care for LEP patients. Working with professional medical interpreters has also been associated with a decrease in communication errors, increase in patient comprehension, increase in patient satisfaction with communication, and improved health outcomes. When a healthcare provider works with a professional medical interpreter, they give their LEP patient the opportunity to effectively communicate their symptoms to them. This in turn, allows the healthcare provider to develop an appropriate plan for treatment that can then be communicated to their LEP patient.

When a patient with LEP is able to effectively communicate with their healthcare provider, they are able to work with their healthcare provider and make an informed decision about their health, which leads to treatment adherence and satisfaction with healthcare. When a patient with LEP does not understand the instructions they are given, they are likely to follow the instructions incorrectly which can result in the patient needing to come in for urgent care. Not only does this result in increased healthcare costs, it also jeopardizes the health and well-being of the patient. However, when a patient with LEP understands their healthcare provider's recommendations, they become active participants in taking care of their health.

It is important for healthcare providers to learn about their LEP patient's cultural healthcare practices. Healthcare providers should ask, in a nonjudgmental way, about their patient's understanding of their health condition. When a healthcare provider shows cultural humility and a genuine interest in learning about their LEP patient, they are better able to earn their patient's trust which leads to improved communication.

Everyone who seeks healthcare has the right to receive that care in a manner that they can understand. Providing the highest-quality and safe care to all patient populations is the responsibility of healthcare providers and healthcare institutions. Research suggests that vulnerable populations, such as patients who have limited English proficiency are at higher risk to suffer from adverse events in hospitals than those who speak English due to communication barriers. It has also been shown that LEP patients may feel embarrassed or intimidated by how they may be perceived by healthcare providers if they advocate for themselves to have a medical interpreter present. Healthcare providers also must address their own biases and other perceived barriers to working with medical interpreters when caring for LEP patients. The authors assert that it is a best practice not to ask family members or bilingual staff to interpreter for LEP patients, even if that option seems more readily available and faster than requesting a medical interpreter.

It is also not appropriate to have children serve as interpreters for their LEP parents. Nor is it adequate for healthcare providers to use limited second-language skills when caring for LEP patients. It is best to partner with a professional medical interpreter. Healthcare providers must also engage LEP patients in sharing their beliefs and cultural concepts about their illness and create an environment where LEP patients feel safe in doing so. Making assumptions about LEP patients' particular belief system or practices can lead to creating barriers and mistrust, which in turn compromises LEP patients' adherence to plans of care. Healthcare providers can empower themselves and their LEP patients by partnering and working with trained medical interpreters. By working together optimal communication can be achieved, treatment outcomes can be improved, and the overall health of our diverse population can be promoted.

References

1. Chen AH, Youdelman MK, Brooks J. The legal framework for language access in healthcare settings: title VI and beyond. J Gen Intern Med. 2007;22 Suppl 2:362–7.
2. IMIA Guide on Working with Medical Interpreters. Available at: http://www.imiaweb.org/uploads/pages/380_5.pdf.

3. A national code of ethics for interpreters in health care. The National Council on Interpreting in Health Care. 2004. Available at: http://www.ncihc.org/assets/documents/publications/NCIHC%20National%20Code%20of%20Ethics.pdf.

4. Humes K, Jones N, Ramirez R. Overview of race and Hispanic origin: 2010. Suitland: Census Bureau; 2011. Available at: www.census.gov/prod/cen2010/briefs/c2010br-02.pdf.

5. Kaiser Family Foundation. A profile of health insurance exchange enrollees. Focus on health reform. 2011. Available at: http://kff.org/health-reform/report/a-profile-of-health-insurance-exchange-enrollees/.

6. Cohen JJ, Gabriel BA, Terrell C. The case for diversity in the health care workforce. Health Aff. 2002;21(5):90–102.

7. Divi C, Koss RG, Schmaltz SP, et al. Language proficiency and adverse events in U.S. hospitals: a pilot study. International J Qual Health Care. 2007;10(2):60–7.

8. Flores G, Laws MB, Mayo SJ, Zuckerman B, Abreu M, Medina L, et al. Errors in medical interpretation and their potential clinical consequences in pediatric encounters. Pediatrics. 2003;111(1):6–14.

9. Schenker Y, Lo B, Ettinger KM, Fernandez A. Navigating language barriers under difficult circumstances. Ann Intern Med. 2008;149(4):264–9.

10. U.S. Department of Health and Human Services. Guidance to federal financial assistance recipients regarding title VI and the prohibition against National Origin Discrimination Affecting Limited English Proficient Persons – Summary. 2006. Available at: http://www.hhs.gov/ocr/civilrights/resources/laws/summaryguidance.html.

11. U.S. Department of Justice and Civil Rights Division. Information and technical assistance on the Americans with disabilities act. 2010. Available at: http://www.ada.gov/2010_regs.htm

12. U.S. Department of Health and Human Services. Your rights under section 504 of the rehabilitation act. 2006. Available at: http://www.hhs.gov/ocr/civilrights/resources/factsheets/504.pdf.

13. Schapiro L, Vargas E, Hidalgo R, Brier M, Sanchez L, Hobrecker K, et al. Lost in translation: integrating medical interpreters into the multidisciplinary team. Oncologist. 2008;13(5):586–92.

14. U.S. Department of Health and Human Services. Improving patient safety systems for patients with limited english proficiency. 2012. Available at: http://www.ahrq.gov/professionals/systems/hospital/lepguide/index.html.

15. Karliner LS, Jacobs EA, Chen AH, Mutha S. Do professional interpreters improve clinical care for patients with limited English proficiency? A systematic review of the literature. Health Serv Res. 2007;42(2):727–54.

16. Lindholm M, Hargraves JL, Ferguson WJ, Reed G. Professional language interpretation and inpatient length of stay and readmission rates. J Gen Intern Med. 2012;27(10):1294–9.

17. Diamond LC, Schenker Y, Curry L, Bradley EH, Fernandez A. Getting by: underuse of interpreters by resident physicians. J Gen Intern Med. 2009;24(2):256–62.

18. Mui AC, Kang SY, Kang D, Domanski MD. English language proficiency and health-related quality of life among Chinese and Korean immigrant elders. Health Soc Work. 2007;32(2):119–27.

19. U.S. Department of Health and Human Services. Chapter 1: Background on patient safety and LEP populations. 2012. Available at: http://www.ahrq.gov/professionals/systems/hospital/lepguide/lepguide1.html.

20. Institute of Medicine (IOM). Crossing the quality chasm. Crossing the quality chasm: a new health system for the 21st century. Washington, D.C: National Academy Press; 2001.

21. Quan K. The high costs of language barriers in medical malpractice. Berkeley: University of California School of Public Health, National Health Law Program; 2010. Available at: http://www.pacificinterpreters.com/docs/resources/high-costs-of-language-barriers-in-malpractice_nhelp.pdf.

22. American Medical Association. An ethical force program consensus report. Improving communication improving care. 2006. Available at: https://accrualnet.cancer.gov/education/

ethical_force_program_consensus_report_improving_communication_improving_care#. VM-1FdE5AuQ.

23. John-Baptiste A, Naglie G, Tomlinson G, Alibhai SM, Etchells E, Cheung A, et al. The effect of english language proficiency on length of stay and in-hospital mortality. J Gen Intern Med. 2004;19(3):221–8.

24. Proskauer's Accessibility and Accommodations Practice Group. United States: New Jersey Jury Awards Deaf Patient $400,000 for physician's failure to provide sign language interpreter. 2009. Available at: http://www.mondaq.com/unitedstates/x/72664/employment+litigation+tribunals/ New+Jersey+Jury+Awards+Deaf+Patient+400000+For+Physicians+Failure+To+Provide+Si gn+Language+Interpreter+.

25. Pijnenburg MA, Gordijn B. Identity and moral responsibility of healthcare organizations. Theor Med Bioeth. 2005;26(2):141–60.

26. Wilmot S. Corporate moral responsibility in health care. Med Health Care Philos. 2000;3(2): 139–46.

27. Emanuel LL. Ethics and the structures of healthcare. Camb Q Healthc Ethics. 2000;9(2): 151–68.

28. Majumdar B, Browne G, Roberts J, Carpio B. Effects of cultural sensitivity training on health care provider attitudes and patient outcomes. J Nurs Scholarsh. 2004;36(2):161–6.

29. Lukoschek P. African Americans' beliefs and attitudes regarding hypertension and its treatment: a qualitative study. J Health Care Poor Underserved. 2003;14(4):566–87.

30. Rose LE, Kim MT, Dennison CR, Hill MN. The contexts of adherence for African Americans with high blood pressure. J Adv Nurs. 2000;32(3):587–94.

31. Spector RE. Cultural diversity in health and illness. Upper Saddle River: Prentice Hall; 2009. Print.

32. Yetter G. Expelling the wind: traditional Cambodian healing practices. Your gateway to Southeast Asia. Latitudesnu RSS. Web. Available at: http://latitudes.nu/expelling-the-wind-traditional-cambodian-healing-practices/.

33. Urrutia RP, Merisier D, Small M, Urrutia E, Tinfo N, Walmer DK. Unmet health needs identified by Haitian women as priorities for attention: a qualitative study. Reprod Health Matters. 2012;20(39):93–103.

34. Hornberger J, Itakura H, Wilson SR. Bridging language and cultural barriers between physicians and patients. Public Health Rep. 1997;112(5):410–7.

35. Chalabian J, Dunnington G. Impact of language barrier on quality of patient care, resident stress, and teaching. Teach Learn Med. 1997;9:84–90.

36. Burbano O'Leary SC, Federico S, Hampers LC. The truth about language barriers: one residency program's experience. Pediatrics. 2003;111(5 Pt 1):e569–73.

37. Baker DW, Hayes R, Fortier JP. Interpreter use and satisfaction with interpersonal aspects of care for Spanish-speaking patients. Med Care. 1998;36(10):1461–70.

38. Bauer AM, Alegria M. Impact of patient language proficiency and interpreter service use on the quality of psychiatric care: a systematic review. Psychiatr Serv. 2010;61(8):765–73.

39. Dang J, Lee J, Tran JH, Kagawa-Singer M, Foo MA, Nguyen TU, et al. The role of medical interpretation on breast and cervical cancer screening among Asian American and Pacific Islander women. J Cancer Educ. 2010;25(2):253–62.

40. Robb N, Greenhalgh T. "You have to cover up the words of the doctor": the mediation of trust in interpreted consultations in primary care. J Health Organ Manag. 2006;20(5):434–55.

41. Crane JA. Patient comprehension of doctor-patient communication on discharge from the emergency department. J Emerg Med. 1997;15(1):1–7.

42. Weech-Maldonado R, Morales LS, Spritzer K, Elliott M, Hays RD. Racial and ethnic differences in parents' assessments of pediatric care in Medicaid managed care. Health Serv Res. 2001;36(3):575–94.

43. Jacobs EA, Agger-Gupta N, Chen AH, Piotrowski A, Hardt EJ. Language barriers in health care settings: an annotated bibliography of the research literature. Woodland Hills: The California Endowment; 2003. p. 1–80. Available at: http://www.calendow.org/uploadedFiles/ language_barriers_health_care.pdf.

44. Flores G. The impact of medical interpreter services on the quality of health care: a systematic review. Med Care Res Rev. 2005;62(3):255–99.
45. Prince D, Nelson M. Teaching Spanish to emergency medicine residents. Acad Emerg Med. 1995;2(1):32–6; discussion 6–7.
46. Chan A, Woodruff RK. Comparison of palliative care needs of English- and non-English-speaking patients. J Palliat Care. 1999;15(1):26–30.
47. Bischoff A, Perneger TV, Bovier PA, Loutan L, Stalder H. Improving communication between physicians and patients who speak a foreign language. Br J Gen Pract. 2003;53(492):541–6.
48. Kuo D, Fagan MJ. Satisfaction with methods of Spanish interpretation in an ambulatory care clinic. J Gen Intern Med. 1999;14(9):547–50.
49. Ngo-Metzger Q, Massagli MP, Clarridge BR, Manocchia M, Davis RB, Iezzoni LI, et al. Linguistic and cultural barriers to care. J Gen Intern Med. 2003;18(1):44–52.
50. Karliner LS, Perez-Stable EJ, Gildengorin G. The language divide. The importance of training in the use of interpreters for outpatient practice. J Gen Intern Med. 2004;19(2):175–83.
51. Price-Wise G. Language, culture, and medical tragedy: the case of Willie Ramirez. Health Affairs Blog. 2008. Available at: healthaffairs.org/blog/2008/11/19/language-culture-and-medical-tragedy-the-case-of-willie-ramirez/.
52. Ring DC, Herndon JH, Meyer GS. Case records of The Massachusetts General Hospital: case 34–2010: a 65-year-old woman with an incorrect operation on the left hand. N Engl J Med. 2010;363(20):1950–7.
53. Schulman KA, Berlin JA, Harless W, Kerner JF, Sistrunk S, Gersh BJ, et al. The effect of race and sex on physicians' recommendations for cardiac catheterization. N Engl J Med. 1999;340(8):618–26.
54. Todd KH, Samaroo N, Hoffman JR. Ethnicity as a risk factor for inadequate emergency department analgesia. JAMA. 1993;269(12):1537–9.
55. Tucker CM, Marsiske M, Rice KG, Nielson JJ, Herman K. Patient-centered culturally sensitive health care: model testing and refinement. Health Psychol. 2011;30(3):342–50.
56. Tervalon M, Murray-Garcia J. Cultural humility versus cultural competence: a critical distinction in defining physician training outcomes in multicultural education. J Health Care Poor Underserved. 1998;9(2):117–25.

Chapter 15
Improving Workforce Diversity in Minority and Majority Institutions

Ed W. Childs, Joel Okoli, and Clarence E. Clark III

Introduction

To improve healthcare workforce diversity in minority and majority institutions, one must not only examine the supply (medical students, nursing students, etc.) but also the forces that may impede progress to healthcare workforce diversity. Here, we will tackle these key elements and then discuss current and future strategies that may provide meaningful solutions to this important dilemma.

How one interprets where we are in the process of diversifying our medical institutions depends on which characteristics of one's personnel are most important such as gender, race/ethnicity, level of experience of faculty, and/or types of disciplines or specialties of teaching faculty, residents, and students. For the purpose of this section, we will focus on gender, race, and ethnicity. We will also define the term underrepresentation using the authors' of the book *In the Nation's Compelling Interest: Ensuring Diversity in the Health Care Workforce* definition [1]: "…racial and ethnic groups that are underrepresented in the health professions relative to their numbers in the general population." Persons that make up this group are

Ed W. Childs, MD (✉)
Department of Surgery, Morehouse School of Medicine, Atlanta, GA, USA
e-mail: echilds@msm.edu

J. Okoli, MD
Morehouse School of Medicine, Atlanta, GA, USA
e-mail: jokoli@msm.edu

C.E. Clark III
Section of Colon and Rectal Surgery, Department of Surgery,
Morehouse School of Medicine, 720 Westview Drive, S.W., Atlanta, GA 30310, USA
e-mail: cclark@msm.edu

© Springer International Publishing Switzerland 2016
R. Parekh, Ed W. Childs (eds.), *Stigma and Prejudice: Touchstones in Understanding Diversity in Healthcare*, Current Clinical Psychiatry,
DOI 10.1007/978-3-319-27580-2_15

African Americans, mainland Puerto Ricans, and Native Americans, including American Indians, Alaska Natives, Asian Americans, Pacific Islanders, Latinos, Native Hawaiians, and women.

The Gender Gap in Medical Institutions

To begin the discussion of diversity, we start with gender and how this characteristic of faculty and students have shaped our institutions over time. The overall faculty makeup in US medical institutions has evolved. Women who reached the rank of full professor (FP) rose from 4.7 % in 1969 to 18.7 % in 2009 [2]. This trend was also seen in the associate professor (AoP) group (10.5 % increased to 30.8 %), the assistant professor (AiP) group (19.4 % increased to 41.7 %), and the instructor/other (Ins) group (32.5 % increased to 51.9 %) according to AAMC data. Interestingly, the authors showed that as women increased in rank, there was a decrease in representation for this cohort as new faculty as well as for faculty continuing in academic medicine. This perceived lack of progress to build the new pool of women in academic medicine may be a result of matriculating student gender trends.

We can prove or disprove this theory by examining enrollment data over the past two decades. Adriole et al., in their work examining associations of variables contributing to suboptimal performance of medical students, report demographic data of US accredited medical schools from 1994 to 1999 [3]. They showed that 56.2 % of the matriculates were male and 43.8 % were female over this time frame. Recently, the AAMC 2014 reported their findings on gender and medical school applicants/matriculates. Of the 731,595 applications, 45.9 % were women and 54.1 % were men. Of these applicants, 20,343 matriculated in 2014 with 47.8 % being women and 52.2 % men. When compared to Adriole et al.'s work published in 2010, there has been an increase in the proportion of women matriculating to medical school over the past two decades. Thus, matriculating female students are following the same pattern of growth as advancing professors. The lack of new faculty or women in academic medicine may be the result of women entering into private practice: a trend that would need to be assessed further to validate.

Despite medical school faculty and student populations being predominantly male, the gender gap is ever decreasing. More faculty members at all levels are increasingly female, but the number of women achieving rank of FP is not keeping pace with the proportional increase in academic positions. This trend may continue to evolve as the number of female students continues to increase over time.

Race/Ethnicity in Majority Medical Institutions

Another variable well studied in the world of diversity is ethnicity or race. As it relates to medical school demographics, the overall faculty makeup of US medical institutions has increased for nonwhite educators similar to the trend seen in women

[2]. Nonwhite FP faculty rose from 4.7 % in 1969 to 14.5 % in 2009. This trend was also seen in AoP (7.8 % increased to 22.6 %), in AiP (11.3 % increased to 33.7 %), and in Ins positions (13.4 % increased to 31.8 %). The authors also showed that nonwhite faculty made up a greater proportion of new academic medicine faculty than continuing faculty over time regardless of rank. In other words, access and pool of providers have improved to help diversify institutions. Is there a similar trend in matriculating students to medical schools? Adriole et al. in 2010 showed in over 97,000 students identified from 1994 to 1999 that 66.1 % were white, 18.2 % Asian/Pacific Islander, 0.8 % other, and 14.9 % underrepresented minorities. Over this same time frame, the ethnic composition of matriculates showed little change: from 15.8 to 19.9 % for Asian/Pacific Islander, 13.9–15.7 % for underrepresented minorities, and 65.3–66.5 % for whites. The authors also found that nonwhite race/ethnicity was one of three independent risk factors associated with greater likelihood of academic withdrawal or dismissal and graduation without first attempting at passing the US Medical Licensing Examination Step 1 and/or Step 2. These findings ultimately impact race demographics when selecting for academic and nonacademic positions in healthcare. Are minority medical institutions such as those affiliated with historically black colleges and universities (HBCUs) filling in the proverbial gab in educating future healthcare workers?

The Minority Institutions

Historically black colleges and universities have several affiliated medical schools such as Morehouse School of Medicine, Howard University School of Medicine, Meharry Medical College, and Charles R. Drew University of Medicine and Science. In 2013, Noonan et al. revealed an interesting trend seen in this cohort of colleges and universities that help shape the dilemma in the workforce debate [4].

The authors found that the number of medical degrees conferred by historically black institutions increased by only 2.8 % compared to 7.4 % for all institutions. In addition, HBCUs make up a very small percentage of overall medical degrees in the United States at 1.37 % in 2008 which has slowly declined from 2000. Similar trends were seen in dental, nursing, and public health students. Therefore, less and less underrepresented healthcare providers are coming from HBCUs. Is this the sign that these institutions are beginning to play a limited role in diversifying the healthcare workforce or are majority institutions gaining more interest in reversing past trends?

Noonan et al. report that minority institutions are not pacing majority institutions in sheer number regarding graduates in healthcare professions who are underrepresented. The existence of minority institutions is therefore important, but if the mission of these schools is to fill the race/ethnicity gap seen in US healthcare systems, more concerted effort must be sought out to aggressively increase the sheer number of matriculants and graduates to keep up with the demand. Furthermore, the class and faculty makeup should also consider the long-term impact of having such a low representation of other races considered majority in medicine.

Barriers That Effect Change and Sledge Hammers for These Barriers

To begin improving the diversity of minority and majority institutions, one must examine the barriers to progress. In 2015 Smith et al. examined the diversity of medical students by region and compared these results to the US national census [5]. The authors showed that the disparity of racial minorities within US allopathic medical schools directly correlates with the limited overall number of applicants for such racial groups. For example, the authors revealed that Black/African American individuals comprise up to 21 % of the population in one region and yet account for only 8 % of medical school applicants. The authors concluded that initiatives targeting underrepresented minorities at an early stage are critical when addressing racial disparity in US medical schools and ultimately in the physician workforce.

Such an initiative is the American College of Surgeons' High School Program that introduces African American, Hispanic American, and other underrepresented minority high school students to careers in medicine and surgery at a point in their lives when they are formulating plans for the future. Another example of such a program is the Vivien Thomas Summer Research Program of Morehouse School of Medicine, an 8-week program established in 2002 to recruit high school students to serve as apprentices in biomedical research laboratories under the mentorship of the research faculty. Since its inception, 190 students have participated and successfully completed the program.

Another program introduced in Atlanta in 2013 to tackle the workforce diversity effort is the Reach One Each One (ROEO) Youth Medical Mentoring Program spearheaded by Morehouse School of Medicine Department of Surgery in conjunction with Grady Memorial Hospital and Emory School of Medicine. This program was designed to introduce and expose high-performing high school students from underrepresented backgrounds who are interested in pursuing medical careers to various specialties during an intensive 10-week course.

Upon completion of its inaugural year in 2013, 17 Atlanta Public Schools and DeKalb County School students successfully completed and graduated from the ROEO program. Several of those graduates went on to become premed students at Columbus State University, Georgia Piedmont Technical College, Georgia Perimeter, Georgia Southern University, Gordon State College, Atlanta Technical College, Atlanta Metropolitan College, The University of Alabama at Birmingham, Tuskegee University, and Xavier University of Louisiana, to name a few. The class size for ROEO has increased to over 30 high school juniors and seniors in 2014 with interest spreading around the Atlanta and Atlanta Metro Area every year.

Outside of the Atlanta community, other programs have been established to join in the fight against poor representation of minorities in the healthcare workforce. Crockett at Michigan State University described an NIH-sponsored Research Education Program to Increase Diversity (REPID) among health researchers in

2014 [6]. The authors/facilitators of this program recruit students/learners from a diverse population of undergraduates, graduates, health professionals, and lifelong learners. The learners receive a scholarship that covers a stipend and housing allowance while engaged in hands-on research experience and attendance of academic conferences. Fifty-one students were enrolled in the first 3 years of the program of which 36 (80 %) have continued their research experiences beyond the program. African American females made the majority of the participants at 30 % followed by Hispanic females (13 %) and those with disadvantaged background (11 %) or an annual income below established low-income thresholds. The lowest enrolled group was reported to be American Indian or Alaska Native at 2 %. Other similar programs such as Training and Education to Advance Minority Scholars in Science (TEAM-Science) program at the University of Wisconsin-Madison work to improve diversity in PhD programs [7], a critical component to the healthcare industry.

Efforts, such as the aforementioned, target students at various levels of education and expose these individuals to future endeavors not commonly seen in their communities. The fight, however, does not stop here. Once these learners have made it through the application and matriculation phase of their education, systems must be in place to continue the progression when formally training in postgraduate residencies and the like.

Improving Workforce Diversity at the Training Level

At the training level, Lightfoote et al. provide a constructive and systematic approach to the lack of diversity in the healthcare system in general using their field of radiology and radiation oncology as an example [8]. The authors first note the greater likelihood of African Americans and Hispanics to attended medical schools affiliated with HBCUs, which interestingly lack radiology and radiation oncology (RRO) training programs. Thus, students at these minority institutions are less likely to be exposed to RRO in clinical rotations or electives or to radiologists or radiation oncologists as faculty and mentors. The authors concluded from this observation that the American College of Radiology should explore ways it can promote accredited residency programs at these institutions. Other initiatives highlighted in this article are providing financial and mentoring assistance to increase the number of applications from women and underrepresented students to residency programs, develop leaders that value diversity, require diverse search committees for new hires, hold leadership accountable for the implementation of diversity and inclusion practices, and require that a 5-year review of the department or practice includes assessment of diversity and inclusion, to name a few. Proposals such as these must be considered at the training level for all disciplines to propel an ever-growing diverse pool of students into careers via clinical and basic science training programs upon successful completion of graduate education.

References

1. Committee on Institutional and Policy-Level Strategies for Increasing the Diversity of the U.S. Healthcare workforce. In the nation's compelling interest: ensuring diversity in the health care workforce. Washington, DC: National Academies Press (US); 2004.
2. Association of American Medical Colleges Facts and Figures. Washington, DC: AAMC. Available at https://www.aamc.org/initiatives/diversity/179816/facts_and_figures.html.
3. Andriole DA, Jeffe DB. Prematriculation variables associated with suboptimal outcomes for the 1994–1999 cohort of US medical school matriculants. JAMA. 2010;304(11):1212–9.
4. Noonan A, Lindong I, Jaitley VN. The role of historically black colleges and universities in training the health care workforce. Am J Public Health. 2013;103(3):412–5.
5. Smith MM, Rose SH, Schroeder DR, Long TR. Diversity of United States medical students by region compared to US census data. Adv Med Educ Pract. 2015;6:367–72.
6. Crockett ET. A research education program model to prepare a highly qualified workforce in biomedical and health-related research and increase diversity. BMC Med Educ. 2014;14:202.
7. Byars-Winston A, Gutierrez B, Topp S, Carnes M. Integrating theory and practice to increase scientific workforce diversity: a framework for career development in graduate research training. CBE Life Sci Educ. 2011;10(4):357–67.
8. Lightfoote JB, Fielding JR, Deville C, Gunderman RB, Morgan GN, Pandharipande PV, Duerinckx AJ, Wynn RB, Macura KJ. Improving diversity, inclusion, and representation in radiology and radiation oncology part 2: challenges and recommendations. J Am Coll Radiol. 2014;11(8):764–70.

Chapter 16
Leveraging Technology for Health Equity

Aida L. Jiménez, Eunice Malavé de León, Ginette Sims,
Celsie M. Hiraldo-Lebrón, Phillip J. Small, and Maged N. Kamel Boulos

Over the last 20 years, information technology (IT) has transformed the way that people all over the world live. From revolutionizing the manner in which society communicates to affecting the way that people acquire and substantiate information [1], IT has changed the way that humans interact with one another and the various systems in which they live. IT also has the potential to transform the way that healthcare providers (HCPs) communicate and deliver services [2, 3] and bridge health disparities.

A.L. Jiménez, PhD (✉)
Department of Psychiatry, Vanderbilt University,
1601 23rd Ave South Room 3050 FA, Nashville, TN 37212, USA
e-mail: aidaljimenez@aol.com

E. Malavé de León, EdD, LCSW
Behavioral Health Department, Southside Medical Center, Atlanta, GA, USA
e-mail: em743@nova.edu

G. Sims, BA
Department of Psychiatry, Massachusetts General Hospital Psychiatry, Center for Diversity,
McLean Hospital, Belmont, MA, USA
e-mail: gsims@partners.org

C.M. Hiraldo-Lebrón, PhD
Behavioral Health Department, NYU Lutheran Medical Center, Brooklyn, NY, USA
e-mail: chiraldo@lmcmc.com

P.J. Small, MA
Department of Psychology, Arizona State University, Tempe, AZ, USA
e-mail: psmall@asu.edu

M.N. Kamel Boulos, MD, PhD
The Alexander Graham Bell Centre for Digital Health, University of the Highlands and
Islands, Inverness, UK
e-mail: maged.kamelboulos@uhi.ac.uk

© Springer International Publishing Switzerland 2016
R. Parekh, Ed W. Childs (eds.), *Stigma and Prejudice: Touchstones in Understanding Diversity in Healthcare*, Current Clinical Psychiatry,
DOI 10.1007/978-3-319-27580-2_16

In today's society, the Internet has become a main source of medical information [4], contributing to a person-centered healthcare system that empowers patients to become active participants in their care by making information more accessible and self-directed learning more common and convenient [5]. Given this reality, HCPs must be competent in using the services the Internet provides to best guide patients towards the appropriate treatment. The purpose of this chapter is to explore ways in which IT can address the health needs of vulnerable populations and reduce prejudice for populations including those discussed in previous chapters. We will discuss current disparities in healthcare, the ways in which IT has changed healthcare, IT tools that have assisted underserved populations today, and ethical and logistical challenges involved with the use of technology in healthcare.

Healthcare Disparities

Health disparities continue to exist in multiple populations [6]. Healthcare services are still distributed inefficiently and unevenly across populations. For example, the literature provides evidence that people with disabilities [7], homeless individuals [8, 9], immigrants [10, 11], and those who struggle with substance abuse [12] face many barriers to treatment and have inadequate access to quality healthcare services. Vast research also shows health disparity among racial and ethnic minorities and rural populations. Even though we don't cover these populations in section one, IT has demonstrated to be a potential tool to increase health equity for these disenfranchised groups. Racial and ethnic minorities often receive poorer quality of care [13, 14], are less likely to seek healthcare services [15], often leave treatment prematurely, and have lower levels of attendance and retention in healthcare than non-Latino whites [16, 17].

Further, more than 20 million people in the United States live in Medically Underserved Areas (MUAs) [7] that have a shortage of physicians to meet their basic healthcare needs [18]. One of the problems with the provision of care in MUAs is the difficulty in recruiting and maintaining health professionals in sufficient numbers to attend the needs of these populations [19]. Throughout the rest of this chapter, the authors will discuss how IT can work as an innovative method for reducing disparities in healthcare.

Prevalence of IT Use

Technology has become a ubiquitous part of life in the twenty-first century. Modern technology influences every aspect of our life from making payments and communicating with friends, family, and coworkers, to searching for health information and scheduling appointments with providers [1]. In 2011, about 30.2 % of the world's population had access to the Internet.[1] In 2014, 90 % of American adults age 18 and older had a cell phone, 57 % had a laptop, and 19 % had a tablet computer; and about six in ten adults (63 %) went wireless with one of those devices [20].

Since 2004, teens have shown the greatest Internet use of any age group [21]. Ninety-two percent of teens report going online daily, and 24 % report going online multiple times each day. Although the primary point of Internet access is through computers, accessing the Internet via smartphone is on the rise. Among teens, texting is the preferred method of communication, and the volume of teen texting has risen from a median of 50 texts a day in 2009 to a median of 60 texts a day in 2012 [21]. Teen girls text more than boys with a median of 100 texts a day compared to 50 texts a day in 2011. This youthful population represents the next generation of HCPs and patients alike.

Social media and social networking now reach at least four out of five active Internet users in the United States.[2] Americans now spend more time on Facebook than on Yahoo, Google, YouTube, Blogger, Tumblr, and Twitter combined. Similar findings have been reported in Europe.[3] In August 2015, Facebook reached a new milestone of a billion users in a single day.[4]

Unlike the commonly held belief that social networking is mainly used by teenagers and young adults, a recent survey reported that use of Facebook and other social networking sites is on the rise among those aged 50–64. Approximately 33 % of Internet users in the 65-plus age group also used such sites [22], which some have described as the "graying of social networking sites." Introductory courses that teach how to use Facebook and Twitter for those aged 60 and older are now available, another testimony of the growing popularity of social networking tools among older generations.[5] IT is clearly a potentially important tool among aging populations.

A survey conducted with people with disabilities resulting from brain and spinal cord injuries found that 73 % of respondents used computers and had access to the Internet. This finding suggests IT tools can be a potential medium for the dissemination of health-related information and services for this underserved population [23].

---

[1] World Internet Usage Statistics News and World Population Stats. Miniwatts Marketing Group, 31 March 2011: http://www.internetworldstats.com/stats.htm. See also http://geography.oii.ox. ac.uk/?page=internet-population-and-penetration.

[2] Nielsen. State of the Media – The Social Media Report 2012: http://blog.nielsen.com/nielsen-wire/social/.

[3] Van Belleghem S. 347 million Europeans use social networks. Posted on 14 September 2011: http://blog.insites.eu/2011/09/14/347-million-europeans-use-social-networks-results-of-a-global-social-media-study/.

[4] BBC News. Facebook has a billion users in a single day, says Mark Zuckerberg. Posted on 28 August 2015: http://bbc.co.uk/news/world-us-canada-34082393.

[5] Toth S. Social media revolution: New courses in Howard County tap into Facebook's growing senior demographic. Posted on 12 December 2011: http://www.baltimoresun.com/explore/howard/publications/howard-magazine/bs-exho-social-media-revolution-20111212,0,6100789.story.

IT can be a potential medium to reach vulnerable and disenfranchised populations who may otherwise go without the care they require. With these new realities in mind, the authors recommend that HCPs become competent in the use of IT and help their patients navigate the new challenges and benefits of IT.

IT Competency

Achieving IT competency is critical for all HCPs. Emerging technology is widely and increasingly becoming an unavoidable part of our services. In fact, telemedicine guidelines encourage HCPs to assume responsibility and obtain relevant professional training, knowledge, and skills on the emerging areas of technology in order to teach and treat patients competently [24]. The youthful population of today has been termed "digital natives" because they have grown up using technology, while those of us who are trying to learn the new language of technology have been termed "digital immigrants" [25]. Digital immigrants retain their language of accessing information in traditional ways while learning a new language with accent [25].

HCPs need adequate digital language or eHealth literacy training for finding, interpreting, and evaluating the usefulness of health and medical-related information on the social web, in order to better serve their patients and the general public [26]. This term "eHealth literacy" ("e" for electronic) refers to the ability of individuals to seek, find, understand, and appraise health information from electronic resources and apply such knowledge to addressing or solving a health problem [26, 27]. Health literacy on the Internet requires computer and Internet literacy and skills for locating and appraising online health information [28].

Having access to the Internet and mastering the essential computer skills does not guarantee that a patient will be able to properly evaluate and understand online health information [26, 29]. There is a need to educate at-risk vulnerable groups to design social media presences in a way that benefits more patients [30]. Accessibility and eInclusion should be adequately addressed in such designs, ensuring "technology accessibility by all" and the participation of older people with lower access rates to the Internet and without the necessary skills to use the various social web tools, as well as the inclusion of other marginalized or disadvantaged groups of the society [31].

Developing eHealth places high demand in multiple competencies, including cognitive and behavioral, that can only be developed through regular education and practice [32]. HCPs need to learn and use the same language patients use, in order to better facilitate clear communications. HCPs also need to consider, for that same purpose, any specific cultural needs and the socioeconomic levels of different ethnic groups in the communities they are serving.[6]

---

[6] See the US National Medical Association's Cultural Competence Primer: http://www.webcitation.org/66BPe3CTo.

IT Tools for HCPs

The integration of technology and health has been termed "telehealth." The term refers to providing healthcare services remotely, via telephone, email, or videoconferencing. Other words used to refer to telehealth include telemedicine, mobile health (mHealth), or eHealth. Telehealth uses telecommunications and information technologies to provide access to health information, assessment, diagnosis, intervention, consultation, supervision, education, and follow-up programs across geographical distance [2, 33, 34]. The technology used in telehealth includes telephones, mobile devices, interactive videoconferencing, email, text, and resources found on the Internet like self-help websites, blogs, online therapy, and social media. Communication may be synchronous, which means having multiple parties communicating in real time (e.g., interactive videoconferencing and telephone), or asynchronous, which refers to time-delayed communication such as email, online bulletin boards, and the storing and forwarding of information. Telehealth was introduced decades ago, but it is gaining in popularity and relevance as VCTs have improved and become more accessible [35, 36].

At present there are many telehealth resources available for providers and patients, but for the purpose of enhancing health equity, the authors will focus on resources that have the potential to enhance healthcare quality for underserved populations. The following resources explained below are social networking, electronic health records (EHRs), videoconferencing technology (VCT), mHealth, and online therapy.

Social Networking

As discussed earlier, the use of social networking has rapidly increased in the last several years, and HCPs can no longer afford to ignore social media as a powerful means for reaching out to their patients. Health organizations should go where people already are online, rather than just build their own isolated web islands of read-only information portals and expect people to visit.

Research demonstrates that Internet use and online social engagement can protect against health literacy decline during aging, independent of cognitive decline [37]. It also offers opportunities for older people to keep healthy and combat social isolation [38]. The city of Barcelona has been a pioneer in developing digital inclusion eHealth programs targeting older and isolated people [38]. Another example of leveraging social networking to bridge health disparities is with racial and ethnic minorities. Researchers showed that Black non-Hispanics and Hispanics access the Internet, send and receive emails, and download applications (apps) more than White non-Hispanics [38].

Creating online tools and educational courses through social networking is an innovative way to decrease health disparities. The US Center for Disease Control (CDC) uses social media extensively in its own public campaigns and outreach activities[7] and offers a number of excellent health literacy, social media, and social marketing training materials, guidelines, and toolkits that can prove very helpful to social media content developers and public health practitioners in general (Fig. 16.1).

The capacity to reach out to many people, quickly and with minimal costs compared to other forms of advertising, is among the strongest aspects of social media and can play an important role in health education, promotion, and outreach programs [39]. Online social networks and participatory communication methods can provide excellent opportunities for peer-to-peer support [40] and thus contribute to reducing the burden on conventional healthcare systems. PatientsLikeMe,[8] a social networking site for patients with various medical conditions, is now a classic example of online patient-to-patient support, and those using it often report a number of perceived benefits from improved disease self-management [41, 42].

Nonetheless, social media content needs to be tailored to suit the preferences of target audiences and their level of understanding. Involving patients in planning, implementing, disseminating, and evaluating online health information and services is of prime importance [43]. A strategy based on shared-audience information sets can be adopted to maximize the efficiencies of content authoring and delivery vs. varying degrees of patient literacy, from the expert patient to the completely illiterate patient [44].

With patients being able to freely text and post comments on an organization's social media, maintainers of social media pages should regularly monitor and moderate their content for any forms of spam or patient privacy violations. Healthcare agencies should develop clear policies regarding what HCPs and staff can post on the agency's social media page [45].[9] Other strategies include connecting social media technologies to evidence-informed online resources, matching new applications with the correct user populations, and integrating health communication best practices, including addressing health literacy issues in the relevant social media content and regularly running the latter through readers' panels[10] representing the full range of patient audiences [43, 46, 47].

EHRs

EHRs are digital versions of patients' paper charts, which contain information about patients' medical history, diagnoses, medications, immunization dates, allergies, and

---

[7] See http://www.cdc.gov/socialmedia/.

[8] PatientsLikeMe: http://www.patientslikeme.com/.

[9] For example, Mayo Clinic (USA) has its own guidelines for its employees and students who participate in social media: http://sharing.mayoclinic.org/guidelines/for-mayo-clinic-employees/.

[10] In the UK, readers' panels are now common across the NHS; the following Google query should retrieve some examples: http://www.google.co.uk/search?q=readers+panels+nhs.

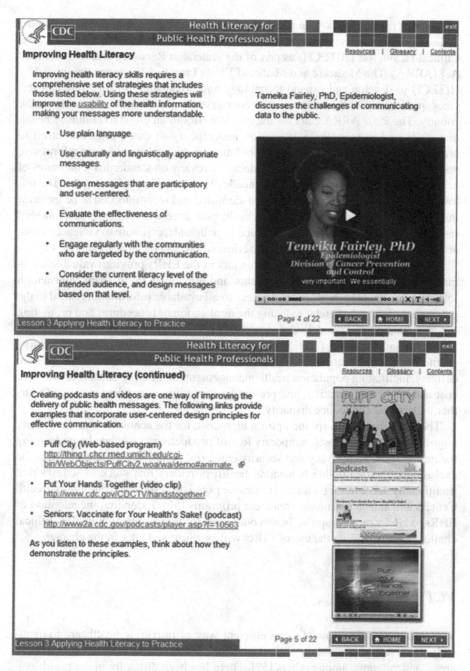

Fig. 16.1 Screenshots of the US CDC (free) online course entitled "Health Literacy for Public Health Professionals" (Source: Kamel Boulos [104])

lab and test results. In 2009, in an effort to eliminate health disparities in the United States, Congress passed the Health Information Technology for Economic and Clinical Health Act (HITECH) as part of the American Recovery and Reinvestment Act (ARRA). The Medicare and Medicaid EHRs Incentive Programs are funded by HITECH to develop and expand technology and broadband infrastructure and services, particularly in low-income and underserved remote communities, across the country. The 2009 ARRA calls for the use of EHRs in an effort to eliminate health disparities and increase the effectiveness and efficacy of care [48]. In an effort to provide better patient care, improved population health, and enable more informative research, the Institute of Medicine conducted a review on standardized measures of key social and health determinants that needed to be recorded in EHRs [49]. The following is social determinant information identified and recommended to be included in EHRs: sociodemographics, access to healthcare, access to healthy foods, financial resource strain, social support, environmental pollutants, exposure to violence, stress, affect (depression, anxiety), housing, discrimination, and racial segregation [49].

The inclusion of these social determinants in the EHRs provides valuable information of the effectiveness of treatments and allows HCPs to share information [50]. Sharing enables HCPs to have access to all available information related to the patient being served, thereby reducing the duplication of procedures and promoting the coordination of care delivery across different sites to reduce healthcare costs. Additional advantages of EHRs include the following: centralizing information, promoting data collection and analytics for evidence-based approaches to care delivery, facilitating population health management, facilitating consumer access to cost and quality information, and promoting the ability to conduct research to further understand and reduce disparity.

The EHR drawbacks are the upfront high cost, for the acquisition of the system, ongoing maintenance costs, temporary loss of productivity associated with learning the new system, and privacy and security concerns. Additional disadvantages is the exclusion of some eligible behavioral health providers that work in settings that traditionally serve immigrant and vulnerable population such as Community Health Centers and substance misuse treatment programs [51]. Extending the adoption of EHRs to HCPs might improve health outcomes for vulnerable populations. Ethical challenges surrounding the use of EHRs will be discussed later in the chapter.

VCT

VCT has been demonstrated as an efficient way of providing healthcare to medically underserved population such as patients in prisons, patients living in remote areas, and veterans, among others [52]. There has been difficulty in the health system in recruiting and maintaining health professionals in remote areas to attend the needs of these populations [19]. Therefore, VCT may have great implications for these underserved populations [53–55].

VCT is not just important for remote communities, but also for any underserved communities that have limited access to care. An example of this is the deaf population, which is one of the most underserved communities [56]. A shortage of culturally and linguistically competent HCPs who can provide healthcare to deaf individuals causes disparity [56–58]. VCT has been an integral part of the deaf community over 10 years, and it has commonly been referred to as the videophone. VCT has been demonstrated as an effective tool for alleviating the barriers to healthcare access for the deaf individuals because it allows for signage [59, 60]. Use of VCT has improved access to care for deaf population, but there is still need for empirical evidence to support its effectiveness [59].

VCT is a proven tool in treating veterans, a special population in need of access to healthcare services and who often underutilize services due to stigma, stoicism, and lack of knowledge. VCT can be leveraged to address this gap in care [61]. Veterans are also overrepresented in the US homeless population (Department of Housing and Urban Development, 2011) and commonly develop medical and mental health disorders [62, 63]. To address the high rates of underuse of healthcare services, the VA has invested in innovative eHealth tools to improve veterans' access to healthcare services [64]. Now health services can be provided to veterans in remote, community-run clinics through closed-circuit video communication between the patient and HCP.

VCT could also prove important for high-profile celebrities like athletes and Hollywood actors who often travel for weeks at a time. Using VCT to access healthcare may help VIPs avoid the trouble of being seen seeking certain healthcare services. There is a particular stigma attached to admitting the need for healthcare in the realm of sports, which makes IT potentially even more important [65].

The research is not robust yet, but the authors' believe that VCT can provide services to other vulnerable populations discussed in section one. IT is going to continue to proliferate and make its way into medicine, and it is likely to reach people that have not been reached before.

Scientific literature pertaining to the use of VCT identifies several barriers. For example, with regard to rural areas, rural cultural beliefs might be a barrier to the implementation of VCT. One value associated with rural cultural beliefs is the preference for social relationships that are face to face and personal rather than impersonal such as relationships developed via computers and telecommunication [66]. Some additional difficulties in implementing VCT in remote areas are lack of computer literacy, lack of technological comfort, lack of funding to provide an appropriate infrastructure, cost of implementation of these technologies, cost and availability of trained health workers and supporting staff, and adaptation of these technologies into the workflow [67]. Since underserved populations tend to have a higher degree of complexity in the management of their health conditions, any effective IT program needs to be tempered with the special characteristics of the populations to be served [68].

mHealth

One prediction in 2010 was that mobile web access via smartphones and other Internet devices, such as the Apple iPads and small touch-screen tablets, would overtake conventional desktop Internet use by 2015.[11] UK mobile Internet use was already nearing 50 %, according to a 2011 Office for National Statistics (ONS) report.[12] The mobile social web is now enabling people to easily share, rate, recommend, and find software apps about almost any topic. A mobile app for trusted and reliable health advice offered by the National Health Service (NHS) in England was downloaded by more than one million persons in its first 6 months after launch in May 2011.[13]

In this age of smartphones and wearable technology, many healthcare providers are using the information available on these devices to track patients' heart rate, exercise, and other health information. This innovation in technology has the capability of benefiting HCPs by using phone apps and even more advanced technology. Such apps could include mood trackers, thought journals, behavioral records, accessible notes, and phone-accessible mindfulness guides. For patients who have insomnia, existing sleep trackers could provide important information for an HCP about when his or her patient is going to sleep and is waking up and how disturbed their sleep cycle is. In healthcare settings, HCPs are often limited to what they see and hear in weekly, 50-min sessions, and encouraging patients to take advantage of the technology that many already own could lead to improved healthcare. Some benefits of mHealth include low start-up cost, potential for real-time data collection, feedback capability, relevance to multiple types of populations, flexible payment plans, and increased dissemination capability.

Smartphones are the most popular mobile devices used in mHealth interventions because they are accessible, inexpensive, convenient, and easy to use. What was once a model for causal communication, cell phone texting has become a valuable tool in clinical settings. Cell phones have also become more widely accessible to low-income populations due to the provision of affordable option plans and unlimited mobile texting [69]. In a study conducted with Medicaid patients and other insurance holders, Medicaid patients were more likely (79 %) to use text messages than those who had private insurance (65–68 %) [70]. This finding reflects that texting might be a promising tool to target the needs of low-income populations and decrease health disparity. The bidirectional sharing of information and dialogue with HCPs facilitates patients playing an active role in their care. This paradigm shift towards patient-centeredness in healthcare is promoted with technologies such as mHealth that encourages patients to engage actively in sharing. Strong patient-provider communication has been associated with increased patient satisfaction, increased compliance, and improved treatment outcomes [71].

In an effort to improve health, the US Department of Health and Human Services (HHS) evaluated existing initiatives of texting and its effectiveness to promote

---

[11] Meeker M, Devitt S, Wu L. Internet Trends. Morgan Stanley, 12 April 2010: http://www.morganstanley.com/institutional/techresearch/pdfs/Internet_Trends_041210.pdf.

[12] Mobile Internet use nearing 50 %. BBC News, 31 August 2011: http://www.bbc.co.uk/news/technology-14731757.

[13] NHS direct mobile app used 1 million times. Posted on 11 November 2011: http://www.nhsdirect.nhs.uk/News/NewsArchive/2011/MobileAppUsed1mTimes.

health. Females, particularly single mothers (30 %), experience higher rates of poverty and disparity of healthcare services [72]. One promising program addressing this disparity has been Text4Baby which provides pregnant and new mothers free health advice text messages in English or Spanish to promote health among mothers and babies. Other programs or initiatives are TXT4Tots, SmokeFreeTXT, QuitNowTXT, SmokeFree Moms, and Health Alerts On-the-Go [73]. Females, particularly single mothers (30 %), experience higher rates of poverty and disparity of healthcare services [72]. Using IT with this population is an innovative way of bridging disparity gaps.

A substantial body of research has shown that text messaging programs can bring about behavior change to improve smoking cessation [74–76], weight loss [77–79], and treatment compliance for both medication adherence [80] and appointment attendance [81, 82]. Some mHealth approaches have also shown success in diet and physical activity interventions in adults and children [83–85]. Literature demonstrates that certain groups have poor treatment compliance [16, 86]. These IT tools might be invaluable to target these populations and close the gap of health disparity, though further research since the evidence is limited [87–89].

Currently, there are many apps available for health prevention and well-being, but the Federal Drug Administration (FDA) has no regulations for these apps and, therefore, most of the services have not been scientifically tested to ensure effective outcomes. Providers should use and promote these apps as self-help resources and take cautionary steps to minimize any type of risk(s) to patients' safety and/or well-being (Table 16.1).

Table 16.1 Mental Health Apps available for smartphone(s)

App Name	Description
AAC Autism myVoiceCommunicator	Autism communication aid
Autism/DTT Colors Full	Autism, attention deficit disorder (ADD), attention deficit hyperactive disorder (ADHD), and discrete trial training (DTT)
Breathing Zone: Relaxing Breathing Exercises	Relaxation and stress relief through therapeutic breathing
Cope with Bereavement	Hypnotherapy, coping
Depressed	Depression
Depression Consultant	Depression
Depression Cure: The Free 12 week course	12-step depression treatment
Depression Test & Tracker	Depression assessment and tracking
Digipill: Change Your Mind	Psychoacoustics to attend to depression, stress, weight, smoking, anxiety, etc.
DOD Self Helpline	Sexual assault
DREAM-e: Dream Therapy	Dreams
Eat, Sleep & Be Thin Hypnosis	(Self) Hypnosis, weight loss
iCBT	Cognitive behavioral therapy, stress, and anxiety

(continued)

Table 16.1 (continued)

App Name	Description
Inner Balance	Stress
Know thyself free psychology	Depression, panic, and emotional evaluation
Live Happy	Depression
Marriage and Counseling	Marriage counseling
Men's Psychology	Men's psychology improvement
Mental Fitness	Subconsciousness
Mental Health Assessments	Mental health assessment (surveys)
Mental Workout	Meditation and stress
Middle School Confidential 2: Real Friends vs. the Other Kind	Emotional and Social Issues
Mood Tuner	Stress
MoodBender	Re-energizing
MoodKit: Mood Improvement Tools	Emotion/well-being through cognitive behavior therapy (CBT)
MyinstantCOACH(TM)	Life coaching
MyPsych	Counseling
Panic Attack Eliminator	Panic attack
Panic Attack TalkDown	Panic attack
Panic Manager	Panic attack relief
Personal Psychology Tests	A variety of simple questionnaires to help determine various psychology disorder
Pocket PCM	Process Communication Model reference
Quit Smoking Now	Smoking addiction
Relax	Relaxation therapy
Senti	Stress
Sleep Now with Dr. Holt HD	Hypnotherapy, sleeping issues
Sport Psychology Focus&Breathe	Sports psychology
Stop Smoking in 5 Days	Smoking addiction
Stop Smoking Now (Pocket Hypnotherapy)	Hypnotherapy, smoking
Stress Free with Deepak Chopra	Stress management
Surviving Depression	Depression
SWS: Grief Support	Grief
Teen2Xtreme	Health literacy for teens
Unstuck	Personal growth
Wee You-Things	Teach diversity to kids
Your Child's Social Health	Surveys and assessments common in psychology and sociology targeting child social health
Your Rapid Diagnosis: Mental Health	Mental health diagnosis
Relax and Sleep Well with Glenn Harold	Hypnotherapy/sleep
CBT-i Coach	Insomnia

Apps can be downloaded through the App Store (i.e., Apple devices) and Google play (i.e., Android devices)

Fig. 16.2 Screenshot of the Plain Language Medical Dictionary iPhone app. The few terms shown in this screenshot of the app, such as "abdomen," "ability," 'absorption," and "accelerate," remind us, clinicians, scholars, and policy makers with a professional background, how such terms that we treat as easy, simple, and self-explanatory can be a source of confusion for many other people, even highly literate people, hence the importance of such online dictionary apps and tools. For example, the word "unsweetened" could cause much confusion to diabetic patients with low reading skills, who may only recognize the "sweetened" part in "unsweetened" and skip the "un" prefix, thus leading to the opposite behavior [43] (Source: Kamel Boulos [104])

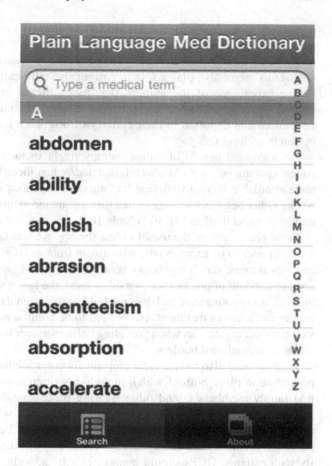

An example of an educational mobile app is the "Plain Language Medical Dictionary" iPhone app.[14] This free app converts medical language into everyday English and could be helpful for people to understand the meaning of medical terms they encounter online (Fig. 16.2).

Online Therapy

During the last decade, experts in the field have published findings that support the rapid development of online services, given their potential to reduce existing gaps between individuals struggling with psychopathology and access to treatment [90]. Currently healthcare among certain groups has been low, due to high

----

[14] Plain Language Medical Dictionary app: http://itunes.apple.com/us/app/plain-language-medical-dictionary/id443405990?mt=8.

premature termination and retention as mentioned earlier [15–17]. Patients avoid seeking healthcare treatment due to stigma; therefore, online therapy might be an innovative way to engage patients into treatment. Legal or citizenship status might also play a role in patient specialty care seeking. It is the collective experience of the authors that many illegal immigrants (individuals without legal citizenship) do not seek health treatment for fear of being denounced and deported to their country of origin. Online therapy might be an option to address this gap.

An additional benefit of online therapy might include cost-effectiveness. For patients paying out of pocket, web-based and/or text therapy applications convey a more affordable alternative to health treatment (i.e., Talkspace rates start at $19 per week). Other benefits for using online therapy are the anonymity, convenience, and uninhibitedness it offers [91, 92] (Table 16.2).

Some challenges on the use of online therapy are similar to those discussed for VCT. A patient who receives online treatment from an HCP who is in the same state can appeal to the state's regulatory board for any violations against either the state code or standard of practice. On the other hand, the law does not protect patients if the HCP is in another state and does not hold a professional license where the patient resides and receives treatment. HCPs need to be familiar and comply with all relevant laws and regulations when providing online services to patients across jurisdictional or international borders.

HCPs should also have a clear consent form for telehealth and an emergency procedure in place both of which include a written authority to contact identified family members(s) and other treating professionals in the patient's local area in case the HCP needs emergency backup. As with VCT, HCPs giving online therapy should use websites compliant with the Federal Health Insurance Portability and Accountability Act (HIPAA) and discuss limits of confidentiality with patients. HCPs should manage risk by adhering to their state standard of care and by using well-documented protocols [93]. See Table 16.3 for guidelines resources.

Education: Supervising Through Internet

According to the 2009 Practice Guidelines for Videoconferencing, supervision of all HCP students can be facilitated by VCT. Allowing for HCP students to obtain quality supervision using videoconferencing would benefit the field of healthcare in two major ways. First, more healthcare trainees would be able to practice in remote areas that generally lack healthcare services. Second, video supervision would allow trainees to travel to other sites to observe and learn from rare cases around the country or state without lacking professional supervision. Video supervision has the advantage of reducing costs of traveling and disseminating clinical training to minority providers that are in remote areas and could thereby increase the range of healthcare.

Table 16.2 Apps/websites providing therapy services in the United States

App/website	Description	URL
Text4Baby	Focuses on promoting maternal and child health. Provides free health text messages to new or pregnant mothers	http://www.text4baby.org
SmokeFreeTXT	Delivers tips, encouragement, and advice about smoking cessation	http://www.smokefree.gov/hp.aspx
MyTherapistNet	Website that presents legitimate therapists to the public	www.MyTherapistNet.com
Concerned Counseling	Network of online therapists based in San Antonio	www.concernedcounseling.com
Metanoia.org	Private nonprofit advocacy site that lists online therapists	www.metanoia.org
PsychCentral	Comprehensive guides to mental health online	http://psychcentral.com/
[a]Online-Therapy.com	Based on researched CBT for diverse presenting problems (i.e., depression, anxiety); includes daily contact with therapist using worksheets plus access to therapist live chat	http://www.online-therapy.com
[a]Lantern	Programs based on cognitive behavioral therapy and are built in partnership with experts at Stanford University, Penn State University and Washington University in St. Louis	https://golantern.com
[a]BetterHelp	Can be used from any device that has a web browser. It can be a computer, tablet, or smartphone. There is no special hardware required and you don't need to install any software	https://www.betterhelp.com
[a]Talkspace	Introduces Unlimited Messaging Therapy™, Video Therapy, and Couples Therapy. Promotes affordable rate(s) and confidential and anonymous therapy via smartphone and/or computer	http://www.talkspace.com

[a]Currently considered *unofficial* Telemental Health and/or mHealth service providers in the United States

Table 16.3 Telemental Health Resources

American Academy of Child and Adolescent Psychiatry	Practice Parameter for Telepsychiatry with Children and Adolescents (2008)	http://www.aacap.org/galleries/PracticeParameters/Telepsychiatry.pdf
American Psychological Association	Ethics Committee, APA statement on services by telephone, teleconferencing, and Internet Telehealth 50-State Review (March, 2010)	http://www.apa.org/ethics/education/telephone-statement.aspx http://www.apapracticecentral.org/advocacy/state/telehealth-slides.pdf
Videoconferencing-Based Telemental Health	Practice guidelines	http://www.americantelemed.org/i4a/pages/index.cfm?pageID=3326
National Association of Social Workers and Association of Social Work Boards	Standards for Technology and Social Work Practice	http://www.socialworkers.org/practice/standards/NASWTechnologyStandards.pdf
Ohio Psychological Association	Telepsychology Guidelines	http://www.ohpsych.org/resources/1/files/Comm%20Tech%20Committee/OPATelepsychologyGuidelines41710.pdf
University of Colorado Denver	Telemental Health Guidelines	http://www.tmhguide.org/
Administration Office of Telehealth	Health Resources and Services	http://www.hrsa.gov/ruralhealth/about/telehealth/
Department of the Army	Utilization of Tele-Behavioral Health Services	https://www.qmo.amedd.army.mil/credentialing/09_042.pdf
American Telemedicine Association (ATA)	Telemedicine Health Guidelines	http://www.americantelemed.org/resources/telemedicine-practice-guidelines/telemedicine-practice-guidelines/clinical-guidelines-for-telepathology#.Vd8M_-kn3wx
British Psychological Society (2009)	Provision of Psychological Services via the Internet and Other Non-direct Means	www.efpa.be
Canadian Psychological Association (2006)	Telemental Health Guidelines for Canada	http://www.cpa.ca/aboutcpa/committees/ethics/psychserviceselectronically/
US Department of Health & Human Services	Centers for Medicare & Medicaid Services	http://www.gpo.gov/fdsys/pkg/FR-2011-05-05/pdf/2011-10875.pdf

Ethical Considerations in Using IT

IT has many advantages in closing the gap in heath disparities but also posits many ethical challenges. HCPs need to develop technology proficiency to discuss risks and ethical controversies that may arise in treatment with patients. HCPs have major responsibility to take all reasonable action not to harm patients. Some general concerns with the use of IT are confidentiality issues, patient safety, informed consent, risk management, and licensure issues. Only programs compliant with the Federal Health Insurance Portability and Accountability Act (HIPAA) should be used when using technology for health services. HIPAA gives patients rights over their health information and sets rules and limitations on who can view and receive their health information. HCPs must take reasonable measures to protect sensitive data and discuss with patients the risks of breach of confidentiality. HCPs should also encourage patients to be cautious and diligent with the information they are able to keep in their personal devices. Security measures should be in place to ensure privacy. Text messaging encryption measures and password protection are recommended to ensure the integrity of the data. HCPs needs to be aware that Skype is not considered HIPAA compliant as it does not provide a secure system to store transmitted information [94, 95]. Most health and medical licensing boards seem to agree that an HCP should be licensed in the jurisdiction where the patient is located. In addition, emergency procedures should be in place for locating a patient's local police and hospitals when providing VCT or online treatments. Healthcare providers should have a backup plan in case there is a connection problem and discuss a protocol for when emergency arises.

Technology is moving more quickly than the research that informs health providers. By the time the research process is ready to support dissemination of the intervention to larger populations, the technology tested may have become obsolete [96, 97]. This posits challenges to regulatory bodies' ability to keep pace with rapid innovations in technology [96, 97]. The code of ethics in different health professions does not directly address specific types of technology, so the professionals themselves are charged with the responsibility of making ethical decisions. Novel ethical dilemmas might be a reflection of the new emerging technologies. Nonetheless, the advantages of using innovative IT tools to increase health equity challenge HCPs to think critically on ways to minimize ethical risks while promoting patients' well-being.

Future Directions

Scientific literature has demonstrated that IT provides the opportunity to bring more services to underserved populations but more research is needed to understand what kinds of services and what technologies are likely to be most useful with specific populations. As this new generation of digital natives moves into the future, we will expect an increase in the use and demand of technology in the healthcare arena. We must navigate this water ethically and responsibly and incorporate technology in professional and academic trainings. The rapid changes and inclusion of new technology tools in the healthcare setting merit constant education from HCPs, researchers, and patients.

In the United States, there is a shortage of bilingual and bicultural HCPs available to serve limited English-proficient patients [98]. The United States is a nation that is increasing in diversity, and by 2050 it is expected that 82 % of US growth will be attributed to Latinos [99]. In 20 years, one in every three persons will be Latino, hence, there is a lack of Latino HCPs [98]. Using distant-learning technology might be a viable way to reduce costs and promote training diverse populations to serve the needs of the country. In many hospitals today, HCPs use translators through a phone call system. Instead, it might be more efficient to use an HCP that has the appropriate training and competencies to treat a patient from distance. Training and supervising HCPs through remote electronic media are an effective way to reduce costs of traveling; increase quality training; increase racial, ethnic, bilingual, and other minority providers; and increase collaboration between HCPs from different state jurisdictions and countries. This can be viable if the field moves towards a national and international worldwide license promoting international health collaborations. IT can be instrumental in promoting international collaboration that can enhance the understanding of diverse populations. Authors suggest that leveraging technology for health is critical for ethnic minorities as well as special populations.

Furthermore, just because we live in a digital era, we cannot assume that all children, adolescents, and adults are literate in technology; literacy seems to be affected by social determinants such as ethnicity, race, gender, and available resources. If we want to promote patient-centered care among the underserved and increase their access to quality services, we need to provide basic education on technology and low-cost access to Internet or technological devices such as smartphones, tablets, or computers. Otherwise, the gap will increase due to lack of education and economic challenges. Technological education should be part of all schools' curriculums, as well as graduate training programs for HCPs.

The lack of technological health literacy in experienced HCPs (digital immigrants), who are often professors, consultants, or supervisors to medical and health trainees, may limit them to adequately address online problems that occur to them or their younger colleagues and trainees. Therefore, in order to proficiently navigate the new technology to better serve the needs of our population, we need to pursue regular continuing education to keep up with the ever-changing landscape, and we also need to include technology literacy in the curriculum of health graduate programs.

Summary

In this chapter the authors make the point that IT can be an innovative way to foster health equity in ethnic and racial minorities, disenfranchised populations, and VIP populations, as well as other populations discussed in previous chapters. As demonstrated in the literature, technology can be instrumental in the improvement of healthcare quality and reduction of health costs, stigma, and health disparities in vulnerable populations [100]. The different IT tools discussed in this chapter can be promising resources in addressing and alleviating the barriers to healthcare access and treatment vulnerable populations face [59, 60].

IT has the ability to reach out for broader audiences, to bridge physical distances and cultural differences, and to make information more accessible. Making information more accessible and self-directed learning more common and convenient can encourage patients to be active participants in their care. By activating and empowering patients, the cultural stigma surrounding healthcare is decreased [101]. As indicated in the literature, the majority of the vulnerable population is characterized by low levels of education, economic challenges, and impoverished environmental conditions [102, 103]. The use of IT tools with underserved populations might be the solution to improve quality of life and health in this and other diverse populations.

Another advantage of IT is the potential to facilitate research through the use of different tools such as EHRs, apps, and social media. Gathering large data sets in systematic ways can improve our understanding of the effect of contextual factors, genetics, and behavioral factors on the health of diverse populations to improve health equity.

On the other hand, IT brings a new language that HCPs who are mainly digital immigrants need to learn and understand. In order for the underserved to understand and use eHealth technology, we need to provide and increase eHealth literacy education among patients and HCPs. Technology has become a ubiquitous part of life in the twenty-first century, and it is our responsibility to become competent in the use of IT and help our patients navigate the new challenges and benefits of IT. Nonetheless, HCPs must also be aware of the ethical and legal challenges of levering technology for health equity. Furthermore, research on the topic of IT and health disparities are limited, but the authors believe that technology is the future bridge in medicine to decrease health disparity in vulnerable populations.

References

1. Purcell K, Rainie L. Technology's impact on workers. Pew Research Center. 2014. Available from: http://www.pewinternet.org/files/2014/12/PI_Web25WorkTech_12.30.141.pdf.
2. Merz Nagel D, Palumbo G. The role of blogging in mental health. In: Anthony K, Merz Nagel D, Goss S, editors. The use of technology in mental health: applications, ethics and practice. Illinois: Charles C. Thomas Publisher; 2010. p. 76–84.
3. Norcross JC, Hedges M, Prochaska JO. The face of 2010: a Delphi poll on the future of psychotherapy. Prof Psychol Res Pract. 2002;33:316–22.
4. Fox S, Duggan M. Health online 2013 [Internet]. Washington, D.C.; 2013. [cited 11 May 2015]. Available from: http://pewinternet.org/Reports/2013/Health-online.aspx.
5. Demiris G, Afrin LB, Speedie S, Courtney KL, Sondhi M, Vimarlund V, et al. Patient-centered applications: use of information technology to promote disease management and wellness. A White Paper by the AMIA Knowledge in Motion Working Group. J Am Med Inform Assoc

[Internet]. 2008;15(1):8–13. Available from: http://jamia.oxfordjournals.org/cgi/doi/10.1197/jamia.M2492.

6. U.S. Department of Health and Human Services. 2012 National Healthcare Quality Report [Internet]. Rockville; 2013. Available from: http://archive.ahrq.gov/research/findings/nhqrdr/nhqr12/2012nhqr.pdf.

7. Kushel MB. Factors associated with the health care utilization of homeless persons. JAMA [Internet]. 2001;285(2):200. Available from: http://jama.jamanetwork.com/article.aspx?doi=10.1001/jama.285.2.200.

8. Department of Housing and Urban Development. HUD supplemental report to the 2009 annual homeless assessment report to Congress. U.S. Department of Housing and Urban Development [Internet]. 2011. Available from: http://www.hudhre.info/documents/2009AHARVeteransReport.pdf.

9. McGuire J, Rosenheck R. The quality of preventive medical care for homeless veterans with mental illness. J Healthc Qual. 2005;27(6):26–32.

10. Edward J. Undocumented immigrants and access to health care: making a case for policy reform. Policy Polit Nurs Pract [Internet]. 2014;15(1-2):5–14. Available from: http://ppn.sagepub.com/cgi/doi/10.1177/1527154414532694.

11. Wallace SP, Torres J, Sadegh-Nobari T, Pourat N, Brown R. Undocumented immigrants and health care reform. UCLA Center for Health Policy Research. Final Report to the Commonwealth Fund; 2012.

12. Gorman A. Barriers remain despite health law's push to expand access to substance abuse treatment [Internet]. Kaiser Health News. 2014 [cited 15 Sept 2015]. Available from: http://khn.org/news/substance-abuse-treatment-access-health-law/.

13. (AHRQ) Agency for Healthcare Research and Quality. National Healthcare Disparities Report [Internet]. 2008 [cited 3 Aug 2011]. Available from: www.ahrq.gov/qual/nhdr05/fullreport/Index.htm.

14. Snowden L, Catalano R, Shumway M. Disproportionate use of psychiatric emergency services by African Americans. Psychiatr Serv [Internet]. 2009;60(12):1664–71. Available from: http://psychiatryonline.org/article.aspx?doi=10.1176/appi.ps.60.12.1664.

15. Scholle SH, Kelleher K. Preferences for depression advice among low-income women. Matern Child Health J. 2003;7:95–102.

16. McCaul M, Svikis DS, Moore RD. Predictors of outpatient treatment retention: patient versus substance use characteristics. Drug Alcohol Depend. 2001;62:9–17.

17. McFarland BR, Klein D. Mental health service use by patients with dysthymic disorder: treatment use and dropout in a 7 1/2-year naturalistic follow-up study. Compr Psychiatry [Internet]. 2005;46:246–53.

18. National Association of Community Health. Health wanted: the state of unmet need for primary health care in America [Internet]. Washington, D.C.; 2012. Available from: http://www.nachc.com/client/HealthWanted.pdf.

19. Brand MK, Mohatt DF. Mental health and rural America: 1994–2005 [Internet]. U.S. Department of Health Human Services Health Resources and Services Administration Office of Rural Health Policy. 2007. Available from: ftp://ftp.hrsa.gov/ruralhealth/RuralMentalHealth.pdf.

20. Duggan M, Ellison NB, Lampe C, Lenhart A, Madden M. Social media update 2014. Washington,D.C: Pew Research Center; 2015. Available from: http://www.pewinternet.org/files/2015/01/PI_SocialMediaUpdate20144.pdf.

21. Lenhart A. Teens, social media & technology overview 2015. Washington, D.C.: Pew Research Center's Internet & American Project; 2012. Available from: http://www.pewinternet.org/2015/04/09/teens-social-media-technology-2015.

22. Madden M, Zickuhr K. 65% of online adults use social networking sites [Internet]. Washington, DC; 2011. Available from: http://www.pewinternet.org/~/media//Files/Reports/2011/PIP-SNS-Update-2011.pdf.

23. Hauber RP, Vesmarovich S, Dufour L. The use of computers and the internet as a source of health information for people with disabilities. Rehabil Nurs [Internet]. 2002;27(4):142–5. Available from: http://doi.wiley.com/10.1002/j.2048-7940.2002.tb02222.x.

24. American Psychological Association. American Psychological Association guidelines for the practice of telepsychology [Internet]. 2013. Available from: http://www.apa.org/practice/guidelines/telepsychology.aspx.
25. Prensky M. Digital natives, digital immigrants Part 1. On the Horizon 2001;9(5):1–6. http://dx.doi.org/10.1108/10748120110424816.
26. Stellefson M, Hanik B, Chaney B, Chaney D, Tennant B, Chavarria EA. eHealth literacy among college students: a systematic review with implications for eHealth education. J Med Internet Res [Internet]. 2011;13(4):e102. Available from: http://www.jmir.org/2011/4/e102/.
27. Ratzan SC, Parker R. Introduction. National library of medicine current bibliographies in medicine: health literacy. In: Seldon CR, Zorn M, Ratzan SC, Parker RM, editors. National library of medicine current bibliographies in medicine: health literacy. NLM Pub. No. CBM 2000-1 ed. Bethesda: National Institutes of Health, US Department of Health and Human Services.
28. Glassman P. Health literacy. US National Network of Libraries of Medicine [Internet]. National Network of Libraries of Medicine. 2011. Available from: http://nnlm.gov/outreach/consumer/hlthlit.html.
29. Knapp C, Madden V, Wang H, Sloyer PSE. Internet use and eHealth literacy of low-income parents whose children have special health care needs. J Med Internet Res. 2011;13(3), e75.
30. Neter E, Brainin E. eHealth literacy: extending the digital divide to the realm of health information. J Med Internet Res. 2012;14(1), e19.
31. Fox S, Purcell K. Chronic disease and the Internet [Internet]. 2010. Available from: http://pewinternet.org/Reports/2010/Chronic-Disease.aspx.
32. Norman CD, Skinner HA. eHealth literacy: essential skills for consumer health in a networked World. J Med Internet Res. 2006;8(4), e27.
33. Glueckauf RL, Pickett TC, Ketterson TU, Loomis JS, Rozensky RH. Preparation for the delivery of telehealth services: a self-study framework for expansion of practice. Prof Psychol Res Pract [Internet]. 2003;34(2):159–63. Available from: http://doi.apa.org/getdoi.cfm?doi=10.1037/0735-7028.34.2.159.
34. Castelnuovo G, Gaggioli A, Mantovani F, Riva G. New and old tools in psychotherapy: the use of technology for the integration of traditional clinical treatments. Psychother Theory Res Pract Train. 2003;40(1/2):33–44.
35. Dixon R. Internet videoconferencing: coming to your campus soon! Educ Q [Internet]. 2000;(4):22–7. Available from: https://net.educause.edu/ir/library/pdf/EQM0043.pdf.
36. Dietrich D, Thomesse JP, Neumann P, editors. Fieldbus systems and their applications. Oxford: Elsevier IFAC Publications; 2003.
37. Kobayashi LC, Wardle J, von Wagner C. Internet use, social engagement and health literacy decline during ageing in a longitudinal cohort of older English adults. J Epidemiol Community Health [Internet]. 2015;69(3):278–83. Available from: http://jech.bmj.com/lookup/doi/10.1136/jech-2014-204733.
38. Kamel Boulos MN, Tsouros AD, Halopainen A. "Social, innovative and smart cities are happy and resilient": insights from the WHO EURO 2014 International Healthy Cities Conference. Int J Heal Geogr [Internet]. 2015;14(3). Available from: http://www.ij-healthgeographics.com/content/pdf/1476-072X-14-3.pdf – HTML: http://www.ij-healthgeographics.com/content/14/1/3.
39. Gosselin P, Poitras P. Use of an internet "viral" marketing software platform in health promotion. J Med Internet Res [Internet]. 2008;10(4):e47. Available from: http://www.jmir.org/2008/4/e47/.
40. Fox S. The social life of health information, 2011: Peer-to-peer Healthcare [Internet]. 2011. Available from: http://pewinternet.org/Reports/2011/Social-Life-of-Health-Info/Part-3/Section-1.aspx.
41. Frost JH, Massagli MP. Social uses of personal health information within PatientsLikeMe, an online patient community: What can happen when patients have access to one another's data. J Med Internet Res [Internet]. 2008;10(3):e15. Available from: http://www.jmir.org/2008/3/e15/.
42. Wicks P, Keininger DL, Massagli MP, la Loge de C, Brownstein C, Isojärvi J, et al. Perceived benefits of sharing health data between people with epilepsy on an online platform. Epilepsy

Behav [Internet]. 2012;23(1):16–23. Available from: http://linkinghub.elsevier.com/retrieve/pii/S1525505011005609.

43. Boulos MN. British internet-derived patient information on diabetes mellitus: is it readable? Diabetes Technol Ther. 2005;7(3):528–35.

44. Kamel Boulos MN, Harvey FE, Roudsari AV, Bellazzi R, Hernando ME, Deutsch T, et al. A proposed semantic framework for diabetes education content management, customisation and delivery within the M2DM project. Comput Methods Programs Biomed [Internet]. 2006;83(3):188–97. Available from: http://linkinghub.elsevier.com/retrieve/pii/S0169260706001635.

45. Kamel Boulos M. Social media and Web 2.0: effect on governance for health. In: Kickbusch I, Gleicher D, editors. Smart governance for health and well-being: the evidence [Internet]. World Health Organization Regional Office for Europe; 2014. p. 106–27. Available from: http://www.euro.who.int/__data/assets/pdf_file/0005/257513/Smart-governance-for-health-and-well-being-the-evidence.pdf.

46. Gibbons MC, Fleisher L, Slamon RE, Bass S, Kandadai V, Beck JR. Exploring the potential of Web 2.0 to address health disparities. J Health Commun [Internet]. 2011;16(sup1):77–89. Available from: http://dx.doi.org/10.1080/10810730.2011.596916.

47. Metzger MJ, Flanagin AJ. Technologies to enhance evidence-based medical information. J Health Commun. 2011;16 Suppl 1:45–58.

48. Corrigan JM, Donaldson MS, Kohn LT, Maguire SK, Pike KC. Crossing the quality chasm: a new health system for the 21st Century. Washington, DC: National Academy Press; 2001.

49. Sanchez K, Chapa T, Ybarra R, Martinez ON. Eliminating disparities through the integration of behavioral health and primary care services for racial and ethnic minority populations, including individuals with limited english proficiency: a literature review report. United States Department of Health and Human Services, Office of Minority Health; 2012.

50. Adler NE, Stead W. Patients in context- HER capture of social and behavioral determinants of health. N Engl J Med. 2015;372(8):698–701. doi: 10.1056/NEJMp1413945.

51. Getz L. EHRs in behavioral health — a digital future? Soc Work Today [Internet]. 2013;13(3):24. Available from: http://www.socialworktoday.com/archive/051313p24.shtml.

52. American Telemedicine Association. Telemedicine Defined [Internet]. 2010 [cited 6 Jan 2015]. Available from: http://www.americantelemed.org/about-telemedicine/what-is-telemedicine#.Ve886WTBzGc.

53. Barnwell SV, Juretic MA, Hoerster KD, Van de Plasch R, Felker BL. VA puget sound telemental health service to rural veterans: a growing program. Psychol Serv. 2012;9(2):209–11.

54. Jerome LW, Zaylor C. Cyberspace: creating a therapeutic environment for telehealth applications. Prof Psychol Res Pract. 2000;31:478–83.

55. Jaglal SB, Haroun VA, Salbach NM, Hawker G, Voth J, Lou W, et al. Increasing access to chronic disease self-management programs in rural and remote communities using telehealth. Telemed e-Health [Internet]. 2013;19(6):467–73. Available from: http://online.liebertpub.com/doi/abs/10.1089/tmj.2012.0197.

56. Kvam MH, Loeb M, Tambs K. Mental health in deaf adults: symptoms of anxiety and depression among hearing and deaf individuals. J Deaf Stud Deaf Educ. 2007;12:1–7.

57. Munro-Ludders B, Simpatico T, Zvetina D. Making public mental-health services accessible to deaf consumers: Illinois Deaf Services. Am Ann Deaf. 2004;148:396–403.

58. Steinberg AG, Sullivan VJ, Loew RC. Cultural and linguistic barriers to mental health service access: the deaf consumer's perspective. Am J Psychiatry. 1998;155:982–4.

59. Wilson JA, Schild S. Provision of mental health care services to deaf individuals using telehealth. Prof Psychol Res Pract. 2014;45(5):324–31.

60. Wilson JA, Wells MG. Telehealth and the deaf: a comparison study. J Deaf Stud Deaf Educ. 2009;14:386–402.

61. Whealing JM, Kuhn E, Pietrzak RH. Applying behavior change theory to technology promoting Veteran Mental Health Care seeking. Psychol Serv. 2014;11(4):486–94.

62. Benros ME. Posttraumatic stress disorder and autoimmune diseases. Biol Psychiatry. 2015;77(4):312–3.

63. Pietrzak RH, Goldstein RB, Southwick SM, Grant BF. Prevalence and Axis I comorbidity of full and partial posttraumatic stress disorder in the United States: results from Wave 2 of the National Epidemiologic Survey on Alcohol and Related Conditions. J Anxiety Disord. 2011;25:456–65.
64. Department of Veterans Affairs. VA hires more mental health professionals to expand access for veterans. Office of Public and Intergovernmental Affairs. U.S. Department of Veterans Affairs. 2013 http://www.va.gov/opa/pressrel/pressrelease.cfm?id=2428.
65. McLean B. Stigma of mental health in sports remains an opponent. NAMI: National Alliance on Mental Health. 2015. Available from: http://www2.nami.org/Template.cfm?Section=Top_Story&template=/ContentManagement/ContentDisplay.cfm&ContentID=166507.
66. Logan JR. Rural America as a symbol of American values. Rural Dev Res Rep [Internet]. 1997;12(1):19–21. Available from: http://webarchives.cdlib.org/sw1bc3ts3z/http://ers.usda.gov/Publications/RDP/rdp1096/RDP1096E.pdf.
67. NORC at the University of Chicago. Assessment of health IT and data exchange in safety net providers. Final report to assistant secretary for planning and evaluation [Internet]. 2010. Available from: http://aspe.hhs.gov/sp/reports/2010/chcit2010/report.pdf.
68. NORC A the U of C. Understanding the impact of health IT in underserved communities and those with health disparities [Internet]. Bethesda; 2010. Available from: http://www.healthit.gov/sites/default/files/pdf/hit-underserved-communities-health-disparities.pdf.
69. Hispanic Institute and Mobile Future. Hispanic broadband access: making the most of the mobile, connected future [Internet]. 2009. Available from: http://www.thehispanicinstitute.net/files/u2/Hispanics_and_Broadband_Access_0.pdf.
70. PwC Health Research Institute. Healthcare unwired: new business models delivering care anywhere. 2010. http://pwchealth.com/cgi-local/hregister.cgi/reg/healthcare-unwired.pdf.
71. Stewart M, Brown JB, Donner A, McWhinney IR, Oates J, Weston W, Jordan J. The impact of patient-centered care on outcomes. J Fam Pract. 2000;49(9):796–804.
72. US Census Bureau Data Integration Division. Educational attainment. 2013. p. 3–5. Available from: http://www.census.gov/hhes/socdemo/education/.
73. U.S. Department of Health and Human Services (HERSA). Health Resources and Services Administration. Using health text messages to improve consumer health knowledge, behaviors, and outcomes: an environmental scan. U.S. HRSA, editor. Rockville: U.S.; 2014.
74. Haug S, Meyer C, Schorr G, Bauer S, John U. Continuous individual support of smoking cessation using text messaging: a pilot experimental study. Nicotine Tob Res. 2009;11(8):915–23.
75. Obermayer JL, Rley WT, Asif O, Jean-Mary J. College smoking-cessation using cell phone text messaging. J Am Coll Health. 2004;53(2):71–8.
76. Whittaker R, Borland R, Bullen C, Lin RB, McRobbie H, Rodgers A. Mobile phone-based interventions for smoking cessation. In: Whittaker R, editor. Cochrane database of systematic reviews [Internet]. Chichester: Wiley; 2009. Available from: http://doi.wiley.com/10.1002/14651858.CD006611.pub2.
77. Haines J, McDonald J, O'Brien A, et al. Healthy habits, happy homes: randomized trial to improve household routines for obesity prevention among preschool-aged children. JAMA Pediatr. 2013;167(11):1072–9.
78. Lang L. Text messaging may help children to fight off obesity. Gastroenterology. 2009;136(1):7–8.
79. Tate EB, Spruijt-Metz D, O'Reilly G, Jordan-Marsh M, Gotsis M, Pentz MA, et al. mHealth approaches to child obesity prevention: successes, unique challenges, and next directions. Transl Behav Med [Internet]. 2013;3(4):406–15. Available from: http://link.springer.com/10.1007/s13142-013-0222-3.
80. Vervloet M, Linn AJ, van Weert JCM, de Bakker DH, Bouvy ML, van Dijk L. The effectiveness of interventions using electronic reminders to improve adherence to chronic medication: a systematic review of the literature. J Am Med Inform Assoc [Internet]. 2012;19(5):696–704. Available from: http://jamia.oxfordjournals.org/lookup/doi/10.1136/amiajnl-2011-000748.
81. Downer SR, Meara JG, Da Costa AC, Sethuraman K. SMS text messaging improves outpatient attendance. Aust Health Rev. 2006;30(3):389–96. http://dx.doi.org/10.1071/AH060389.

82. Gurol-Urganci I, de Jongh T, Vodopivec-Jamsek V, Atun R, Car J. Mobile phone messaging reminders for attendance at healthcare appointments. In: Car J, editor. Cochrane database of systematic reviews [Internet]. Chichester: Wiley; 2013. Available from: http://doi.wiley.com/10.1002/14651858.CD007458.pub3.

83. Hurling R, Catt M, Boni MD, et al. Using internet and mobile phone technology to deliver an automated physical activity program: randomized controlled trial. J Med Internet Res. 2007;9(2), e7.

84. Shapiro JR, Bauer S, Hamer RM, Kordy H, Ward D, Bulik CM. Use of text messaging for monitoring sugar-sweetened beverages, physical activity, and screen time in children: a pilot study. J Nutr Educ Behav. 2008;40(6):385–91.

85. Zhu FQ, Mariappan A, Boushey CJ, et al. Technology-assisted dietary assessment. Conference on computational imaging VI. San Jose: Proc SPIE. 2008 Mar 20; 6814: 681411. doi: 10.1117/12.778616; 2008.

86. Alegría M, Vallas M, Pumarriega AJ. Racial and ethnic disparities in pediatric mental health. Child Adolesc Psychiatr Clin N Am. 2010;19(4):759–74.

87. Boncana H. "mHealth Evidence Database." Presentation at the mHealth working group meeting [Internet]. 2013. Available from: http://www.mhealthworkinggroup.org/resources/presentation-about-mhealth-evidence-database.

88. Nilsen W, Santosh K, Shar A, Varoquiers DC, Wiley T, Riley WT, Pavel M, Atienza A. Advancing the science of mHealth. J Health Commun Int Perspect. 2012;17(suppl): 5–10.

89. Tamrat T, Kachnoswki S. Special delivery: an analysis of mHealth in maternal and newborn health programs and their outcomes around the world. Matern Child Health J. 2012;16(5): 1092–101.

90. Reynolds DJ, Stiles WB, Bailer AJ, Hughes MR. Impact of exchanges and client–therapist alliance in online-text psychotherapy. Cyberpsychol Behav Soc Netw [Internet]. 2013;16(5):370–7. Available from: http://online.liebertpub.com/doi/abs/10.1089/cyber.2012.0195.

91. Barak A, Grohol JM. Current and future trends in internet- supported mental health interventions. J Technol Hum Serv. 2011;29(3):155–96.

92. Suler J. The online disinhibition effect. Cyber Psychol Behav. 2004;7:321–6.

93. Maheu MM, Gordon BL. Counseling and therapy on the internet. Prof Psychol Res Pract. 2000;31:484–9.

94. Luxton DD, Kayl RA, Mishkind MC. mHealth data security: the need for HIPAA-compliant standardization. Tlemed E-Health. 2012;18(4):284–8.

95. Maheu MM, Pulier ML, et al. The mental health professional and the new technologies. Mahweh: Erlbaum; 2005.

96. Dickey R. Perceived risks and benefits of emerging technologies in professional psychology. http://digitalcommons.georgefox.edu/psyd/74. George Fox University; 2011.

97. Taylor L, McMinn MR, Bufford RK, Chang KBT. Psychologists' attitudes and ethical concerns regarding the use of social networking websites. Prof J Psychol Res Pract. 2010;41(2):153–9. http://psycnet.apa.org/doi/10.1037/a0017996.

98. Aguilar-gaxiola S, Loera G, Mendez L, Sala M. Community-defined solutions for latino mental health care disparities: California reducing disparities project, Latino Strategic Planning Workgroup Population Report. Sacramento: UC Davis; 2012.

99. Johnson KM, Lichter DT. Growing diversity among America's children and youth: spatial and temporal dimensions. Popul Dev Rev. 2010;36(March):151–75.

100. Chaudhry B, Wang J, Wu S, Maglione M, Mojica W, Roth E, et al. Systematic review: impact of health information technology on quality, efficiency, and costs of medical care. Ann Intern Med. 2006;144:742–52.

101. Holden KB, Xanthos C. Disadvantages in mental health care among African Americans. J Health Care Poor Underserved. 2009;20:17–23.

102. Treadwell H, Xanthos C, Holden K, editors. Social determinants of health among African-American men. San Francisco: Jossey-Bass/Wiley; 2012.

103. Zuvekas SH, Taliaferro GS. Pathways to access: health insurance, the health care delivery system, and racial/ethnic disparities, 1996–1999. Health Aff [Internet]. 2003;22(2):139–53. Available from: http://content.healthaffairs.org/cgi/doi/10.1377/hlthaff.22.2.139.
104. Kamel Boulos MN. On social media in health literacy. WebmedCentral HEALTH INFORMATICS. 2012;3(1): WMC002936.

Chapter 17
Advances and Challenges in Conducting Research with Diverse and Vulnerable Populations in a Healthcare Setting: Reducing Stigma and Increasing Cultural Sensitivity

Louise Dixon, Manisha Salinas, and Luana Marques

Introduction

Health research of diverse and vulnerable populations has been historically under-emphasized and overlooked. This is, in part, due to inadequate methodological and ethical practices, which can contribute to persistent health disparities across groups. Currently, studies continue to demonstrate that co-occurring psychosocial factors can synergistically increase an individual's risk for acquiring one or more health problem [1], and diverse and vulnerable populations have worse health outcomes than their counterparts [2–5]. Additionally, these groups have less access to evidence-based treatments, which can further exacerbate health problems [6–10]. Research is needed to determine best practices and increase access to care in these populations, reduce stigma, and increase cultural sensitivity. For example, one of the most prominent barriers to care is societal stigma around mental health and lack of cultural sensitivity among researchers and clinicians [11]. Research may help clinicians and investigators alike in understanding ways to overcome stigma and increase cultural sensitivity, which in turn results in better patient outcomes and increased access to care.

L. Dixon, BA (✉)
Department of Psychology, University of California Los Angeles, Los Angeles, CA, USA
e-mail: ldixon7891@ucla.edu

M. Salinas, MA
Department of Psychiatry, Massachusetts General Hospital, Boston, MA, USA

Department of Public Health, Texas A&M Health Science Center, School of Public Health, Round Rock, TX, USA

L. Marques, PhD
Department of Psychiatry, Massachusetts General Hospital, Boston, MA, USA

Department of Psychiatry, Harvard Medical School, Boston, MA, USA

© Springer International Publishing Switzerland 2016
R. Parekh, Ed W. Childs (eds.), *Stigma and Prejudice: Touchstones in Understanding Diversity in Healthcare*, Current Clinical Psychiatry,
DOI 10.1007/978-3-319-27580-2_17

However, conducting research can be challenging, as many socially disadvantaged groups have a history of experiencing maltreatment in research. Although there are safeguards in place to protect diverse and vulnerable groups from unethical research practices, recruitment and retention in research continues to pose a significant barrier. In turn, these barriers deter many researchers from conducting studies that could potentially improve health outcomes and access to care.

This chapter will review the literature on the advances and challenges in conducting research with diverse and vulnerable populations in a healthcare setting. The aim of this chapter is to aid researchers across diverse health-related fields in understanding ethical challenges in conducting research with diverse and vulnerable populations in the context of history in addition to discussing some of the methodological challenges of working with these groups. In addition to focusing broadly across diverse and vulnerable populations, we will also highlight concerns that are population specific across the following domains: (1) racial and ethnic minorities, (2) sexual orientation and gender minorities (i.e., lesbian, gay, bisexual, trans*, queer [LGBTQ]), (3) prisoners, and (4) individuals with chronic illnesses or limitations. Specifically, we will answer the following two questions: (1) what are important historical and ethical considerations for research with diverse and vulnerable populations and (2) what are important methodological considerations for research with diverse and vulnerable populations? Finally, we will provide suggestions for future research based on the literature presented in the chapter.

What Are Important Historical and Ethical Considerations for Research with Diverse and Vulnerable Populations?

Racial and Ethnic Minorities

Racial and ethnic minorities in this chapter refer to Latinos, Asians, African Americans, and American Indians or Alaskan Natives. While there are a vast array of groups and subgroups within these categories, this section will focus on a broad scope of underlying principles in health research with these particular groups. Racial and ethnic minorities overall have high prevalence of health problems and diseases, as well as less availability and accessibility of healthcare than whites in the USA [12]. Historically, ethnic minorities have been largely marginalized in health research and have been subject to exploitation, discrimination, and underrepresentation due to language barriers, low socioeconomic status, differences in communication styles, and mistrust of medical professionals [13]. This history has resulted in significant challenges in conducting the necessary research to adequately address observed health disparities. Today, the National Institutes of Health insists that clinical trials include a participant sample consisting of a diverse population of volunteers [11]. Building trusting relationships and ensuring ethical treatment of research participants have been greatly prioritized in contemporary health research; however, much is still needed to be considered [14].

Steps taken to ensure a more ethical approach for these groups are based on respect and awareness on part of the researcher, with the goal of promoting social justice and advocacy to improve health outcomes and reduce disparities [15–17]. For example, Rugkåsa and Canvin [17] examined the HealthTalkOnline collection, an online resource consisting of narratives from a diverse group of individuals with a wide array of health conditions. The purpose of the diversity of these narratives is to ensure that anyone who accesses the site will have access to an account from a person of a similar race, age, or ethnicity. While there are certain considerations shared across ethnic minority groups, the unique ethical considerations of major racial and ethnic groups in the USA are highlighted below, focusing on Latinos, Asians, African Americans, and American Indian or Alaskan Natives.

As a result of immigration, Latino and Asian groups share considerable similarities in the application of ethical practice to health research. Important research considerations for these groups involve understanding cultural values and beliefs which may present as barriers, including immigration status, language, or other sociocultural characteristics. For example, Latino immigrants may be more likely to have an undocumented status, as the majority of undocumented individuals in the USA have been from Latin-American countries, and may be excluded from potentially beneficial health research [18]. Moreover, the fear of deportation or other political ramifications from being "exposed" may be present, so ensuring confidentiality for these individuals is of utmost importance [19].

Though Asian groups are also rapidly growing in the USA, health data is limited, and negative attitudes toward Asian immigrants have persisted for decades [20]. Racial discrimination can impair social mobility and contribute to mortality in minority groups [21]. Researchers have found the prevalence of stereotypes including that Asians are seen as docile or speak with heavily accented English [20]. Continued discrimination can negatively impact accessing health services, and limited health research for these groups point toward the need for increasing participation in studies [20, 22]. Asian groups overall may face more stigma in expressing issues, such as mental health problems, so cultural norms and values should be taken into consideration in communicating purposes of health research in these communities [23]. Studies should clearly outline goals and be presented in a respectful manner with the unique characteristics of the targeted group in mind. For those with limited English proficiency or other cultural barriers, human subject's protection statements may not be clearly outlined and trust with researchers can be significantly affected. Additionally, immigrant groups in general may also be particularly vulnerable as they are newcomers faced with an unfamiliar healthcare system or may have limited communication abilities to seek treatment. As a result, the purpose and intent of health research studies may be misunderstood or misinterpreted by participants [19]. These groups are less likely to participate in health research, so sensitivity toward immigrant and cultural characteristics should be taken into consideration.

African Americans also generally have low participation in health research [15]. The mistrust of authoritative persons and institutions, such as those in research, is rooted in historical and persistent discrimination faced by African Americans in society. The Tuskegee syphilis study, for example, is well known for its exploitation and abuse of African-American research participants and contributes to the feelings of distrust in these communities [14, 24].

The Tuskegee study was federally funded and conducted in 1932 in Macon County, Alabama. In this area, syphilis had become an epidemic, and the US Public Health Service was called in to help with the issue, as untreated syphilis can lead to serious health problems and even death. Participants in the study were all poor African-American men and were uninformed of the actual intentions of the research; they vaguely were told they were being treated for "bad blood" [25]. The participants were treated as inferior and were given substandard care compared to the treatment of syphilis in other parts of the country. The men ended up being tested for procedural and disease-related complications rather than being treated for syphilis itself. The lack of informed consent, voluntary participation, and poor treatment of the African-American participants led to a call for mandatory ethics committees to standardize appropriate treatment of human subjects in health research [25].

Decades later, research assessing African-American perspectives on health research participation found many group members continue to believe researchers were dishonest and unclear in aspects of research such as informed consent and did not provide enough information about the purpose or benefits of the research study [26]. Many participants felt that being involved in medical trials makes them a "guinea pig" and may fear the actual research trials could lead to medical conditions or infectious diseases [27]. Ethical considerations with these groups include awareness for reasons of mistrust and importance of full disclosure in research.

Finally, American Indian and Alaskan Natives suffer from significant historical abuse and exploitation as a result of early European colonization, with health inequalities persisting even today. After land being forcefully taken by governmental authorities, languages and practices prohibited, and sovereign rights violated, mistrust and suspicion within these groups toward "outsiders" understandably occurred [28, 29]. Clinical misconduct has continued even within the past few decades, as medical researchers have misused data or conducted research that has negatively contributed to stigma among these communities by reinforcing negative stereotypes [28]. The historical maltreatment, societal discrimination, and unethical research practices have continued over the course of hundreds of years still affecting these communities, and considerations for the context of these communities should inform ethical practices for health researchers [28, 30].

Sexual Orientation and Gender Minorities

Sexual orientation and gender minority groups (i.e., LGBTQ) are also particularly vulnerable due to societal stigma and mistreatment. This population has also historically been mistreated or overlooked in health research [31, 32]. In the past, for example, homosexuality was considered deviant behavior or seen as a psychological disorder by researchers [32, 33]. In the early twentieth century, homosexuality was even considered a biological deficiency by scientists, and those who exhibited this type of behavior faced imprisonment or physical harm, such as castration [34]. It was not until the 1970s that the American Psychiatric Association formally removed homosexuality as a mental disorder [35]. While this began a paradigm shift regarding the perception of homosexuality, social attitudes continue to be negative and stigmatizing toward these groups [32, 33, 35].

Societal acceptance of sexual minorities is an ongoing struggle. For this reason, ethical considerations involving participant protection and confidentiality are essential. Sexual behavior in general is considered a very sensitive and private topic, so research focusing on sexual minority health may be viewed as overly intrusive [36]. This calls for building trust within the sexual orientation and gender minority community and making motives for research clear, ensuring results from studies will not harm or otherwise negatively impact individuals or their communities [36]. Research with these groups should promote social justice to help eliminate stigma and improve access to resources [35]. Research should also ensure confidentiality and anonymity of information, so that individuals are not "outed" because of participation in sexual orientation-focused or gender minority-focused research [35, 37].

Prisoners

In the USA, the US Department of Corrections supervises seven million individuals, which is almost 25 % of the world's prison population [38, 39]. Prisoners lose their autonomy upon incarceration and experience marginalization, which increases their vulnerability to maltreatment in healthcare research [40]. Like other vulnerable populations, prisoners have a history of exploitation and marginalization that raises several ethical concerns when using prisoners as research subjects in healthcare. In 1948 in light of the Nuremberg trials, the *Journal of the American Medical Association* published regulations for conducting research with prisoners. These new protections allowed researchers to conduct research with prisoners, and research on prisoners became widespread. Yet, since there were no regulations to ensure disclosure of risks, prisoners became a heavily studied population in various research studies that involved potentially life-threatening consequences throughout the 1950–1980s [41]. For example, prisoners were often used as subjects in drug toxicity trials and pharmaceutical research, in addition to being in studies involving the introduction of infectious diseases to otherwise healthy individuals [41–43]. Additionally, many research studies involved coercion and lack of informed consent [42].

The Common Rule (1991) finally identified prisoners as a vulnerable population and thus deserving of particular protections in research. For example, only minimal risk research is allowed, and certain types of research are permitted if the research is funded by a federal agency [41]. Most recently in 2006, the Institute of Medicine (IOM) issued the Ethical Considerations for Research Involving Prisoners, which contained five components: (1) expansion of the definition of "prisoner"; (2) insurance of universal, consistent ethical protection; (3) a shift from a category-based to a risk-benefit approach to research review; (4) an update to the ethical framework to include collaborative responsibility; and (5) enhancement of the systematic oversight of research with prisoners [41, 42, 44].

International regulations agree on several components of research with prisoners: (1) prisoners should have access to research that provides direct benefits, and (2) prisoners are in a vulnerable state that could interfere with the process of informed consent and should be protected [45]. In order to protect prisoners during the process of consent, more attention should be paid to assure non-coerced consent, and there should be restrictions on the type of research performed in prison settings. Participation in research should not come with any financial incentive, nor should influence length of sentence. Restrictions for research include limitation of risk for all research, and no research should afford the possibility of physical or moral injury [45]. Given that there are many restrictions on conducting research with prison populations, many researchers now question whether prisoners are now an overprotected group, meaning protections limit the potential benefits of research [42, 46]. Finding a way to conduct safe, beneficial research with the prison population that has the potential to influence health outcomes is an essential next step in the field; although regulations and protection for researches allow ethical investigations, learning how to better serve and treat the health needs of this population is essential to improving health outcomes – which is why research is desperately needed.

Individuals with Chronic Illnesses or Limitations

Individuals with chronic illnesses or limitations (e.g., Alzheimer's, substance use disorders, HIV, etc.) have a history of maltreatment in science [47, 48]. Since World War II, there have been several safeguards aimed at protecting individuals with these limitations, for which the biggest challenge in research has been and remains the informed consent process. The Helsinki Declaration (1964) stated that all individuals involved in research must have sufficient information about a study to make an informed choice about participation, must be able to make a decision, and must be able to make the decision autonomously and voluntarily. Today, there is lack of consensus in the literature about what criteria should be used to determine if someone is able to consent to research. However, researchers have agreed that at a minimum, a participant should be able to indicate his or her preference between participation and nonparticipation and should be able to communicate these options to researchers [48].

Researchers have raised several questions about how one should obtain consent from an individual with chronic illnesses or limitations. One proposed method of obtaining consent is by using a patient advocate during the consent process or obtaining consent by proxy [49, 50]. If researchers are gathering consent by proxy, it is essential to identify the people who would be most appropriate to give consent.

However, consent by proxy is not without limitations; determining what is in the participant's "best interest" cannot be measured objectively [49]. Some argue that using proxies does not empower individuals with chronic illnesses, in particular intellectual, cognitive, or developmental limitations, because of application of this principle would only allow others to make decisions on their behalf. Some researchers have argued that assent is sufficient in the context of clinical research with individuals with these conditions, which relies on knowledge of participants' facial expressions, vocalizations, and behaviors [49].

There are also ethical considerations for confidentiality in research in which third parties (such as parents, proxies, etc.) are involved in study participation and treatment. Researchers and clinicians may have difficulty determining how much personal health information they should share with these parties. Duncan, Drew, Hodgson, and Sawyer (2009) report difficulty maintaining confidentiality in research with adolescents with chronic illness who are noncompliant with medication and experiencing negative health outcomes; although the researchers promised the adolescent confidentiality, they felt a moral obligation to report the noncompliance to his parents.

Lastly, research with individuals with chronic illnesses or limitations can be difficult because many trials involve more than minimal risk [51]. In particular, in many pharmaceutical or treatment trails, side effects of a given intervention may constitute more than minimal risk, especially if the research is with otherwise healthy individuals [51]. In these cases, it is critical for researchers and ethics committees to determine the best ways of obtaining consent for such research, given the pressing need for advancement of research in conditions such as Alzheimer's disease, HIV, and other chronic medical conditions.

Moving Forward: Ethical Principles for Research with Diverse and Vulnerable Populations

Although the needs of each group discussed here vary widely, the authors' collective expertise support the application of five core principles in conducting research in all healthcare settings, specifically with diverse and vulnerable populations:

- First, it is important to ensure safety and that no harm will come to participants. Unethical clinical trials specifically targeting minorities in the past have consequently deterred participant involvement in health studies [52, 53]. While benefits should greatly outweigh risks, it is essential to explicitly state any potential risks involved in the study, as well as subsequent measures taken for participant protection [54].
- Second, there is a possibility that groups may be unable to read or understand projects outlining informed consent and confidentiality of studies. This can lead to further barriers of misinterpretation of actions and intent [55]. Transparency throughout the research process can help ensure maximum benefit with least

possible harm [56]. Finding new strategies to conduct study for informed consent that are transparent as possible is essential to research with diverse and vulnerable populations.

- Third, researchers should be aware of the sociocultural context of their communities. As mentioned, each community is different and carries its own history, culture, values, customs, and language. Researchers should be sensitive to the social environment and characteristics so that community members may feel more respected and encouraged to participate in research [52, 53, 57].
- The purpose of research is to guide clinicians' future work. There needs to be education about research, specifically in order to increase cultural sensitivity among clinicians in order to increase treatment efficacy.
- Finally, the overall purpose of health research in ethnic minority communities should always be to build and maintain relationships while working alongside the community for their advancement [53, 55]. Collaborating directly with community leaders and liaisons can help give a voice to the minority group and provide adequate representation in research [58, 59]. Additionally, employing researchers and other personnel with matching backgrounds of the minority groups is critical to help build trust and maintain relations with the community [60]. Increasing ethical practices involves empowering groups and mutually beneficial research and practice [16]. Ultimately, participants and community members should be involved throughout the research process, and the dissemination impact should continue even after study completion [56]. Increasing community-based participatory research has the potential to reduce health disparities among the patients that need care most by translating science into practice [61].

Consideration for historical and ethical principles of conducting research with diverse and vulnerable populations is critical for researchers, as many of these principles are at the core of developing appropriate methodologies for use in healthcare settings [36]. Using ethical research methodologies in healthcare research with diverse and vulnerable populations is important given that there is a dearth of beneficial research findings that could be used for implementation in healthcare settings.

What Are Important Methodological Considerations for Research with Diverse and Vulnerable Populations?

Methodological considerations in health research are closely tied to ethical approaches, as research methodology should be practiced ethically to prioritize the protection of participants while addressing their needs through advancing science. Issues arising from sampling, measurement, and participant recruitment are important to consideration with health research. As noted, many diverse and vulnerable populations have past experiences of mistreatment and discrimination with healthcare researchers and institutions [62–64]. While the number of racial and ethnic minority groups is increasing, their representation in health research does not always reflect this reality [17, 59]. Inadequate representations of minority groups in preventative interventions ultimately ignore the population which benefits most by treatment [59, 65].

Issues with sampling can also lead to barriers with data measurement within these groups. Some of these challenges in measurement of data for minority groups can include rigid measurement tools and language issues. For example, measurement tools such as surveys or interview questionnaires are more effective if they are flexible and can adapt to the group being studied [65]. This can involve terminology familiar with the group or allow for in-person interviews if participants do not have a phone. Moreover, conducting research in the appropriate language and adjusting content for cultural and contextual differences are considerations which should be prioritized in health research with diverse and vulnerable populations.

Finally, sampling and measurement are dependent on effective recruitment and retention of participants in health research. Frequently, culturally and linguistically appropriate recruitment materials are not well integrated into intervention material and so participants in diverse or vulnerable groups are likely to be overlooked [14, 65]. To maximize recruitment and retention, the sociocultural context of the study setting should be taken into consideration, and investigators should educate populations of interest on the purpose of research [17]. Social and cultural characteristics can include norms (e.g., doctor-patient relationship), customs, values (e.g., *familismo*), and language of the groups being studied. In areas with limited resources, common characteristics to take into consideration include difficulties in transportation to research site, lack of child care, or time off rigid work schedules. Participant attrition in health research studies can be partly alleviated by researchers taking these multiple demands of participant's everyday life into consideration by allowing flexibility in study protocol [14, 65]. Thus, research methodology should involve an appreciation and understanding of the characteristics and environment of the community in which studies are conducted.

A culturally sensitive approach can help researchers maintain awareness and sensitivity toward the social and cultural context of which studies are being implemented. For example, cultural competency in health studies has been shown to increase patient satisfaction and improve providers' knowledge and skills when treating patients of a different culture [66]. Factors such as having formally trained medical interpreters, utilizing trusted community members with shared history and values in the planning and implementation of interventions, and approaching participants with respectful awareness of their current practices, norms, and values can all help contribute to a culturally sensitive approach in health research [61, 66].

Cultural sensitivity emphasizes both cultural and linguistic sensitivity in health research to better reach a population in the most relevant and appropriate manner [67]. While this concept has proven to be difficult to both measure and operationalize, its core principles emphasize the acknowledgement and recognition of unique characteristics of a given group by an "outsider" [67]. Culturally competent research involves awareness and respect of the community's social and cultural context on the part of the provider, institution, or health researcher [67, 68]. Research that does not prioritize the perspective of the vulnerable group essentially perpetuates health inequalities in these communities and silences the voices of the marginalized group [69]. Cultural competence is necessary in all phases of research, from study design and participant recruitment and retention to program implementation [16]. Across all minority groups, cultural competent methodological approaches are crucial, and furthermore, since an increasing portion of the US population is minorities [11], clinicians and researchers alike need to be more culturally sensitive.

Racial and Ethnic Minorities

Latinos Though Latinos in the USA are among the fastest-growing minority group, their presence in scientific research continues to be underrepresented [70]. The term "Latinos" encompass a large, heterogeneous group and can refer to individuals from Latin-American countries and who may be both US and foreign born [70]. This may be problematic in terms of sampling and generalization, as each group has their own background and specific characteristics which should be taken into consideration when conducting research. Since mainstream research studies have been designed primarily for white, middle class, English-speaking Americans, it is important to examine some of the unique characteristics seen in Latino groups to gain a basic understanding of conducting research in these groups [71].

While Latino groups are diverse, some of the cultural values can be applied across groups for initial research within Latino communities. For example, the ideas of *confianza*, *respeto*, and *familismo* are important to consider. These concepts include trust between participants and researchers (*confianza*), appropriate treatment and respect toward individuals who hold power (*respeto*), and an understanding of the importance of the central role played by family within the community (*familismo*) [70, 72, 73]. In addition, employing bilingual and bicultural staff from the community being studied has been shown to have a positive effect in health research conducted in with Latinos [70, 73–75]. Incorporating community input and values can help build and maintain long-term relationships with researchers and has shown to have a positive effect on common methodological concerns such as recruitment and retention across various health studies [70, 72, 73].

African Americans African Americans suffer with disproportionately poorer health compared to the white majority in the USA, such as higher rates of obesity and hypertension [72, 76, 77]. Some of the significant considerations with research in African-American communities are understanding issues of mistrust of research and medicine, as well as experience of continued discrimination and racism [78]. Continued negative experiences of discrimination within the general healthcare system act as barriers to research within this community. For example, common issues such as perceived discrimination has shown to have adverse effects on individual health [79]. It is necessary on the part of the researcher to work to decrease medical mistrust by implementing appropriate and respectful relationships within the community [80]. Sensitivity and awareness toward the social conditions and context of African-American groups in health research is crucial for encouraging participation in health studies and improving disparities among this population [72].

Since African Americans experience systematic racial discrimination, which has contributed to adverse affects on health, it is important to gain appropriate access into the community [81]. For example, churches may be central to certain African-American communities; working through these community-based organizations has been shown to help with recruitment and retention of African-American participants [59]. Collaborating with key community members that are trusted and respected in the community can help health researchers maintain cultural awareness within this group. On a broader scale, the National Center on Minority Health and Health Disparities (NCMHD) takes a patient-centered approach to emphasize prioritization in African-American health research [82]. NCMHD programs center around research, community outreach, knowledge dissemination, and cultural competence for minority groups.

American Indians and Alaskan Natives American Indians and Alaskan Natives are vulnerable groups often underrepresented in research studies [30]. Many American Indian groups suffer greatly from high rates of poverty, poor health status, and highly stigmatized mental health and substance use disorders [30, 83]. Unfortunately, obtaining a statistically significant sample size can prove to be difficult in health research [30, 84]. Issues with sampling, measurement, and overgeneralization of results in research are in part due to the small number of geographically dispersed groups, as well as the mistrust stemming from the legacy of mistreatment by outsiders [14].

To overcome common methodological challenges, Caldwell et al. [85] discuss the 20 guiding principles set forth by the American Indian research and program evaluation methodology (AIRPEM; Table 17.1), which directly address methodological challenges of research with indigenous groups in the USA. The guidelines can also be applicable to interdisciplinary health research. These principles underscore the importance of a community-based, collaborative approach, which should fundamentally be culturally and linguistically appropriate. The AIRPEM concepts also take the communal society of many indigenous groups into account by involving community members throughout the research process [14]. Although they were developed for use with American Indian/Alaskan Native populations, the AIRPEM principles may also apply to other minority groups.

Researchers in the past have been criticized for exploiting the American Indian communities for their personal benefit rather than for community development [84]. Therefore, conducting research focusing on community empowerment through a participatory approach, and keeping in line with the AIRPEM guidelines, can help give more power and control to local members [85]. These guidelines can assist researchers in building local capacity and promoting solutions to problems specifically identified by the community [85].

Table 17.1 AIRPEM guidelines

Guideline number	Description
1	Research with AI/ANs should be done in a community-based, collaborative, and participatory way and should be informed by understanding dynamics of postcolonial trauma and stress
2	Research with AI/AN communities must be relational research
3	Research should be authentic partnerships
4	AI/AN community partners should be involved in the oversight of research
5	Researchers should be informed and directed by existing ethical guidelines and research codes
6	The factors of tribal, cultural, and linguistic diversity need to be taken into account in the development of research designs.
7	Research design, instrumentation, data collection, and interpretation, dissemination, and other post-research activities should give prominent attention to the strengths and cultural protective factors of Native communities
8	Research should involve culture-specific interventions and locally meaningful constructs
9	Researchers must explicitly identify how the research findings will benefit the tribe and its members
10	Training and employment of tribal members as research or evaluation project staff should be a priority
11	Research must be concerned that the research protocol does not harm the tribe, its members, and the environment
12	Research participants must be guaranteed confidentiality and anonymity
13	Tribal or community review of all research findings is essential
14	Active tribal or community involvement in data interpretation is essential
15	Community control of the data throughout the research process can help ensure its appropriate uses from the viewpoint of community or tribal representatives
16	Researchers need to work with Native communities and tribes to define culturally appropriate standards for excellence in research design, reporting, and methods of demonstrating research success
17	Capacity building for research and program evaluation should be part of every research project in Indian Country
18	Research scientists working in Indian Country may increasingly need to accept responsibility to support tribes and communities by advocating for solutions to problems identified in their studies
19	Linkages, networking, and multidisciplinary approach
20	Research that focuses on individual tribes, Native villages, or communities can be essential for local participation in research for community relevance and for community action planning

Adapted from Ref. [85]

Asians Similar to other minority groups, the category of "Asian" is a methodological challenge as an all-encompassing term for a geographically large, vastly heterogeneous group [23]. For health researchers, lack of recognition of these differences can lead to overgeneralization, stereotyping, and erroneous sampling data [23].

Specificity, in study sampling and design, studies should examine the distinctions and unique needs of the group before a program is implemented [86]. The challenge to obtaining data and information on the health of these groups is in part due to the discrimination faced by groups with an Asian cultural background.

Discrimination facing Asian or Asian-American groups especially stems from the existing "model minority" stereotype. The model minority stereotype attempts to universalize the Asian-American experience, maintaining the idea that Asians are well adjusted to American culture, good at math and science, and compliant with authority [87]. While seeming positive, research has shown this stereotype has adverse health effects on Asian individuals, including their mental health [23, 88]. The model minority stereotype perpetuates the myth of Asian Americans surpassing the health disparities faced by other minorities and successfully assimilating in the American system [20]. This stereotype also assumes discrimination has been eliminated based on merit and societal integration [20, 88, 89]. As a result, Asian groups are perceived as having fewer, if any, health problems compared to other minority groups and are less recognized as being a vulnerable population for health research [20, 22, 88].

Though data is emerging which indicate Asians suffer from serious mental health issues such as depression and anxiety disorders, the model minority stereotype is one way that research may be limited on prevalence of health issues [88, 90]. Some of these issues include high risk for poor physical and mental health, underutilization of services, and cultural stigma of seeking treatment [87]. Overall, misleading stereotypes and overgeneralization of groups are important to consider when conducting research with Asian-American groups.

Sexual Orientation and Gender Minorities

There are several important methodological considerations with sexual orientation and gender minorities [91], which include clearly defining the population to be studied and sampling issues with a "hidden" population. First, explicitly defining the population of interest is crucial. Understanding appropriate terminology based on individual preferences in such a diverse group is important early in the research process. In other words, language and terminology used by researchers should reflect how the participant identifies themselves [35]. This should occur early in the research process so as not to be misleading or have intentions misinterpreted.

The labeling and definitions used to describe various aspects of sexual orientation or sexual identity has gone through significant changes in research. For example, the notable Kinsey studies demonstrated sexuality and sexual orientation was not a static, dichotomous variable, but fluid and changing throughout the life course [32]. Sexual fluidity was also confirmed in recent longitudinal research on same-sex attractions in women [91]. This was important in that it shifted the way sexuality was studied and allowed for more variation in research.

Appropriateness of terminology and labeling is also important to take into account with contemporary research, as many sexual minorities are increasingly self-identifying as simply "queer." This term has been reclaimed by sexual minority groups and encompasses a range of those who feel discriminated based on sexual status or behavior [92]. Furthermore, the operationalization and measurement of sexual orientation have been inconsistent in research, as the tendency is to oversimplify or inaccurately represent participants [93]. For example, studies have suggested researchers should consider conceptual distinctions among commonly used terminology, such as sexual orientation, attraction or preference, identity, and behavior [93, 94]. Sexual orientation and gender minorities may be inaccurately represented in health research without taking these factors into consideration, so recognizing within-group diversity can help prevent overgeneralization [91].

Representative sampling may further be challenging since sexual minorities are considered more of a "hidden minority" than others. Sexual minority status may not be readily visible, and researcher investigators often do not include questions regarding sexual minority status [32, 95]. Reasons behind staying "hidden" may be due to self-guilt or shame based on internalized feelings of heterosexism. Internalized heterosexism is "individual's self-stigmatization as a consequence of accepting society's negative attitudes toward nonheterosexuals" [33]. This is important to consider in health research so the researcher may be aware of sexual cultural competency and the complexity of interpersonal challenges faced by participants [35, 95, 96]. This will lead to more culturally sensitive research in health, which then results in treatments for individuals who identify as a sexual orientation or gender minority that are more sensitive to their culture and experiences.

Prisoners

Adults in prison are at a higher risk than the population at large for a range of health problems [43, 97]. A majority of prisoners report chronic health conditions, ongoing mental illness, and substance use disorders (SUDs; 42). Further, individuals who are recently released from prison are at a higher risk of death due, often from suicide or drug overdose [39]. Outside of prison, some subgroups of offenders (e.g., sex offenders) are highly stigmatized and often face challenges associated with their criminal past in the "real world," such as establishing support and social networks [40], and have higher death rates in the years following release [98]. More evidence is needed to establish best medical practices in correctional settings, which can only be accomplished through research [42, 45]. However, prisoners are an overprotected population, which can make conducting research challenging. Yet, efforts are being made by academic and other research-based institutions to establish relationships with prisons in order to engage in collaborative research projects [97]. Therefore, it is essential to address several methodological considerations when conducting healthcare research in prison settings.

First, researchers must keep in mind the interests and missions of corrections professionals, as they are often misaligned. Researchers are focused on publications and objective assessment whereas corrections professionals are often more concerned with the safety and security of inmates and staff. One first step to merging these separate interests is establishing relationships with individuals working in multiple roles and identifying key stakeholders to inform every phase of the research [42, 43, 97, 99]. An agreement should also be made early in the research process about publication of results; some personnel that work in correctional settings may have strict rules around publishing seemingly unfavorable research outcomes [42]. This may be aided by choosing research topics that are important to the institution itself [42, 43, 97].

There are several logistical considerations for conducting research with prisoners. Each time a prisoner is physically moved for research purposes, risks are present. As such, all research processes should be implemented in a way that minimize burden to corrections staff and minimizes movement of prisoners. In order to facilitate logistics, it would behoove researchers to have a prison-researcher liaison, who is responsible for organization of the study, scheduling, recruitment, etc. [43]. Additionally, each prison has its own unique characteristics, and as such more time should be spent designing recruitment, consent, and procedures according to the specific prison's system. Usually, studies in correctional settings often take much longer than they may otherwise [42, 43]. In order to maintain confidentiality, researchers should have strict privacy guidelines at the outset of their research study. For example, researchers in prisons may want to consider how subject ID numbers are connected to patients' names in the event that the research data is subpoenaed [40]. Researchers should be careful that their questions do not provoke answers that may violate "inmate code." In previous studies, some prisoners have stated that their fellow inmates questioned their motives in participating in research (e.g., asking if they were a "snitch"), which could potentially have negative consequences for the participant. Finally, prisoners have very high dropout rates for research due to a variety of factors (e.g., transfers or releases), which makes participant retention difficult [42, 43].

In addition to considerations for participants, researchers should consider several methodological issues in order to protect themselves. Blagden and Pemberton [40] particularly stress the importance of protections for researchers, including identification of secondary traumatization, separation of personal feelings (e.g., disgust, anger) from their professional role, and an awareness of how gender may impact the way prisoners relate to the researcher. The authors also stress the importance of never confirming nor challenging prisoners' distorted views (e.g., rape myths) if they ask questions like, "Do you know what I mean?" Research procedures should reflect these protections.

Moving forward, researchers will face many challenges in research in health in prison settings. First, because of the hierarchical, structured nature of prisons, it is very difficult to incorporate changes due to research findings into the system [42, 43]. As a result, many beneficial or positive research findings are unable to be integrated due to the existing structure [43]. Second, there is a need for implementation and dissemination research in correctional settings. Very few prisons use evidence-based mental health practices; lack of resources and acuity of patients are often cited as the reasons for lack of use of EBTs [42]. Third, there is a need to identify which subgroups of the prison population are at greatest risk of death upon release and to minimize the risk of death or poor health for these groups [39].

Individuals with Chronic Illnesses or Limitations

In many ways, participating in research is a rewarding experience for individuals with chronic illnesses or limitations. Research participants with severe illnesses (e.g., HIV/AIDS, muscular dystrophy, substance use disorders, etc.) usually are socially isolated and have limited access to professional care. As such, participation has the potential to enrich their lives in addition to the other direct or indirect benefits they may gain [49, 100]. However, ethical research practices are essential to maintaining subject safety.

As stated earlier, the most important methodological consideration for researchers working with this population is the process of obtaining informed consent. One strategy researchers have used is incorporating visuals in the consent process for individuals with intellectual or cognitive limitations [50, 101]. In one study, researchers prepared a consent book that contained all of the information necessary for consent. The words were printed in a large font and were supported by colorful pictures and diagrams. The researchers used simple language and explained each component point-by-point. The researchers also assured that there was enough time to complete the consent process [50]. Making arrangements for individuals with chronic health conditions based on individual differences is essential for involving them in research [100].

Moving forward, researchers should involve individuals with chronic illnesses or limitations in research. Participatory research is important in developing methodology that empowers individuals with chronic health problems and allows this vulnerable population to have a voice in research as advisors, leaders, and/or collaborators of research of all types [102, 103]. However, researchers should be aware that it is often individuals with the best communication skills whose voices are heard in research. Efforts should be made to involve individuals with various abilities and limitations [103].

Summary

For health researchers, it is essential to form relationships with community members throughout all phases of research with diverse and vulnerable populations. Effective ways to build trust and facilitate participation in a relevant and appropriate manner can be through consistent and open communication with local gatekeepers, leaders, and stakeholders [17, 59]. Close collaboration is crucial to understand shared beliefs and values of the community, which in turn can help overcome pitfalls in methodological challenges with vulnerable groups.

Bonevski et al. [65] suggest a "participant-centered approach" which prioritizes individual needs and tailors research methodology to address concerns. It is also important to establish a relationship of trust and communicate the importance of participants' meaningful role in the research [59]. Providing useful incentives, keeping in contact regularly, and emphasizing the benefits of the research for both the participant and the larger community are ways which can help take into account the barriers to be presented [65, 104].

Challenges for the Future

In conclusion, researchers should keep in mind the historical contexts from which ethical principles arose for diverse and vulnerable populations and use these ethical principles to conduct methodologically sound research. There is an increasing need for evidence-based interventions for health for these groups, and research is necessary to determine how evidence-based treatments should be used and implemented. Researchers should always (1) provide assurance that no harm will come to study participants, (2) obtain consent in a way that subjects may make an informed decision, (3) remain aware and sensitive to the sociocultural context of the community with which they are working, and (4) make sure that they are working alongside the community for mutual advancement of health.

Moving forward, researchers' biggest challenges will be largely in the field of dissemination and implementation research. For most health concerns, there are evidence-based treatments available. However, they frequently do not reach diverse or vulnerable populations. There is an increasing need to close the gap between science and practice, especially for these groups given their overall poorer health and limited access to evidence-based care. In other words, researchers should not be asking the question, "What works?" but "What works *where*, and *why*?" Addressing these questions of dissemination and implementation will allow for greater access to evidence-based treatments and better overall health.

References

1. Singer M, Clair S. Syndemics and public health: reconceptualizing disease in bio-social context. Med Anthropol Q. 2003;17(4):423–41.
2. Betancourt JR, Green AR, Carrillo JE, Ananeh-Firempong 2nd O. Defining cultural competence: a practical framework for addressing racial/ethnic disparities in health and health care. Public Health Rep. 2003;118(4):293–302.
3. Cutcher Z, Degenhardt L, Alati R, Kinner SA. Poor health and social outcomes for ex-prisoners with a history of mental disorder: a longitudinal study. Aust N Z J Public Health. 2014;38(5): 424–9.

4. Hart D. Toward better care for lesbian, gay, bisexual and transgender patients. Minn Med. 2013;96(8):42–5.
5. Ouellette-Kuntz H. Understanding health disparities and inequities faced by individuals with intellectual disabilities. J Appl Res Intellect Disabil. 2005;18(2):113–21.
6. Call KT, McAlpine DD, Garcia CM, Shippee N, Beebe T, Adeniyi TC, et al. Barriers to care in an ethnically diverse publicly insured population: is health care reform enough? Med Care. 2014;52(8):720–7.
7. Erdley SD, Anklam DD, Reardon CC. Breaking barriers and building bridges: understanding the pervasive needs of older LGBT adults and the value of social work in health care. J Gerontol Soc Work. 2014;57(2–4):362–85.
8. Hunt JB, Eisenberg D, Lu L, Gathright M. Racial/ethnic disparities in mental health care utilization among U.S. College Students: applying the Institution of Medicine Definition of Health Care Disparities. Acad Psychiatry. 2014;39(5):520–6.
9. Krauss MW, Gulley S, Sciegaj M, Wells N. Access to specialty medical care for children with mental retardation, autism, and other special health care needs. Ment Retard. 2003;41(5):329–39.
10. Wilper AP, Woolhandler S, Boyd JW, Lasser KE, McCormick D, Bor DH, et al. The health and health care of US prisoners: results of a nationwide survey. Am J Public Health. 2009;99(4):666–72.
11. Office of the Surgeon General. Mental health: culture, race, and ethnicity: a supplement to mental health: a report of the Surgeon General. Rockville; 2001.
12. Mullins CD, Onukwugha E, Cooke JL, Hussain A, Baquet CR. The potential impact of comparative effectiveness research on the health of minority populations. Health Aff (Millwood). 2010;29(11):2098–104.
13. Giuliano AR, Mokuau N, Hughes C, Tortolero-Luna G, Risendal B, Ho RCS, et al. Participation of minorities in cancer research: the influence of structural, cultural, and linguistic factors. Ann Epidemiol. 2000;10(8 Suppl):S22–34.
14. George S, Duran N, Norris K. A systematic review of barriers and facilitators to minority research participation among African Americans, Latinos, Asian Americans, and Pacific Islanders. Am J Public Health. 2014;104(2):e16–31.
15. Corbie-Smith G, Thomas SB, St. George DM. DIstrust, race, and research. Arch Intern Med. 2002;162(21):2458–63.
16. Minkler M. Ethical challenges for the "outside" researcher in community-based participatory research. Health Educ Behav. 2004;31(6):684–97.
17. Rugkåsa J, Canvin K. Researching mental health in minority ethnic communities: reflections on recruitment. Qual Health Res. 2011;21(1):132–43.
18. Ortega AN. Health care access, use of services, and experiences among undocumented Mexicans and other Latinos. Arch Intern Med. 2007;167(21):2354–60.
19. Bauer HM, Rodriguez MA, Quiroga SS, Flores-Ortiz YG. Barriers to health care for abused Latina and Asian immigrant women. J Health Care Poor Underserved. 2000;11(1):33–44.
20. Gee GC, Gee A, Ro S, Shariff MD. Racial discrimination and health among Asian Americans: evidence, assessment, and directions for future research. Epidemiol Rev. 2009;31(1):130–51.
21. Karlsen S, Nazroo JY. Relation between racial discrimination, social class, and health among ethnic minority groups. Am J Public Health. 2002;92(4):624–31.
22. Islam NSP, Khan SMDP, Kwon SD, Jang DJD, Ro MD, Trinh-Shevrin CD. Methodological issues in the collection, analysis, and reporting of granular data in Asian American Populations: historical challenges and potential solutions. J Health Care Poor Underserved. 2010;21(4):1354–81.
23. Leong FL, Lau AL. Barriers to providing effective mental health services to Asian Americans. Ment Health Serv Res. 2001;3(4):201–14.
24. Eiser AR. Viewpoint: cultural competence and the African American experience with health care: the case for specific content in cross-cultural education. Acad Med. 2007;82(2):176–83.
25. Daugherty-Brownrigg B, editor. Tuskegee syphilis study. New York: Springer; 2013.

26. Corbie-Smith G, Thomas SB, Williams MV, Moody-Ayers S. Attitudes and beliefs of African Americans toward participation in medical research. J Gen Intern Med. 1999;14(9): 537–46.
27. Farmer DF, Jackson SA, Camacho F, Hall MA. Attitudes of African American and low socio-economic status white women toward medical research. J Health Care Poor Underserved. 2007;18(1):85–99.
28. Pacheco CM, Daley SM, Brown T, Filippi M, Greiner A, Daley CM. Moving forward: breaking the cycle of mistrust between American Indians and researchers. Am J Public Health. 2013;103(12):2152–9.
29. Waiters KL, Simoni JM. Decolonizing strategies for mentoring American Indians and Alaska natives in HIV and mental health research. Am J Public Health. 2009;99:S71–6.
30. Gryczynski J, Johnson JL. Challenges in public health research with American Indians and other small ethnocultural minority populations. Subst Use Misuse. 2011;46(11):1363–71.
31. Boehmer U. Twenty years of public health research: inclusion of lesbian, gay, bisexual, and transgender populations. Am J Public Health. 2002;92(7):1125–30.
32. Fassinger RE. The hidden minority – Issues and challenges in working with lesbian women and gay men. Couns Psycho. 1991;19(2):157–76.
33. Herek GM, Garnets LD. Sexual orientation and mental health. Annu Rev Clin Psychol. 2007;3(1):353–75.
34. Byne W. Ethical implications of scientific research on the causes of sexual orientation. Health Care Anal. 1997;5(2):136–48.
35. Bettinger T. Ethical and methodological complexities in research involving sexual minorities. New Horiz Adult Edu Hum Res Dev. 2010;24(1):43–58.
36. Elam G, Fenton KA. Researching sensitive issues and ethnicity: lessons from sexual health. Ethn Health. 2003;8(1):15.
37. Diclemente R, DiClemente M, Ruiz J. Barriers to adolescentsÊ¼ participation in HIV biomedical prevention research. J Acquir Immune Defic Syndr. 2010;54(1):S12–7.
38. Glaze LE, Herberman EJ. Correctional populations in the United States, 2012. In: Justice USDo, Bureau of Justice Statistics. 2013.
39. Kinner SA, Forsyth S, Williams G. Systematic review of record linkage studies of mortality in ex-prisoners: why (good) methods matter. Addiction. 2013;108(1):38–49.
40. Blagden N, Pemberton S. The challenge in conducting qualitative research with convicted sex offenders. Howard J Criminal Just. 2010;49(3):269–81.
41. McDermott BE. Coercion in research: are prisoners the only vulnerable population? J Am Acad Psych Law. 2013;41(1):8–13.
42. Cislo AM, Trestman R. Challenges and solutions for conducting research in correctional settings: the U.S. experience. Int J Law Psychiatry. 2013;36(3–4):304–10.
43. Wakai S, Shelton D, Trestman RL, Kesten K. Conducting research in corrections: challenges and solutions. Behav Sci Law. 2009;27(5):743–52.
44. Crane CA, Hawes SW, Mandel D, Easton CJ. Informed consent: an ethical issue in conducting research with male partner violent offenders. Ethics Behav. 2013;23(6):477–88.
45. Elger BS. Research involving prisoners: consensus and controversies in international and european regulations. Bioethics. 2008;22(4):224–38.
46. Moser DJ, Arndt S, Kanz JE, Benjamin ML, Bayless JD, Reese RL, et al. Coercion and informed consent in research involving prisoners. Compr Psychiatry. 2004;45(1):1–9.
47. Feudtner C, Brosco JP. Do people with intellectual disability require special human subjects research protections? The interplay of history, ethics, and policy. Dev Disabil Res Rev. 2011;17(1):52–6.
48. Iacono T, Carling-Jenkins R. The human rights context for ethical requirements for involving people with intellectual disability in medical research. J Intellect Disabil Res. 2012;56(11): 1122–32.
49. Calveley J. Including adults with intellectual disabilities who lack capacity to consent in research. Nurs Ethics. 2012;19(4):558–67.

50. Taua C, Neville C, Hepworth J. Research participation by people with intellectual disability and mental health issues: an examination of the processes of consent. Int J Ment Health Nurs. 2014;23(6):513–24.
51. Pierce R. Complex calculations: ethical issues in involving at-risk healthy individuals in dementia research. J Med Ethics J Insti Med Ethics. 2010;36(9):553–7.
52. Cacari-Stone L, Avila M. Rethinking research ethics for Latinos: the policy paradox of health reform and the role of social justice. Ethics Behav. 2012;22(6):445–60.
53. Killien M, Bigby JA, Champion V, Fernandez-Repollet E, Jackson RD, Kagawa-Singer M, et al. Involving minority and underrepresented women in clinical trials: the national centers of excellence in women's health. J Womens Health Gend Based Med. 2000;9(10):1061–70.
54. Loue S. Ethical issues in a study of bipolar disorder and HIV risk among African-American men who have sex with men: case study in the ethics of mental health research. J Nerv Ment Dis. 2012;200(3):236–41.
55. Williams RL, Willging CE, Quintero G, Kalishman S, Sussman AL, Freeman WL. Ethics of health research in communities: perspectives from the Southwestern United States. Ann Fam Med. 2010;8(5):433–9.
56. Baumann A, Rodríguez MD, Parra-Cardona JR. Community-based applied research with Latino immigrant families: informing practice and research according to ethical and social justice principles. Fam Process. 2011;50(2):132–48.
57. Egharevba I. Researching an-'other' minority ethnic community: reflections of a black female researcher on the intersections of race, gender and other power positions on the research process. Inter J Soc Res Metho Theory Pract. 2001;4(3):225–41.
58. Lantz PM. Can communities and academia work together on public health research? Evaluation results from a community-based participatory research partnership in Detroit. J Urban Health. 2001;78(3):495–507.
59. Yancey AK, Ortega AN, Kumanyika SK. Effective recruitment and retention of minority research participants. Annu Rev Public Health. 2006;27:1–28.
60. Elliott JR. Ethnic matching of supervisors to subordinate work groups: findings on "bottom-up" ascription and social closure. Soc Probl. 2001;48(2):258–76.
61. Wallerstein NB, Duran B. Using community-based participatory research to address health disparities. Health Promot Pract. 2006;7(3):312–23.
62. Bayoumi A, Hwang S. Methodological, practical, and ethical challenges to inner-city health research. J Urban Health. 2002;79(1):S35–42.
63. Blumenthal DS. Recruitment and retention of subjects for a longitudinal cancer prevention study in an inner-city black-community. Health Serv Res. 1995;30(1):197–205.
64. Martínez MA, Eiroá-Orosa FJ. Psychosocial research and action with survivors of political violence in Latin America: methodological considerations and implications for practice. Interven Int J Mental Health Psycho Work Couns Areas Armed Conflict. 2010;8(1):3–13.
65. Bonevski B, Bonevski M, Randell C, Paul K, Chapman L, Twyman J, et al. Reaching the hard-to-reach: a systematic review of strategies for improving health and medical research with socially disadvantaged groups. BMC Med Res Methodol. 2014;14(1):42.
66. Beach MC, Price EG, Gary TL, Robinson KA, Gozu A, Palacio A, et al. Cultural competence: a systematic review of health care provider educational interventions. Med Care. 2005;43(4):356–73.
67. Vega WA, Lopez SR. Priority issues in Latino mental health services research. Ment Health Serv Res. 2001;3(4):189–200.
68. Howard CA, Andrade SJ, Byrd T. The ethical dimensions of cultural competence in border health care settings. Fam Community Health. 2001;23(4):36–49.
69. Wilson D. Culturally safe research with vulnerable populations. Contemp Nurse J Aust Nurs Prof. 2009;33(1):69–79.
70. Bernal G, Bernal B. Barriers to research and capacity building at Hispanic-serving institutions: the case of HIV/AIDS research at the University of Puerto Rico. Am J Public Health. 2009;99(S1):S60–5.

71. Haack LM, Gerdes AC, Lawton KE. Conducting research with Latino families: examination of strategies to improve recruitment, retention, and satisfaction with an at-risk and underserved population. J Child Family Stud. 2014;23(2):410–21.
72. Mays VM, Cochran SD, Barnes NW. Race, race-based discrimination, and health outcomes among African Americans. Annu Rev Psychol. 2007;58:201–25.
73. Villarruel AM, Jemmott LS, Jemmott JB, Eakin BL. Recruitment and retention of Latino adolescents to a research study: lessons learned from a randomized clinical trial. J Spec Pediatr Nurs. 2006;11(4):244–50.
74. Hinton L, Carter K, Reed BR, Beckett L, Lara E, DeCarli C, et al. Recruitment of a community-based cohort for research on diversity and risk of dementia. Alzheimer Dis Assoc Disord. 2010;24(3):234–41.
75. Skaff MM, Chesla CA, Mycue VS, Fisher L. Lessons in cultural competence: adapting research methodology for Latino participants. J Community Psychol. 2002;30(3):305–23.
76. Hussaini K, Hamm E, Means T. Using community-based participatory mixed methods research to understand preconception health in African American Communities of Arizona. Matern Child Health J. 2013;17(10):1862–71.
77. National Center for Health Statistics. Health, United States, 2013: with special feature on prescription drugs. Hyattsville: National Center for Health Statistics; 2014.
78. Tillman LC. Culturally sensitive research approaches: an African-American perspective. Educ Res. 2002;31(9):3–12.
79. Penner LA, Dovidio JF, Edmondson D, Dailey RK, Markova T, Albrecht TL, et al. The experience of discrimination and black-white health disparities in medical care. J Black Psychol. 2009;35(2):10.
80. Hammond W. Psychosocial correlates of medical mistrust among African American Men. Am J Community Psychol. 2010;45(1–2):87–106.
81. Williams DR, Mohammed SA. Discrimination and racial disparities in health: evidence and needed research. J Behav Med. 2009;32(1):20–47.
82. Snowden LR. Health and mental health policies' role in better understanding and closing African American-white American disparities in treatment access and quality of care. Am Psychol. 2012;67(7):524–31.
83. Grandbois D. Stigma of mental illness among American Indian and Alaska native nations: historical and contemporary perspectives. Issues Ment Health Nurs. 2005;26(10):1001–24.
84. Manson S, Manson D. Enhancing American Indian and Alaska native health research: a multifaceted challenge. J Interprof Care. 2007;21(2):31–9.
85. Caldwell JY, Davis JD, Du Bois B, Echo-Hawk H, Erickson JS, Coins RT, et al. Culturally competent research with American Indians and Alaska natives: findings and recommendations of the first symposium of the work group on American Indian Research and Program Evaluation Methodology. Am Indian Alsk Native Ment Health Res. 2005;12(1):1–21.
86. Hays P, Iwamasa G. Culturally responsive cognitive-behavioral therapy. Washington, DC: American Psychological Association; 2006.
87. Cheryan S, Bodenhausen GV. When positive stereotypes threaten intellectual performance: the psychological hazards of 'model minority' status. Psycho Sci (Wiley-Blackwell). 2000;11(5):399.
88. Sue S, Cheng JKY, Saad CS, Chu JP. Asian American mental health: a call to action. Am Psycho. 2012;67(7):532–44.
89. Lee S, Juon H-S, Martinez G, Hsu C, Robinson ES, Bawa J, et al. Model minority at risk: expressed needs of mental health by Asian American young adults. J Community Health. 2009;34(2):144–52.
90. Lee SS-J. Lessons learned from the U.S. Public health service syphilis study at Tuskegee: incorporating a discourse on relationships into the ethics of research participation among Asian Americans. Ethics Beha. 2012;22(6):489–92.

91. Diamond LM. New paradigms for research on heterosexual and sexual-minority development. J Clini Child Adolesc Psychol Official J Soc Clini Child Adolesc Psychol Am Psychol Asso Divi 53. 2003;32(4):490–8.
92. Warner D. Towards a queer research methodology. Qual Res Psychol. 2004;1(4):321–37.
93. Korchmaros J, Korchmaros C, Powell S. Chasing sexual orientation: a comparison of commonly used single-indicator measures of sexual orientation. J Homosex. 2013;60(4): 596–614.
94. Bostwick W, Bostwick C, Boyd T, Hughes S. Dimensions of sexual orientation and the prevalence of mood and anxiety disorders in the United States. Am J Public Health. 2010;100(3): 468–75.
95. Moradi B, Mohr JJ, Worthington RL, Fassinger RE. Counseling psychology research on sexual (orientation) minority issues: conceptual and methodological challenges and opportunities. J Couns Psychol. 2009;56(1):5–22.
96. Newcomb ME, Mustanski B. Internalized homophobia and internalizing mental health problems: a meta-analytic review. Clin Psychol Rev. 2010;30(8):1019–29.
97. Apa ZL, Bai R, Mukherejee DV, Herzig CTA, Koenigsmann C, Lowy FD, et al. Challenges and strategies for research in prisons. Public Health Nurs. 2012;29(5):467–72.
98. Ellem K, Wilson J, Chui WH, Knox M. Ethical challenges of life story research with ex-prisoners with intellectual disability. Disabi Soc. 2008;23(5):497–509.
99. Innes C. Learning lessons and lessons learned: the National Institute of Justice's Research Demonstration Project Strategy. Annual meetings of the Academy of Criminal Justice Sciences, Boston; 2003.
100. McDonald KE, Kidney CA. What is right? Ethics in intellectual disabilities research. J Poli Pract Intellect Disabi. 2012;9(1):27–39.
101. Boxall K, Ralph S. Research ethics and the use of visual images in research with people with intellectual disability. J Intellect Dev Disabil. 2009;34(1):45–54.
102. Bigby C, Frawley P, Ramcharan P. Conceptualizing inclusive research with people with intellectual disability. J Appl Res Intellect Disabil. 2014;27(1):3–12.
103. Northway R, Jenkins R, Jones V, Howarth J, Hodges Z. Researching policy and practice to safeguard people with intellectual disabilities from abuse: some methodological challenges. J Policy Prac Intellec Disabil. 2013;10(3):188–95.
104. Kim R, Hickman N, Gali K, Orozco N, Prochaska JJ. Maximizing retention with high risk participants in a clinical trial. Am J Health Promot. 2014;28(4):268–74.

Chapter 18
Building Diversity Initiatives in Academic Medicine

Derrick J. Beech and Omar K. Danner

Introduction

The changing landscape in the healthcare environment has presented unique challenges for Academic Medical Centers (AMCs) to transition to "value-based" health services. Shifting demographics with increased ethnic, religious, and gender diversity have made the need for enhancing programs focused on diversity essential in academic medicine. Identifying and replicating effective programs of this nature will be of vital importance as we move into the next generation of healthcare delivery. The value proposition of enhanced diversity in healthcare and academic medicine has been outlined in previous chapters. This overview will focus on initiatives that promote diversity within and associated with AMCs and their ultimate objective of addressing the needs of the present day community. In this chapter, we will explore the importance of diversity in modern healthcare, review the innovative role of pipeline programs in helping to create a diverse healthcare workforce, and discuss the vital impact diversity mentoring in AMCs can have on the development of future healthcare trainees and practitioners.

Importance of a Diverse Health Services Workforce

The traditional pillars of academic medicine – teaching, research, and clinical service – remain critical in the path toward accomplishing the mission of AMCs to optimize and transform healthcare delivery and the health services workforce [1].

D.J. Beech, MD, FACS (✉) • O.K. Danner, MD, FACS
Department of Surgery, Morehouse School of Medicine,
720 Westview Drive, SW, Atlanta, GA 30310, USA
e-mail: dbeech@msm.edu; odanner@msm.edu

© Springer International Publishing Switzerland 2016
R. Parekh, Ed W. Childs (eds.), *Stigma and Prejudice: Touchstones in Understanding Diversity in Healthcare*, Current Clinical Psychiatry,
DOI 10.1007/978-3-319-27380-2_18

However, a relatively new but equally important component of workforce development is the implementation of diversity training which moves beyond the idea of enhancing underrepresented racial and ethnic minorities in the workplace but recognizes the increasing need of inclusion of gay, lesbian, and transgender students, faculty, and providers [1, 2]. In order to sculpt a healthcare delivery system that reflects and meets the needs of modern-day society, AMCs may have to rethink traditional approaches to medical education and make greater efforts to teach trainees and healthcare students inclusiveness and respect for diversity [3].

There have been decades of dedicated effort to promote diversity in the medical profession and academic medical training environment. Diversity initiatives have been endorsed by Association of American Medical Colleges (AAMC), American Medical Association (AMA) Association of American Medical Colleges (AAMC), American Medical Association (AMA) multiple national and regional medical societies [4]. Nevertheless, the need for enhanced and ongoing diversity training remains vital to the success of our new reality in healthcare delivery [5, 6]. With the advent of value-based purchasing and certain provisions of the Affordable Care Act, patients now have greater freedom in choosing healthcare systems and medical providers. Consequently, the medical profession and academic medical training institutions will have to adjust in order to remain competitive in the modern healthcare environment.

Currently, 35 % of the US population is considered to be underrepresented minorities. Furthermore, trends in the US census data and shifting demographics suggest a growing Hispanic population. In fact, Hispanic, African American, and Native American racial groups (and others designated as underrepresented minorities) account for more than 25 % of the US population, but less than 6 % of practicing physicians in the USA. Also, trends in underrepresented minorities matriculating in US medical school, schools of public health, and the allied health professions over recent times suggest continued challenges in access to qualified applicants, pipeline programs, and matriculating health professional students as it relates to promoting a diverse training environment and ultimately a diverse workforce [6].

The primary rationale for developing a diverse health services workforce is the compelling evidence that supports improved diversity will enhance access and quality of care. Data suggest that African American and Hispanic healthcare providers are more likely to see minority patients as well as those that are economically disenfranchised [6]. Therefore, there is great sense of urgency to create a diverse workforce with regard to the health services and a critical need to assure that diverse perspectives and opinions permeate every aspect of the higher education environment [7]. This should be evident in the training process and extend well beyond simply the foundation of equity and fairness. Undoubtedly, everyone deserves the right and should be afforded the opportunity to reach beyond social and historic boundaries and fully engage in the health profession, regardless of their race, ethnicity, religion, gender, or sexual orientation [7]. As it is projected that by 2050, that 50 % or more of the US population will be "people of color" (non-Caucasians), the need for greater diversity in the healthcare environment will become all the more apparent [4, 5].

Extensive studies and countless publications have documented that a disproportionate number of African American and Hispanic patients are uninsured and underinsured [3, 4]. Further, disproportionate access to health services for minority patients combined with the documented disparities in health service delivery throughout every aspect of the healthcare delivery system and significantly poorer outcomes have made approaches to addressing these challenges even more a priority [8]. Although black and other minority physicians may be involved in the care of African American patients at a higher rate than most majority physicians, evidence suggests ethnic minority patients seek and receive care from physicians of the same race more frequently than they seek services from physicians of other racial groups [9, 10]. Similarly, Hispanic physicians care for Hispanic patients at a higher rate than non-Hispanic minority or Caucasian doctors [10].

There are multiple other potential benefits of increasing diversity in the provision of health services, including varying the opinions of critical AMC committees, improving curricula design, diversifying research project formation and execution, enhancing community engagement, and edifying health services policy recommendations. Differing perspectives are very important in developing the structure needed for the most innovative work environment [9, 11].

The Role of Pipeline Programs

Critical to this is better understanding of the essential roles of pipeline programs, which will help to shape the comprehensive outline of the educational continuum. Numerous studies have documented challenges in this continuum. For example, there is extensive geographic variability in the quality of elementary and secondary education [12, 13]. This variability also exists among schools in urban, suburban, and rural locations. There are also challenges in academic advising, professional mentoring, and career development along this continuum [14].

Innovative pipeline programs that address community challenges and barriers have been pioneered by several non-AMC and non-governmental organizations [15]. These agencies provide structured programs that address deficiencies in early childhood development in underserved communities. One example of such is the Super Star Literacy Program, developed by the Junior League of Oakland, California, which collaborated with AmeriCorps members to provide tutorial and afterschool sessions to enhance the literacy competency for kindergarten and first- and second-grade students at the local elementary school in the area, Brookfield Elementary School [16]. A similar program was created and conducted in Providence, Rhode Island, which focused on approaches to enhancing overall performance and developing a strong academic foundation for at-risk preschool students. This program represents a collaboration between Robert L. Bailey, IV elementary school and the YMCA. This holistic approach will occasionally include parents (particularly in families where English is not the first language) to enhance parental engagement and communication [16].

Critical to the success of enrichment programs, throughout the educational continuum, but particularly during the early childhood development phase, is the need for a collaborative approach to strengthening the social and family network combined with improving the students' skills [16]. The Annie E. Casey Foundation, Making Connections Program, is an example of a multi-site, long-term program that has demonstrated success in mentoring at-risk students in which the family is involved in the pipeline process. Lessons learned from the Making Connections Program include that approaches to measuring the outcomes should be implemented early in the process and structuring comprehensive community initiatives is an important component for program success [16]. The Annie E. Casey foundation and their work with at risk children, families, and neighborhoods, is an example of an organization key to achieving the goal in early component of the educational curriculum. They partner with academic entities in the early pipeline programs focused on improving diversity of all aspects along the educational continuum including a diversified workforce [16].

The pipeline programs of Morehouse School of Medicine begin in the early phase of the educational continuum [14]. Our pipeline programs have demonstrated decades of success in addressing the shortage of students interested in health services careers. The two major programs focused on K-12 group include the Benjamin Carson Science Academy and the Vivian Thomas Summer Research Programs.

The Benjamin Carson Science Academy recruits students that are finishing the third grade and supports them via a longitudinal curriculum that extends to the eighth grade year. Named after the famed neurosurgeon, the premise of the program is embodied in this quote from Dr. Carson:

> If we choose to see the obstacles as hurdles, we can leap over them. Successful people don't have fewer problems. They have determined that nothing will stop them from going forward.
>
> -Benjamin Carson, "Gifted Hands"

This program provides a 4-week long summer enrichment experience combined with a year-long Saturday academy for students between grades 4 and 8. The purpose of the pipeline program is to assist at-risk students to enhance their knowledge in science, mathematics, health, and communication skills. This program has been active at Morehouse School of Medicine since 1995. There have been 1337 participants since the inception of this program.

Similar to the Benjamin Carson program for elementary school students, the Vivian Thomas Summer Research program focuses on the high-school student from vulnerable communities with an interest in the STEM disciplines (science, technology, engineering, and math). Students enrolled in the program serve as an apprentice in biomedical research laboratories with assigned mentors. The mentored immersion program was established in 2002. Since the program's inception, 190 students have completed the Vivian Thomas Research program. A significant number of the 190 students have graduated from high school with many entering college, technical school, or an institution for higher education. True to the program's mission is a strong focus on increasing the number of minority students interested in pursuing a career in the biomedical sciences.

Other pipeline programs offered at Morehouse School of Medicine include the Short Term Education Program for Underrepresented Persons (STEP-UP), Promoting Our Worth as Entrepreneurs and Researchers in Innovative Technology (Power- IT), and Student Initiative on Recruitment (SIR) program. These are also three pipeline programs focused on the undergraduate and post-baccalaureate students offered at Morehouse School of Medicine.

Similar to the early childhood development and social support community programs, it is critical that high-school pipeline efforts are coupled with social support networks which address the environmental challenges of the students. The Dukes Foundation, based in Atlanta, Georgia, is a youth mentoring program that provides academic coaching, career development counseling and workshops, and motivational and personal development initiatives for "at-risk" teenage male from urban environments. Founded in 2003 by Horace Dukes, the original aim of providing underprivileged, at-risk young men haircuts, uniforms, and cultural exposure has expanded to the comprehensive personal and professional development program aimed at transforming the lives of disenfranchised minority men.

Physicians, nurses, and scientists with a focus on healthcare services comprise the end products of the training microcosm produced by academic medical centers [15, 17]. Recognizing that the majority of underrepresented minorities will be cared for by nonminority providers and nurses, the majority of community, clinical, and bench research in the medical arena still most commonly originates from and is conducted by nonminority faculty [13, 18–20]. As such, it is critical that there is a diverse faculty and staff to perform these tasks and educate the diverse array of future healthcare providers [21].

Recruitment and Retention of Minority Faculty Members

Hence, the environment itself at academic medical centers must create innovative ways to recruit and retain talented minority faculty members [21]. Historically black colleges and universities (HBCU) are uniquely positioned to lead innovation with regard to health equity policies, practices, and research.

The post-Flexner training environment reduced the number of HBCU academic medical centers to four – Morehouse School of Medicine, Meharry Medical College, Howard University School of Medicine, and King Drew Medical School [3]. Of the four HBCU schools focused on the biomedical sciences, all award the doctor of medicine degree (MD) and only two award doctoral degrees in dentistry (Meharry Medical College in Nashville, Tennessee, and Howard University in Washington, D.C.).

Many nonminority institutions have developed programs designed to enhance faculty, staff, and trainee diversity and created pipeline programs to further diversify the workforce [15]. At Harvard Medical School, the office of Diversity and Inclusion and Community Partnership recognizes the critical need for academic medical centers to engage and include the community in efforts designed to enhance workforce diversity [22]. The mission of the office of Diversity and Inclusion and Community Partnership "is to advance diversity inclusion in healthcare, biomedical, behavioral, and STEM fields that build individual and institutional capacity to achieve excellence, foster innovation and ensure equity in healthcare delivery locally, nationally and globally."

Mounting evidence has suggested that diversity development training programs have the potential to positively impact psychosocial growth and maturation in medical trainees and providers [21]. Several diversity training programs are capitalizing on patients' natural gravitation toward technology as well. Research has shown that patients view technology and technologic literacy as positive and empowering and that patients who master technology have increased self-esteem and better health improvement prospects than their counterparts. Enduring and supportive diverse healthcare provider-patient relationships can powerfully influence the course and quality of patients' lives [22]. As diversity mentoring continues to expand, community agencies and AMCs should consider implementing alternatives to traditional training and begin the initiative early on in pipeline programs. These kinds of efforts may help to reach patients and individuals who might feel disenfranchised and otherwise fall through the cracks.

A unique component of the climate at Morehouse School of Medicine is that of promoting entrepreneurial innovative energy with all of the faculty and staff. Grass roots programs focused on pipeline initiatives and culturally sensitive, patient-centered care have been developed. One such program evolved from the MSM's Division of Trauma and Surgical Critical Care. Dr. Omar Danner, Associate Professor of Surgery, believed that structured exposure to the clinical setting for motivated high-school students with a strong interest in the STEM areas of study could lead to early career decisions to pursue careers in medicine. The Reach One Each One youth mentoring and medical exposure program has as its core objective to stimulate interest in healthcare careers with an emphasis on providing care to the socioeconomically disadvantaged patients in the state of Georgia.

The Reach One Each One Program is a hospital-based youth mentoring and medical exposure initiative designed to encourage high-school students from diverse backgrounds and interested in science, technology, and mathematics to carefully explore career opportunities in the healthcare field. After an initial orientation period, the students are divided into small groups and allowed to spend a half day with different medical disciplines under the supervision of the attending faculty over the next 6-week period. Each service provides a unique experience for its diverse group of students. For example, the surgical section provides an overview of the path to medical school, a hands-on surgical skills lab, and intraoperative exposure. Part of the power of the ROEO enrichment is the direct interaction with medical and surgical attending faculty, residents, hospital personnel, and medical students from diverse background and genders. The final sessions consist of a graduation/awards ceremony with certificate of program completion and a white coat ceremony to plant a seed for what is yet to come.

   Effective mentorship is arguably one of the most important factors needed to shape and influence the success of diversity initiatives [23]. The effects of mentoring relationships on underrepresented adolescents' academic outcomes have been shown to improve perceived scholastic competence in a number of educational settings. Mounting evidence supports that mentoring programs hold great promise in fostering competency among disadvantaged children and adolescents [23]. The impact of exposure of youth from diverse backgrounds to medical professionals and personnel in the hospital setting is intriguing. Based on our preliminary experience with the Reach One Each One Program, medical mentoring by a cohesive group of multidisciplinary professionals has significant potential to positively influence the future career choices of underrepresented adolescents and young adults. Hospital-based youth mentoring programs are therefore a feasible and effective strategy to encourage diverse youth to pursue careers in the healthcare field via pipeline programs in AMCs. These types of programs can give underrepresented youths the opportunity to be exposed to career opportunities in the healthcare arena, of which they may not have otherwise been privy. Working collaboratively with members of the clinical faculty and hospital personnel from various disciplines enhances the quality of the interaction and broadens the overall experience between mentors and mentees [21].

The Power of Mentoring in Academic Medical Centers

Literature suggests that enduring and supportive mentoring relationships in AMCs can powerfully influence the course and quality of training in diversity [22, 24]. As the role of mentoring continues to expand, academic medical centers and community agencies should continue to partner to finds ways to expand beyond the traditional educational model. These innovative relationships provide the potential to reach diverse youth who might otherwise fall through the cracks with early identification and interaction. Studies have shown that adolescents are, in particular, amendable to non-parental, culturally sensitive adult mentors as they strive to create an identity for themselves as well as live more independently from their parents. Acquiring the time to develop these relationships has traditionally presented a dynamic challenge. The Reach One Each One Program presents a unique avenue to help academic medical centers overcome this common challenge through multi-institutional partnerships and capitalizing on exposure to representative minority faculty, trainees, and ancillary healthcare professionals. However, efforts such as ROEO can be effective only when the need for greater diversity and levels of inclusiveness have been fully realized.

   Hospital-based youth mentoring programs provides one example of how academic medical centers can address the growing requirement for increased diversity in our ever-changing healthcare delivery system. Based on our review and understanding of similar programs, AMCs are uniquely situated to provide high-quality and consistent diversity training services to help develop and promulgate an appropriately diverse medical community. In fact, hospital-based mentoring programs emanating from academic medical centers should become an active part of diversity enhancement initiatives and resident training. In order to be successful, concerted efforts by all physicians, administrators, and academic medical center stakeholders will be of vital importance. Skillful diversity role modeling and mentoring of trainees and healthcare students are essential for producing the next generation of culturally sensitive healthcare providers, leaders, scientists, and teachers.

Fully assessing the quality of diversity mentoring relationships requires understanding the characteristics and processes of individual relationships, which are the underpinning for successful diversity mentoring [25]. In addition, the programmatic components that support diverse healthcare professional development must be taken into consideration as well. Several factors have been shown or are thought to influence the quality of diversity mentoring relationships, such as frequency and consistency of contact, the mentor's style and/or approach, and the feelings of connection between protégé and mentor [26]. In order to develop these types of strong interconnections, AMCs should seek to provide quality relationships through proper mentor screening and diversity training and ongoing mentor-mentee contact.

Cultivating Successful Diversity Mentoring Relationships

Although it has become increasingly well accepted that successful diversity mentoring relationships can promote a range of positive professional developmental outcomes, it is equally important to recognize that relationships that fail or are not followed through can lead to decrements in junior minority faculty member development, performance, and overall ability to function [21]. Consequently, strong consideration should be given to the assessment of the quality of the mentor-protégé relationship as it is forming and attempts should be made to identify individuals that may need additional support before those relationships and mentoring efforts fall short of desired goals and expectations [26].

The expansion of diversity training programs and organizations over the past two decades demonstrates the value our society places on developing diverse relationships between vulnerable patients and caring, supportive healthcare providers [27]. However, practitioners and care providers must continue to focus on and assure the effectiveness of this intervention through repetitive, consistent positive interaction with patients under their care. A better understanding of current research-based evidence on diversity training, including review findings, evaluations, and meta-analyses, will provide a basis for a more informed, practically applicable approach to strengthening culturally sensitive medical mentoring programs, interventions, and interactions [28].

The study of diversity spans a wide range of disciplines including psychology, organizational behavior, education, surgery, medicine, and social work, in addition to others. However, there has been a paucity of interdisciplinary dialogue among diversity experts until recently. Greater effort needs to be dedicated to the further development of a multidisciplinary perspective and approach on diversity [29].

Why are mentors important for the transition to a more diverse healthcare system? A mentor may serve as a role model, counselor, and advocate for an under-represented protégé or trainee. These general attributes of successful mentors are not foreign to academic medicine faculty, who staff many of the American medical centers, which may require deliberate cultivation to optimize mentorship capability in the context of diversity training [30]. Moreover, the characteristics required for productive diversity mentoring may be counterintuitive to the learned adaptive behaviors and instinctive personality traits of some even very accomplished academic medical faculty [30]. Accordingly, fostering effective diversity mentoring relationships to reduce the burden of healthcare disparities will require a concerted effort to develop appropriate behaviors and attitudes conducive to the modern healthcare delivery process. The personal and professional growth of our medical trainees and student as well as the succession planning for our future generations of medical providers, healthcare organizations, and the medical profession as a whole will be dependent upon our ability to successfully create an environment conducive to diversity of opinion in the field of medicine.

Researchers have shown that our present conceptualization of diversity should be expanded to include three types of mentoring relationships: direct (diversity) mentoring, collegial interaction to support diversity mentoring, and indirect mentoring (role modeling and role playing) [31]. These types of mentoring relationships may extend and have a profound impact on a large number of healthcare students and emerging trainees. These relationships are capable of changing over time from one type to another, depending on the environment and situation.

Diversity mentoring is usually construed more as responsible medical faculty and healthcare professionals training young trainees and medical students. However, studies have suggested that mentees can potentially mentor each other trainees and students based on the knowledge gained in their diversity mentoring and medical training programs as well as through sharing experiences with their own mentors [32]. The value of this strategy includes building relationships among diverse healthcare team members; creating opportunities for collaboration on community service, teaching, and/or research projects; and developing camaraderie among peer group members from an array of racial and ethnic backgrounds that might not otherwise develop. In one example, the mentors involved in the Monitored Youth Mentoring Program (MYMP) demonstrated that their participation in the program positively enhanced their own formal pedagogy training and teaching ability [33]. Through hands-on practice, they gained expertise and experience that they would not have otherwise received through their traditional academic programs. They were provided with vital exposure to a preventative program and managed to gain insight into the possibilities of introducing earlier intervention and prevention strategies into a vulnerable, at-risk population of adolescent students. Their research showed significant success in two measured variables, learning success and decreasing truancy and disciplinary misdemeanors ($P < 0.05$) [33].

The quality of diversity mentoring relationships seriously matters. In a study of the quality of relationships between adult prevention service providers and young participants in enhancing social skills and strengthening prevention outcomes by the Center for Substance Abuse Prevention, analysis showed that the quality of provider-participant relationships and enhancement of young people's socials skills were vital parts of mentoring program success [34]. Other researchers have shown that patients who perceive a higher level of trust, mutuality, and empathy in their relationship with healthcare providers experienced greater improvements in medical recovery, general well-being, and social skills (i.e., cooperation, self-control, assertiveness, and empathy) than medical patients who perceived a lower quality relationship with their medical providers [35]. These findings underscore the importance of diverse recruitment, training, and maintenance of supervisory practices that promote staff and volunteer diversity skills in order to achieve high-quality relationships with customers of the healthcare system regardless of the specific intervention strategy or medical need.

Over the past two decades, disease prevention as a science has emerged as a discipline built on the integration of life course skill development, research, community epidemiology, and preventive intervention trials. Prevention science is based on the premise that empirically verifiable precursors (risk and protective factors) predict the likelihood of undesired (and/or favorable) behavioral and clinical outcomes, including substance abuse and dependence. It also postulates that negative health outcomes like alcohol abuse and drug dependence can be prevented by reducing or eliminating risk factors and enhancing protective factors in individuals and their environments during the course of medical treatment and preventative maintenance [35]. In order to reach these individuals and get them to truly open up, healthcare provider must be able to relate to them as individuals and connect to their lives and realities at a fundamental level. Diversity initiatives help to begin building the proper foundation for the culturally sensitive conversation and communication needed to address the current and future healthcare need of our ever-changing and diverse society [35].

During the past two decades, comprehensive community-based interventions have been widely implemented in the USA to prevent adolescent health and behavior problems with both federal and foundation support. Translating prevention science into community prevention systems has emerged as a priority for prevention research [35]. AMCs that embrace the focus efforts on diversity training will be at the forefront of the healthcare transformation.

Conceptual and empirical work on diversity mentoring naturally tends to focus on the relationship between mentor and mentee [36]. However, the parent/guardian, guidance counselor, healthcare personnel, and/or social worker may also contribute to the success or failure of the diversity mentoring interventions, and the program's effect size may be partially or significantly influenced by the AMC' and hospital staff's interaction with trainees and patients. Numerous studies illustrate pathways and patterns of communication in the context of more holistic models of mentoring. A systematic model of diversity mentoring could serve to remind researchers and practitioners that mentoring resides within a mutually reinforcing (and inhibiting) network of other pro-social relationships [36]. Through diversity initiative efforts, various types of mentoring relationships can develop between a mentor and a protégé, which may span the mentoring spectrum from role model to preceptor and coach to advisor, among others. When diversity mentors also serve as coaches, they generally are able to improve the overall quality of their mentee's performance and may also have a personal stake in their protégé's success [37]. However, as an advisor, a diverse mentor may have a broader perspective in mind for their understudy and guide their protégé toward more advanced academic and healthcare career development and professional growth. Furthermore, after personal trust has been earned, such a mentor can become a confidant and serve as a sounding board for more sensitive and personal matters [37]. Nevertheless, this requires a directed and concerted effort on the part of the diversity mentor. Finally, an ethnically sensitive counselor can reach the summit of mentoring and become a guide, thus providing the full range of direction typically associated with the mentor archetype. Through understanding of the different kinds of diversity mentoring relationships, mentors and protégés can better select the type of partnership that is the best fit for the given situation [37].

Effective mentorship is arguably one of the most important determinants of success in academic medicine, research, and medical student development [38]. Although numerous published data focus on mentoring from the perspective of mentors, few provide guidance to mentees to help forge these critically important relationships. Based on the corporate concept of "managing up," protégés can learn to take responsibility for his or her part in the collaborative alliance. In addition, they can gain knowledge and insight of how to be the leader of the relationship by guiding and facilitating the mentor's efforts to create a satisfying and productive relationship for both parties [38]. This can only be accomplished by planting the seeds of diversity in the minds of healthcare trainees and students at the early stages of their training as we make this cultural shift in healthcare system delivery. Effective mentorship has the potential to play a critical role in professional and personal growth, career development, as well as academic success. Excellent mentors can provide a distinct vision and guide their protégés to achieve the goals associated with their visions [39]. There is growing evidence that formal mentoring programs have an overall positive impact on minority medical faculty development and may assist in their retention at medical facilities in AMCs [15]. Successful mentors take protégés under their wings for guidance, inspiration, and encouragement and in the process have the potential to create motivated, productive, and successful teachers, practitioners, and future leaders, thus leaving a legacy of diversity and cultural sensitivity as we transition to "value-based" health service delivery [40].

As we function in our everyday lives, all healthcare professionals should remember that we never know when and how our acts of kindness, humility, and graciousness to another will be remembered and acknowledged. This is why diversity mentoring presents such a unique opportunity for people to make a difference in the life of others. Mentors should always continue to be mindful, or conscious of the present opportunity, as they direct young trainees toward their future goals and endeavors [41]. However, as role models, we must also practice empathy and be mindful, which gives us the ability to connect our differences to the experiences of others. Lastly, healthcare providers charged with diversity training should learn to recognize the effects of stress in order to not bring the associated emotions and resulting coping skills into our diversity mentoring and training experience as we help to manage and mold other impressionable minds [42]. Understanding the factors that contribute to high-quality mentoring relationships is critical to developing and sustaining effective diversity training programs. Hierarchical regression models suggest that mentees' academic performance and behavior risk status, parental involvement, and mentoring interaction quality all help to explain the variance demonstrated in mentor-perceived relationship quality. Consequently, diversity program coordinators and participants can benefit from the knowledge that if mentors feel empowered and efficacious and if the mentoring relationship is strong, mentors will more likely persist and carry through on diversity initiatives at AMCs. Through discipline and effort, a diversity mentor can learn to actively listen to others. This type of listening fosters empathy. By working in a positive, caring environment, personal growth in emotional intelligence can be enhanced (McMullen 2003). Through the development of emotional intelligence, the mentor and mentee can improve personally and professionally, creating a win-win situation for all involved.

Conclusion

In closing, healthcare reform has changed the way we will practice and deliver medical care for generations to come. The changing landscape of the healthcare environment is driving Academic Medical Centers (AMCs) to transition to "value-based" health services. Furthermore, shifting demographics along with increased ethnic, religious, and gender diversity have made the need for the development of a diverse workforce essential in academic medicine. Identifying and replicating effective diversity mentoring programs will be of vital importance as we move into the next generation of healthcare delivery.

References

1. Sánchez JP, Castillo-Page L, Spencer DJ, Yehia B, Peters L, Freeman BK, Lee-Rey E. Commentary: the building the next generation of academic physicians initiative: engaging medical students and residents. Acad Med. 2011;86(8):928–31.
2. Merchant J, Omary MB. Underrepresentation of underrepresented minorities in academic medicine: the need to enhance the pipeline and the pipe. Gastroenterology. 2009;138(1): 19–26.
3. Steinecke A, Terrell C. Progress for whose future? The impact of the Flexner report on medical education for racial and ethnic minority physicians in the United States. Acad Med. 2010;85(2):236–45.
4. Steinert Y. Faculty development in the new millennium: key challenges and future directions. Med Teach. 2000;22(1):44–50.
5. Brief A. Diversity at work. New York: Cambridge University Press; 2008.

6. Belcher HM, McFadden J. Rise: promoting diversity among public health professionals. J Public Health Manag Pract. 2014. Retrieved from http://www.ncbi.nlm.nih.gov/pubmed/24419368.
7. Travis E, Doty L, Helitzer D. Sponsorship: a path to the academic medicine C-suite for women faculty? Acad Med. 2013;88(10):1414–7. doi:10.1097/ACM.0b013e3182a35456.
8. Toney M. The long, winding road: one university's quest for minority health care professionals and services. Acad Med. 2012;87(11):1556–61. doi:10.1097/ACM.0b013e31826c97bd.
9. Satcher D. Diverse and dynamic leaders. 2009;83(7):84. Retrieved from http://www.ncbi.nlm.nih.gov/pubmed/19708617.
10. Saha S, Taggart SH, Komaromy M, et al. Do patients choose physicians of their own race? Health Aff. 2000;19:76–83.
11. Satcher D. The importance of diversity to public health. Public Health Rep. 2008;123(3):263.
12. Rust G, Kondwani K, Martinez R, Dansie R, Wong W, Fry-Johnson Y, Woody Rdel M, Daniels EJ, Herbert-Carter J, Aponte L, Strothers H. A crash-course in cultural competence. Ethn Dis. 2006;16(2 suppl 3):S3-29-36.
13. Jeffe DB, Andriole DA, Hageman HL, et al. Reaping what we sow: the emerging academic medicine workforce. J Natl Med Assoc. 2008;100:1026–34.
14. Rust G, Taylor V, Herbert-Carter J, Smith QT, Earles K, Kondwani K. The morehouse faculty development program: evolving methods and 10-year outcomes. Fam Med. 2006;38(1):3–9.
15. Nivet M. Striving toward excellence: faculty diversity in medical education. Washington DC: Association of American Medical Colleges; 2009.
16. Grossman JB, Bulle MJ. Review of what youth programs do to increase the connectedness of youth with adults. J Adolesc Health. 2006;39(6):788–99.
17. Straus SE, Straus C, Tzanetos K. International campaign to revitalise academic medicine: career choice in academic medicine: systematic review. J Gen Intern Med. 2006;2:1222–9.
18. AAMC. Underrepresented in medicine definition. Available from http://www.aamc.org/meded/urm/start.htm.
19. Nunez-Smith M, Curry LA, Bigby J, et al. Impact of race on the professional lives of physicians of African descent. Ann Intern Med. 2007;146:45–51.
20. AAMC. America needs a more diverse physician workforce. Available from http://www.aamc.org/diversity/aspringdocs/toolkit/diversity.pdf.
21. Association of American Medical Colleges. The Diversity Research Forum: the importance and benefits of diverse faculty in academic medicine: implications for recruitment, retention, and promotion, 2008. Available from: www.aamc.org/publications.
22. Saha S, Komaromy M, Koepsell TD, et al. Patient-physician racial concordance and the perceived quality and use of healthcare. Arch Intern Med. 1999;159:997–1004.
23. Rhodes JE, Grossman JB, Roffman J. The rhetoric and reality of youth mentoring. New Dir Youth Dev. 2002;93:9–20.
24. Rao V, Flores G. Why aren't there more African-American physicians? A qualitative study and exploratory inquiry of African-American students' perspectives careers in medicine. J Natl Med Assoc. 2007;99:986–93.
25. Forehand RL. The art and science of mentoring in psychology: a necessary practice to ensure our future. Am Psychol. 2008;63(8):744–55.
26. Deutsch NL, Spencer R. Capturing the magic: assessing the quality of youth mentoring relationships. New Dir Youth Dev. 2009;121:47–70.
27. Rhodes J, Reddy R, Roffman J, Grossman JB. Promoting successful youth mentoring relationships: a preliminary screening questionnaire. J Prim Prev. 2005;26(2):147–67.
28. Rhodes JE. Improving youth mentoring interventions through research-based practice. Am J Community Psychol. 2008;4(1–2):35–42.
29. Eby LT, Allen TD. Moving toward interdisciplinary dialogue in mentoring scholarship: an introduction to the special issue. J Vocat Behav. 2008;72(2):159–67.
30. Pelligrini Jr VD. Mentoring during residency education: a unique challenge for the surgeon? Clin Orthop Relat Res. 2006;449:143–8.

31. Morse JM. Deconstructing the mantra of mentorship: in conversation with Phyllis Noerager Stern. Health Care Women Int. 2006;27(6):548–58.
32. Jacelon CS, Zucker DM, Staccarini JM, Henneman EA. Peer mentoring for tenure-track faculty. J Prof Nurs. 2003;19(6):335–8.
33. Boras S, Zuckerman ZI. Influence of the monitored youth mentoring program for adolescents with behavior problems and behavior disorders. Coll Antropol. 2008;32(3):793–806.
34. Sale E, Bellamy N, Springer JF, Wang MQ. Quality of provider-participant relationships and enhancement of adolescent social skills. J Prim Prev. 2008;29(3):263–78.
35. Hawkins JD, Catalano RF, Arthur MW. Promoting science-based prevention in communities. Addict Behav. 2002;27(6):951–76.
36. Keller TE. A systemic model of youth mentoring intervention. J Prim Prev. 2005;26(2): 169–88.
37. Melanson MA. The mentoring spectrum. US Army Med Dep J. 2009; 37–9.
38. Zerzan JT, Hess R, Schur E, Phillips RS, Rigotti N. Making the most of mentors: a guide for mentees. Acad Med. 2009;84(1):140–4.
39. Schrubbe KF. Mentorship: a critical component for professional growth and academic success. J Dent Educ. 2004;68(3):324–8.
40. Dickey J, Ungerleider R. Managing the demands of professional life. Cardiol Young. 2007;17 Suppl 2:138–44.
41. Karcher MJ, Nakkula MJ, Harris J. Developmental mentoring match characteristics: correspondence between mentors' and mentees' assessments of relationship quality. J Prim Prev. 2005;26(2):93–110.
42. Reeves A. Emotional intelligence: recognizing and regulating emotions. AAOHN J. 2005; 53(4):172–6.

Chapter 19
Looking Outward and Inward: The Role of Introspection in Expanding and Consolidating Our Understanding of Diversity

Sophia L. Maurasse

Living on Both Sides of the Fence: A Personal Account

"Well, for you, Sophia, as an African American it would be different compared to a real African who was from Africa…" His words trailed off into some explanation, or maybe I thought they evaporated without completing a thought. I had stopped listening after the words African American. Yes, it is true that I am Black and I speak English with an accent that very few would ever characterize as anything other than American. So, of course, what else could I possibly be? There was not a hint of uncertainty in his assertion. These two words, African American, each by themselves carried some truth about my ethnic background and nationality but together they referred to a culture very different from the one I identified most closely with. My ease with words had permitted me to blend in very well and people had stopped asking about where I was from. Sometimes, this was a good thing. As a physician and especially a psychiatrist, I guarded with great care the space my patients' work occupied and I was wary of my own identity becoming too entangled in it. But this time, it simply was not a good thing. He was not a patient. He was a physician who was also very well versed in cultural diversity and had traveled quite extensively. How was this possible? And what does it mean to be a "real" African? I have had a number of patients, completely unaware of my ethnic background, tell me how relieved they were since they had had a difficult relationship with their previous physicians who were "not from here." I was thought to be from Tennessee, Florida, or Kentucky, among other states. And, given my last name, surely even if my parents were foreigners, my supervisors and patients frequently thought I was likely born in the USA.

S.L. Maurasse, MD
Department of Psychiatry, McLean Hospital, Belmont, MA, USA
e-mail: smaurasse@partners.org

© Springer International Publishing Switzerland 2016
R. Parekh, Ed W. Childs (eds.), *Stigma and Prejudice: Touchstones in Understanding Diversity in Healthcare*, Current Clinical Psychiatry,
DOI 10.1007/978-3-319-27580-2_19

Introduction

Why Look In and Out?

Maintaining one's gaze in both places works on several levels in that it serves the purpose of obtaining a general impression as well as an in-depth assessment of patients. It is going beyond the initial generalities that cultural knowledge provides to the deeper appreciation of the individual aspects of the patient within the broader, cultural context. This bifocal vision benefits health professionals when they turn it on themselves and consider the context of their cultural perspectives born of their own native and professional identities that are no less real or influential in their understanding of diversity. This analysis cannot be done without recognition that the cultural distance needs to be bridged within as well as between individuals. In turn, what becomes prominent is the real challenge of accurately gauging that distance while discerning the potentially universal principles from those that are culturally or individually specific.

In this chapter, concordance, the expectations of patients and caregivers, its limits and outcomes, social concordance in particular and expanded view of culture, caregivers as members of that culture, the skills involved in the process of understanding cultural humility, curiosity, and competency are explored. Within this frame, studies including those that have been done with various clinical disciplines, including nursing, medicine, psychology, social work, as well as training and management of practitioners in these respective fields, will be reviewed. Concordance is addressed first and what it reveals about the role of various factors including education and income in contributing to culture. And given the limits of concordance, the importance of discordance on a much more fundamental level, that of patient and healthcare professional, is also examined with the assumption that cross-cultural care entails not just the healthcare professional interacting with various cultures as if he or she were operating in a vacuum devoid of culture but that every encounter is a cross-cultural encounter, between that of the patient and of the provider. The hope is that this chapter will provide healthcare professionals an innovative way to understand cultural diversity and bridge those differences.

So Why Consider the Culture of Medicine?

The culture of medicine by its very nature and existence is the thing that must be acknowledged to fully engage in any purposeful attempt to understand and educate others about cultural diversity in healthcare. By virtue of being a culture, it encompasses many factors including shared beliefs and attitudes that influence and mediate the learning of and acceptance of diversity. Secondly, it is a reminder to practitioners to acknowledge their own lack of neutrality, due in part to professional enculturation, which may impact important decision-making. This exploration is a means of tapping in the "hidden curriculum" to fundamentally change how diversity is understood and dealt with in training and practice. Lastly, this awareness allows practitioners to focus on honing lifelong learning skills around maintaining cultural humility and curiosity that are dynamically engaged in their clinical experiences beyond prior knowledge and conceptions.

Learning Objectives

1. Armed with more "information," how does one maintain cultural curiosity about patients? How does *cultural humility* fit in?
2. How much *awareness* do healthcare professionals have about their own preconceived notions as well as their attitudes toward the idea of cultural sensitivity and understanding diversity?
3. In this setting, an incorrect assumption is made based on race and accent as if it were a fact. How does race become a proxy for culture?
4. What does research suggest about *concordance* between patient and healthcare provider and how does this factor into satisfaction and outcomes?
5. What can this reveal about the impact of knowledge, experience, and training on the understanding and acceptance of diversity? And, how is the cultural distance that may persist despite the recommended training gauged and bridged?
6. What factors must be taken into account with increasing investment in understanding cultural diversity?
7. How does understanding diversity expand the view of culture in general? And, how is the culture of medicine accounted for as an important mediator in cross-cultural training and care? Within the culture of medicine, how can training, evaluation, and practice of culturally sensitive care be optimized?
8. How does the increasing diversity within the ranks of caregivers and patient population influence expectations of the more historically common dyad of majority physician and minority patient?
9. How does an understanding of diversity challenge the idea of caregivers being neutral?
10. Finally, how does this relate to caregivers as learners and patients as teachers? How does this change in the dynamics address the gap and work in concert with the principles of looking outward in cultural competence? And how is this dynamic a necessary component in encouraging both introspection and greater curiosity for caregivers?

Looking Outside Ourselves at Others

Concordance

Concordance is most often defined as "similarity or shared identity between physician and patient, based on demographic attributes such as race, sex or age" [1]. Studies in concordance suggest that cultural distance between caregivers and patients is lessened in concordant dyads, where the pair shares an important attribute. For instance, African American patients reported higher levels of satisfaction in their clinical encounters with African American physicians but these patients also showed high rates of satisfaction with physicians classified as Hispanic or "other" [2]. This satisfaction was not linked to the actual outcome of the encounter but to the perception of respect and dignity, the patients' sense of having their concerns taken seriously, as well as the physician making sure that patients understood what was being told to them [2]. Visits between race concordant pairs are longer, both physician and patients speak more slowly, and positive affect of patients is higher [3]. Physicians are also rated as more participatory during visits with race concordant dyads [3].

Concordance: Expectations of Patients and Caregivers

Expectations and choice are also important mediating factors. Regardless of race, if given a choice, patients are more likely to be race concordant [4]. Patients with a preference for concordance who are also in concordant pairs are more likely to be satisfied with their clinical encounters [5]. This is important given that patients not only tend to prefer physicians they perceive as knowledgeable, invested in their concerns, as well as having good interpersonal skills [6] but that they are also more likely to attribute these qualities to physicians of their own racial or ethnic group [7]. When looking at expectations among Whites, Blacks, and Latinos, while all three believed that racism would be less likely in concordant dyads, Blacks and Latinos were more likely than Whites to believe that racism occurred in discordant dyads [5]. Though Whites regardless of preference were most likely to be in concordant dyads, they were also least likely out of the three groups studied to have a preference for concordance. Most importantly, this preference varied with trust as well as fears around unfair treatment. When Blacks had more trust in physicians, there was a decrease in preference for concordance. In both Blacks and Latinos, fear of unfair treatment was positively correlated with preference for concordance. And while both groups were more likely to attribute unfair treatment to their racial or ethnic background, Whites were more likely to attribute this to the kind of treatment they needed on the day of their clinical visit [5].

Patients are not the only ones affected by concordance. Physicians are more likely to perceive patient as less intelligent and compliant if the patient is a minority [4]. And, unfortunately, this perception may not go unnoticed as Blacks, Latinos, and non-Latino Whites reported that class differences between patients and physician could negatively impact the relationship between the two [8]. Specific examples from this sample included patients reporting that physicians did not provide them with adequate explanations because they did not believe the patients would understand [8].

Concordance: Limits and Outcomes

There are limits to the benefits of concordance. It does not necessarily impact outcome or quality measures despite a significant influence on overall satisfaction. Physicians in White concordant pairs were less likely to screen male patient's cholesterol than White physicians in discordant pairs while those in Black concordant pairs were less likely to engage in tobacco cessation counseling [9]. Spanish-speaking patients in language concordant pairs were less likely to be screened for colorectal cancer [10]. These discrepancies further complicate the health disparity picture as far concordance is concerned. And, they suggest that the impact of concordance may also vary with the type of treatment or procedure. Spanish-speaking primary care providers were more likely to explain procedures and complications of colonoscopy or the side effects of vaccines than the English speakers who were ordering the tests without detailed explanations [10]. Yet, they also provide more clarity on what patients, regardless of race, value in their experience of the patient-caregiver relationship while expanding the concept of culture. Certain measures thought to assess patient-centered communication, including physician verbal dominance and patient-centered interviewing scores, did not vary significantly with concordance while patient positive affect, rate of speech, and length of visit did [3]. These last two measures take into account the relative amount of social and emotional exchange relative to physician biomedical agenda-driven exchange between patient and physician [3]. The lack of concordance effect on these measures suggests the importance of focusing on the affective dimension aside from the specific behaviors emphasized in patient-centered communication training [3].

Regular physicians were more likely to be seen as asking enough questions, explaining things clearly, providing needed tests, and paying attention to concerns. Factors like choice, income, age, and whether English was patient's native language were also important in determining satisfaction [4]. Furthermore, concordance is important for those who prefer it but seems to have little importance for those who do not; Blacks and Latinos with no concordance preference, in discordant dyads, have similar rates of satisfaction as Whites in concordant dyads [5]. Concordance is also not necessarily preferred by some groups as seen in one sample where Latinos with private insurance were less likely to prefer Latino physicians than those without insurance [3]. And, as shared in one physician's personal account, his own personal history of being profiled or subjected to stereotypes did not make him immune to the risk of stereotyping or profiling his patients, even when they were seemingly race concordant (Sapien, 2010). In the primary care setting, African American physicians were more likely to check blood pressure as well as ask about tobacco usage than White physicians [9] and Hispanic doctors were more likely to check male patient's cholesterol but less likely to check that of female patients compared to White physicians [9], while Asian physicians were less likely than Whites to check blood pressure and also less likely to check female patient's cholesterol [9].

Social Concordance

Social concordance includes "dimensions that are clearly visible" such as gender, ethnicity, and age as well as less obvious identity characteristics such as education [11]. Patients can rate their physician as being very socially similar to them while also acknowledging that they are ethnically dissimilar. White patients were more likely to report being socially similar to their physicians than Black patients [11].

And in terms of communication as well a perception of care, there seems to be a graded response from low to medium to high levels of social concordance, where positive patient affect and satisfaction increased as social concordance do, suggesting the importance of the cumulative effect of multiple characteristics. This reinforces the point that like Hispanic and Asian groups, African Americans and Whites represent "a broad array of cultural groups" [11].

Social Concordance and an Expanded View of Culture

Concordance studies allow for the expansion of the understanding of culture and diversity. In fact, in a one-time focus group composed of African American, Latinos, and non-Latino Whites, 25% of what was described as text units, defined as "identifiable continuous verbal utterances," contained value systems, followed by customs in 17% of the text units, self-identified ethnicity in 15%, and stereotypes at 4% [8]. In order of decreasing text unit percentages, sensitivity to complementary medicine, health insurance-based discrimination and social class discrimination, ethnic concordance, and age-based discrimination were all cited by this group as factors influencing the quality of medical encounters [8].

Dimensions of culture include a value system which encompass shared norms, values, and beliefs that define a group, as well as a general sense of morals of what is right and wrong, and manifest customs and observable aspects of culture that symbolize a group, including food, music, clothing, and television shows; self-indentified ethnicity; shared experiences, including common experiences that create a sense of membership and bonding; and stereotypes, simplified archetypes of a particular ethnic group that ignores intragroup heterogeneity [8]. With this in mind, the fundamental discordance between caregiver and patient is considered as well as how it informs the awareness of the culture of medicine, what it says about its relationship to other cultures, and, most importantly, how it can be influenced to engender greater cultural sensitivity in trainees and already practicing caregivers.

Looking In: Caregivers as Members of a Culture

A Personal Account

"Well, that is truly a waste of time," my colleague, a psychiatrist, balked as I told him about this chapter. He did not skip a beat as he immediately searched more background information on the sushi menu options. The waitress, who had identified herself as Chinese American, when he had asked her about the proper etiquette in pouring sake, told us how she would do it based on her culture but was not entirely certain about how it was done in Japan. "Seriously, it's either about generalities or specifics you can't use. Every time I have sat through one of those lectures on cultural diversity, it felt like a waste of time," he continued, a little exasperated, wondering how one would even measure what we were teaching, how would we know what we were doing, and what did the research say and, half-jokingly, asked if I was making all this up while he took nothing for granted as he reviewed the menu despite having himself traveled to Japan. Instead, when he was unsure, he appropriately asked questions of the waitress and seamlessly went back and forth between the menu and his smartphone, absorbing and integrating the new knowledge he gathered. I was at a loss for words. His evident openness to international experiences seemed strange when juxtaposed with his reaction to didactics on cultural diversity. At some point, I asserted that an appreciation of the culture of medicine afforded us an opportunity to identify ways in which it hindered or nurtured our understanding of diversity.

Years of medical training had taught us to listen very well. Increasing cultural sensitivity was not about having a different set of ears. To some extent, it was using the same set to listen to another tune with greater awareness of how this set affected our willingness to hear, what we heard, and how we interpreted it. My colleague was pointing out an obvious dilemma: Given that we could not know about each and every culture in depth, what could we accomplish by looking at a select few? How was this not contributing to stereotypes? And given my own international background, would I or would I not need this training? Would he, given his extensive international travel? How would formal didactics account for these personal experiences? For better or worse, his reaction captured what has been studied in terms of the attitude of trainees toward curricula aimed at improving cultural sensitivity.

The Dilemma

Ironically, healthcare professionals deal with this very same dilemma in the realm of illness without becoming hopelessly overwhelmed. Health professionals apply their knowledge and experience, consult with each other, and use a common language in characterizing observed and reported phenomena. They learn about patterns in order to recognize them when they appear. Clinicians also learn about specific conditions, fully aware that their knowledge is limited, that these categories are constructs subject to changes, and that they must remain lifelong learners. During clinical encounters, healthcare professionals are able to hold the generalities while remaining receptive to the details only the individual can provide. This curiosity, in spite and because of a provider's prior knowledge, is crucial as it increases the accuracy of an assessment and the chances that subsequent interventions will be efficacious. Furthermore, healthcare providers are also vigilant in not adhering too rigidly to these thoughtful formulations or treatment plans. They accept that with greater knowledge of their patients, initial impressions may prove to be inaccurate or, at the very least, require some modification to better represent their patient's conditions and to optimize the treatment. Healthcare professionals do not refuse to learn about illnesses because there are so many variations in how individuals present with them.

Instead, they welcome each individual presentation as an opportunity to expand their knowledge base about familiar and unfamiliar conditions.

In and Out: An Old Skill Revisited

This idea of a looking inward and outward is not new; in earlier discussions on "learning to value diversity" [12], the focus was clearly on "changing behavior and informing attitude" instead of the mastery of specific culture or reaching a predetermined goal, which highlighted the following: general skills and principles useful in dealing with a variety of groups, emphasis on valuing the individual including proper contextualization (an integration of not only knowledge of the patient's culture as guideline but also awareness of the context, the social, economic, political, geographic realities of the individual's experience) vs. teaching about specifics, whether they be conditions or mores associated with a specific group, and a self-awareness around the clinicians' own attitudes and beliefs [12]. However, many of the then present and the predictable obstacles, skepticism, warnings, and questions around proper inclusion into training curricula and concerns around evaluation, continue in one way or another to plague the effective development of curriculum or at least attitude toward it [12].

Training healthcare professionals to value diversity "validates the legitimacy and worth of other people's backgrounds and provides a more effective basis for better communication and ultimately, more accessible, appropriate and effective health care" [12]. Many of the skills and attitudes that can be learned and promoted in the context of valuing diversity are generic and will enhance doctor-patient interactions regardless of setting [12]. Examples include increased self-awareness and reflective practice, appreciating the importance of health beliefs and particular cultural perspectives of individuals, avoidance of stereotyping, and more communication skills [12].

It is important to beware of tokenism and consider the context in which training is provided, where the diversity training is added on at the end of another topic or covered as a one-off, risking the health issues being covered out of context within a diverse society; increasing the likelihood of greater focus on differences, especially when centering on culture or disease specific to a particular ethnic group, at the risk of reinforcing stereotypes rather than exploring the learners' own awareness and attitudes; and maintaining a focus on the patient as an individual [12]. Through tokenism, ethnic health issues may "become even more marginalized, losing their relevance to other aspects of training" [12].

There may also be resistance from learners who prefer "recipe" approach with emphasis on passive acquisition of knowledge about how a behavior or disease might be different in an ethnic minority group rather than a "person-centered" that may prompt reflection and examination of their own attitudes [12]. Similarly, it may be easier for teachers to avoid this challenge, especially if they experience a lack of support from colleagues or lack of practical suggestions to facilitate training in ways that are appropriately interactive [12].

Teachers need support. Since this may involve, like the students, challenging their preconceived beliefs and attitudes as well as expose areas of weakness [12]. Evaluation poses its own challenges, especially given that the broad aims of teaching and learning about diversity are increasing awareness, informing attitudes, and encouraging reflective practice; the goal is to "inform attitudes" as attitude is seen as a "construct that is inferred from behavior" [12].

Looking In and Out: As a Way of Accurately Gauging the Distance and Considering Universal Principles

Though trainees cannot be expected to know the many cultures of their patients in depth, they can be expected to be culturally sensitive [13]. With the rise in diversity in caregivers as well as patients, this recognition means that understanding cultural diversity requires that a provider understand his or her culture and that of the patient receiving care [13]. Kai et al. [12] called for both a broad, dynamic sense of the individual's culture including prior health experiences and values, while acknowledging the following "given the increasing ethnic diversity of our societies, no training can prepare learners for all the issues that arise [12]. But they can be "sensitized" to "the importance of diversity" and can develop generic skills to "respond flexibly to diverse patients populations, becoming aware of their own attitudes and prejudices and avoiding stereotyping and responding to patients as individuals [12].

A second-generation Mexican American physician may not truly grasp the perspective of a recent Mexican American immigrant [13]. The need for this bifocal vision is evident in both the recognition of potential obstacles and familiarity with techniques for optimal cross-cultural care. Below are common fallacies in cross-cultural interactions and the learning opportunity they represent [14]:

(a) Everyone believes as we do. This fallacy is a reminder that caregivers need to strike a balance between the tendencies to assume similarity with the need to be aware of the difference of those we encounter [14].
(b) Other cultures are homogeneous. While generalizations can to some degree be used to orient us, we must also recognize that within a culture, there may be certain non-core values shared by enough members to create a subculture [14].
(c) Cultures never change. We must use caution in assuming that past characterizations are valid [14].
(d) All differences between people of different cultures are cultural differences. "Differences shared by others in a given community that has some history and that demonstrate some resilience over time are more likely to be cultural" [14].

A discussion of ethical consultation includes [14] the LEARN model [15], which includes Listening to patient with sympathy, Explaining one's own perception to patient, Acknowledging similarities and differences among perceptions, Recommending a plan with patient's input, and Negotiating whenever necessary to develop mutually acceptable options; the ecological model as described which stress that knowledge of the social and environmental settings of the individual are necessary to understand that individuals behavior and health states [16]; and the Kleinman Explanatory model as a way of helping providers to obtain social and cultural information as well as data on the patient's understanding and interpretation of the situation [17].

If the "fundamental unit of medical care is the doctor-patient/family dyad," then effective cross-cultural communication during a clinical encounter requires that the clinician integrate multiple cultures including his own, that of the patient and the patient's family, and that of the healthcare institution [18]. Cultural competence here is defined as "a skill set that enables a physician in a culturally discordant encounter to respectfully elicit patient and family information needed to make an accurate diagnosis and negotiate a mutually satisfactory goals for the treatment" [18]. Expertise here is driven more by knowledge than a specific skill as it would entail that the provider attains a multicultural or bicultural status, wherein he or she has sufficient knowledge about his or her own culture as well as that of about "one or two cultures of the patients that the provider treats to recognize the differences, understand what they mean, and translate or bridge those differences to accomplish clear communication of information and caring" [18]. Each person within the dyad comes from a different culture and within the healthcare professional, there is an identity arising from the intersection of his or her own culture as well as that stemming from professional training [18]. The provider's cultural concept of health and the patient's own culture intersect with the patient's cultural concept of health. There is an explicit recognition of the healthcare provider's own "natal culture" as well as the influence of his or her professional development [18].

There are three alternatives: the first where the physician works solely within the biomedical paradigm, the second where the patient and healthcare professional work exclusively within each of their native cultures, and the third where the physician works within the patient's cultural framework [18]. And though these three may provide some advantages, another option would be to have the physician and patient negotiate between their concepts of the etiology of disease and the most appropriate means of treatment to reach a mutually desirable goal. Healthcare professionals can still use their knowledge about particular cultural beliefs, values, and practices as hypotheses about individual beliefs, but they must assess the degree to which an individual patient or family adheres to their cultural background, if at all [18]. As a result, RISK reduction assessment to elicit information about a patient's Resources, Identity, Skills, and Knowledge is recommended [18].

Though "everywhere a group's stereotype follows from perceived status and competition with other groups," culture influences group status and perceived group competition [19]. Hence, specific group stereotypes vary cross-culturally [19]. Despite the devastating social and political impact of racism and prejudice, race and ethnicity cannot be discarded as irrelevant to healthcare in the spirit of freeing ourselves from stereotyping or bias. For example, where biological links exist to certain ailments such as sickle cell anemia in those of African ancestry or Tay Sachs disease in Ashkenazi Jewish populations, it has long been accepted that race and ethnicity must be retained as relevant to healthcare. Moreover, ethnicity can be used as "an initial proxy for history, language and culture, and health beliefs, so long as individualization of care is rapid" [20]. It is recommended that healthcare professionals have knowledge of the basic ethnic history, language usage, and customs of ethnic groups of patients that they see frequently [20]. This knowledge can orient clinicians to factors that may impact medical care. However, given the significant risk for negative connotations as well as potential for abuse, race and ethnicity cannot be used as proxies for socioeconomic status or behavior [20]. These last two can be clarified during the clinical interview [20].

Ways of Maintaining Bifocal Vision

The more knowledge healthcare providers gain about diversity, the more likely they are to appreciate the challenge of maintaining genuine self-awareness of their own cultural experience as individuals and as clinicians as well as sincere curiosity around that of their patients in all health encounters. The changing nomenclature, shifting from cultural competence to humility, curiosity, and sensitivity, points to a dynamic conceptualization of how best to approach diversity and culture in healthcare. This approach necessitates but cannot be limited to self-awareness, as it is by no means a disavowal of the responsibility clinicians have to be educated about the political, social, and economic context in which patients live. Rather, it is an appreciation of the complexity of culture and the ever-present challenge of effectively providing optimal healthcare.

The intersectionality perspectives allow for the idea of positionalities, where individuals "simultaneously occupy multiple positions within the socio-cultural, political, and structural fabric of society" and that these positionalities intersect and affect behavior in different settings or contexts [21]. Hence, individuals "may respond differently depending on their gender, age, ability, gender identity or sexual orientation [21]." Within this framework, cultural humility approach would favor incorporating multicultural and intersectional understanding and analysis to improve practice, since together these concepts draw attention from the diversity of the whole person to power differences in relationships to different past and present life experiences including micro aggressions and potential resources or gaps [21].

Cultural Sensitivity, Humility, and Competency

While clinicians do not have to be experts of their patients' culture, they have the task of cultivating self-awareness which among many things serves two major purposes: the identification of personal learning barriers and the understanding of power imbalances within the clinical relationship [21]. This is with the understanding that self-knowledge by itself is not enough and, in fact, cultural humility places clinician in learning mode [21]. The skills needed to achieve this include active listening, reflecting, reserving judgment, entering the client's world, and the following principles: embracing the complexity of diversity, knowing thyself and critically challenging one's openness to learn from others, accepting cultural differences, and relating to children and families in ways that are most understandable to them [21].

Amy Levi's [22] discussion on the ethics of international clinical experiences, in the context of "clinical tourism," for nurses also supports this dual vision, stating that not only do "nurses have an ethical duty to provide good care wherever they are" but that in that vain, reflecting on their own values and beliefs about cultural differences is an "integral part to developing cultural humility." Understanding the political, economic, and social condition of their patients is vital to their ability to contextualize both their experiences of those patients and the resources that they will utilize in the care of those patients [22]. This includes the economic and political situation as well as the availability of resources as they significantly impact not only the care of the patients but also the response from providers as the well-intentioned nurses realized in a resource-depleted system, teams affected by "compassion fatigue" and a high rate of stillbirths in the Dominican Republic as part of an exchange program [23]. That work in the Dominican Republic emphasized how "long term partnerships promotes bilateral cultural humility" [23].

Where cultural sensitivity is helpful in providing a way for approaching individuals with health beliefs different from clinicians, cultural competence is centered on the ability to interact effectively and cultural humility is a "continual process of self-reflection and self-critique that overtly addresses power inequities between providers and clients" [24], as cultural humility "becomes not a goal but an active process, an ongoing way of being in the world and being in a relationship with others and self" [24]. Alsharif [25] suggests that "sensitizing students to the other members of the healthcare team could be incorporated as part of the framework for culturally competent practice" as a means of "embracing the cultural differences that characterize patients, populations and the healthcare team" [25]. Humility as with other virtue or attitude is hard to instill in individuals and is best taught by role models and narrative examples [25].

Conclusion

Where cultural competency "implies that one can function with thorough knowledge of the mores and beliefs of another culture," cultural humility "acknowledges that it is impossible to be adequately knowledgeable about cultures other than one's own" [22]. This stance does not absolve healthcare providers of making the effort to gain as much knowledge about the realities that their patients face [23]. Rather, it is a dilemma that this chapter addressed by exploring a vision that maintains a commitment to curiosity and awareness around the self and the culture of the healthcare provider as well as that of the patient in his or her care in the face of a daunting task of balancing increasing knowledge and experience with skillful open-mindedness. This was explored in a detailed view of concordance between patient and caregivers and what it revealed in terms of its limitations, the expectations, the outcomes, and the impact an expanded view of culture.

References

1. Street RL, O'Malley KJ, Cooper LA, Haidet P. Understanding concordance in patient-physician relationships: personal and ethnic dimensions of shared identity. Ann Family Med. 2008;6(3):198–205.
2. LaVeist TA, Carroll T. Race of physician and satisfaction with care among African-American patients. J Natl Med Assoc. 2002;94(11):937–43.
3. Cooper LA, Roter DL, Johnson RL, Ford DE, Steinwachs DM, Powe NR. Patient-centered communication, ratings of care, and concordance of patient and physician race. Ann Intern Med. 2003;139(11):907–15.
4. LaVeist TA, Nuru-Jeter A. Is doctor-patient race concordance associated with greater satisfaction with care? J Health Soc Behav. 2002;43:296–306.
5. Schnittker J, Liang K. The promise and limits of racial/ethnic concordance in physician-patient interaction. J Health Polit Policy Law. 2006;31(4):811–38.
6. Hill CJ, Garner SJ. Factors influencing physician choice. Hosp Health Serv Adm. 1991;36(4):491–503.
7. Saha S, Taggart SH, Komaromy M, Bindman AB. Do patients choose physicians of their own race? Health Aff. 2000;19(4):76–83.
8. Nápoles-Springer AM, Santoyo J, Houston K, Pérez-Stable EJ, Stewart AL. Patients' perceptions of cultural factors affecting the quality of their medical encounters. Health Expect. 2005;8(1):4–17.
9. Strumpf EC. Racial/ethnic disparities in primary care: the role of physician-patient concordance. Med Care. 2011;49(5):496–503.
10. Eamranond PP, Davis RB, Phillips RS, Wee CC. Patient-physician language concordance and primary care screening among Spanish-speaking patients. Med Care. 2011;49(7):668.
11. Thornton RLJ, Powe NR, Roter D, Cooper LA. Patient–physician social concordance, medical visit communication and patients' perceptions of health care quality. Patient Educ Couns. 2011;85(3):e201–8.
12. Kai J. Valuing ethnic diversity in primary care. Br J Gen Pract. 1999;49(440):171.
13. Zweifler J, Gonzalez AM. Teaching residents to care for culturally diverse populations. Acad Med. 1998;73(10):1056–61.
14. Carrese JA, Perkins HS. Ethics consultation in a culturally diverse society. Public Aff Q. 2003;17:97–120.
15. Berlin EA, Fowkes Jr WC. A teaching framework for cross-cultural health care—application in family practice. West J Med. 1983;139(6):934.
16. Galazka SS, Eckert J. Clinically applied anthropology: concepts for the family physician. J Fam Pract. 1986;22(2):159–65.
17. Kleinman A, Eisenberg L, Good B. Culture, illness, and care: clinical lessons from anthropologic and cross-cultural research. Ann Intern Med. 1978;88(2):251–8.
18. Kagawa-Singer M, Kassim-Lakha S. A strategy to reduce cross-cultural miscommunication and increase the likelihood of improving health outcomes. Acad Med. 2003;78(6):577–87.
19. Cuddy AJ, Fiske ST, Kwan VS, Glick P, Demoulin S, Leyens JP, et al. Stereotype content model across cultures: towards universal similarities and some differences. Br J Soc Psychol. 2009;48(1):1–33.

20. Chin MH, Humikowski CA. When is risk stratification by race or ethnicity justified in medical care? Acad Med. 2002;77(3):202–8.
21. Ortega RM, Faller KC. Training child welfare workers from an intersectional cultural humility perspective: a paradigm shift. Child Welfare. 2011;90(5):27.
22. Levi A. The ethics of nursing student international clinical experiences. J Obstet Gynecol Neonatal Nurs. 2009;38(1):94–9.
23. Foster J. Cultural humility and the importance of long-term relationships in international partnerships. J Obstet Gynecol Neonatal Nurs. 2009;38(1):100–7.
24. Miller S. Cultural humility is the first step to becoming global care providers. J Obstet Gynecol Neonatal Nurs. 2009;38(1):92–3.
25. Alsharif NZ. Cultural humility and interprofessional education and practice: a winning combination. Am J Pharm Educ. 2012;76(7):120.

Chapter 20
Pharmacology: Cultural and Genetic Considerations

Anne Emmerich, Anthony Fatalo, and Bijay Acharya

Ms. A, a 65-year-old Asian woman, is hospitalized with injuries sustained in a motor vehicle accident. Despite escalating doses of codeine pain medication, she continues to report severe pain during scheduled daily interviews through an interpreter. In the next room, her 40-year-old Ethiopian friend with similar injuries is sedated by even small amounts of codeine. The team thinks Ms. A is "medication seeking" and psychiatric consultation is requested.

Introduction

Until late in the twentieth century, a "one-size-fits-all" approach to medication safety and efficacy was the norm, with little attention paid to whether diversity existed in the human response to medication [1]. Discussion of culture in the context of pharmacologic treatment was primarily limited to whether a patient was receiving care from an

A. Emmerich, MD, MA (✉)
Department of Psychiatry, Massachusetts General Hospital,
15 Parkman St., Boston, MA, USA

Harvard Medical School, Boston, MA, USA
e-mail: aemmerich@partners.org

A. Fatalo, RPh, MS, BCPS
Department of Pharmacy, Massachusetts General Hospital, Boston, MA, USA

B. Acharya, MD
Harvard Medical School, Boston, MA, USA

Edward P. Lawrence Center for Quality and Safety, Boston, MA, USA

Department of Medicine, Massachusetts General Hospital, Boston, MA, USA

© Springer International Publishing Switzerland 2016
R. Parekh, Ed W. Childs (eds.), *Stigma and Prejudice: Touchstones in Understanding Diversity in Healthcare*, Current Clinical Psychiatry,
DOI 10.1007/978-3-319-27580-2_20

353

alternative provider, such as a folk healer using plant-derived treatments passed through generations in an ethnic group or other forms of treatment such as magic, dance, or prayer [2]. Cultural changes occurred in the United States in the second half of the twentieth century including legislation which sought to decrease stigma and prejudice and increase integration of racial and ethnic groups. In the scientific arena, legislative efforts were made to reduce the lack of diversity among research participants in clinical medical trials. At the same time, advances in research techniques allowed scientists to map the human genome [3, 4]. These changes expanded the consideration of culture as a factor in the diagnosis and treatment of disease.

Research is rapidly changing the way scientists think about the interaction of illness, genetics, and cultural/environmental factors. It now appears that both cultural/environmental factors and genetic vulnerability are necessary for many illnesses to occur and can significantly impact the interaction between the body and drugs when patients undergo treatment. Provision of appropriate pharmacological (medication) treatment for an individual requires a broad definition of, and understanding of, culture, which includes concepts such as age, race, gender, sexuality, size, health status, dietary preferences, alternative or home health remedies, use of tobacco or substances, exposure to pollutants, and history of trauma and stress.

This chapter aims to give readers a wide-ranging overview of concepts relevant to the emerging understanding of culture, genetics, and pharmacology.

The first section focuses on the interaction of drugs and the body through discussion of (a) pharmacogenomics, (b) population medicine, and (c) environmental factors. We discuss FDA box warnings related to cancer medicine, general medicine, and mental health, areas in which it has been demonstrated that genetic differences can influence illness treatment, safety, and outcome. We discuss examples of research on variation in treatment safety and outcome due to gender, race, and age using examples of population-based medicine that offer clinical utility. Lastly, we consider environmental factors which can influence response to medication.

The second section focuses on factors relevant to decision making by patients and providers: patient-provider interaction, clinician genetic competency, availability of useable information, and protection from genetic discrimination. A case scenario is also provided.

The available information on this topic could fill an entire book, and this chapter does not attempt to mention every treatment regimen or cultural group. The examples chosen for this chapter represent some of the innovative ways in which modern science is bridging differences by expanding our knowledge of the interaction between medication and the human body across diverse genetic and cultural groups. These efforts are giving clinicians and patients new tools as they work together toward the goal of optimal health outcomes.

Section 1: Drugs and the Body

Drug interaction can occur in every tissue of the body. Once a medication is taken (orally, intravenously, subcutaneously, inhaled, etc.), the drug must reach its target tissue(s) and exert its effect before being inactivated or eliminated. The most important known method by which the body metabolizes chemicals is the cytochrome P450 enzyme system. The Human Genome Project, completed in 2003, identified 57 human genes which code for 18 families of cytochrome P450 enzymes [5].

In order to understand cultural, environmental, and genetic variations, and the impact of these on drug treatment, scientists ask specific questions:

1. What part of the drug/body interaction is affected by a genetic, cultural, or environmental variation?
2. If the variation's impact is relevant to a drug, is it the pharmacokinetics (metabolism of the drug by the body) or pharmacodynamics (impact of the drug on the body) that is altered?
3. If the variation is relevant to a disease, does it increase or decrease the likelihood of response to medication treatment?
4. Who is affected by the variation? Caucasians, Asians, men, women, children, elders? At what frequency are they impacted?

Pharmacogenomics

Pharmacogenomics is defined by the Food and Drug Administration (FDA) as the study of "variations of DNA and RNA characteristics related to drug response" [6]. It is estimated that 20–95% of drug disposition and impact has a genetic basis [7].

A central issue underlying the understanding of pharmacogenomics is the concept of polymorphism. This term refers to variations within the genetic structure that lead to variation of traits within the population. Unlike mutations which are rare and sporadic, polymorphisms occur with at least 1 % frequency within the population [8]. An example of a trait influenced by polymorphism is eye color. Modern genetic techniques show that in many cases it is a combination of several polymorphisms that leads to the visible or experienced expression of a trait. Polymorphisms influence the interaction between an individual human body and a medication. Some polymorphisms occur with greater frequency in some groups of people than others, and they can be expressed at various times across the life span.

The FDA Table of Pharmacogenomic Biomarkers in Drug Labeling lists over 100 drugs for which labeling has been updated to provide information on biogenic markers, in the event that genetic testing information is available [9]. The majority do not contain box warnings or information on when testing should be done, however, as there is not enough evidence available as to whether testing is associated with clinically relevant outcomes compared to standard practice.

An example is warfarin. Warfarin is a widely used anticoagulant with a narrow therapeutic window. Too much can cause bleeding; too little can put the patient at risk of thrombosis. Studies show there are at least 30 different CYP2CP9 alleles for warfarin metabolism, some of which cause loss of function and several of which show ethnic variability in the percentage of people who carry loss-of-function alleles. Genes VKORC1 and CYP4F2 are also important and have shown ethnic variability [10]. Approximately 30 % of dose variation in Caucasians is accounted for by these genes, while only 10 % of the dose variation in African Americans is

[11, 12]. However, many nongenetic variables also cause alterations in warfarin drug levels, including diet, smoking status, alcohol, body weight, age, and other drugs or herbal remedies. Many groups have tried to develop dosing guidelines for warfarin based on genetic data, recommending lower starting doses for Asians and higher for African Americans compared to Caucasians and Hispanics [13]. However, while the FDA has included labeling indicating that genetic variation is a factor in warfarin activity, it has not issued specific box warning recommendations as studies have not proven whether more specific testing leads to clinically different outcomes, compared to the current practice of frequent blood testing of anticoagulation status.

One of the cytochrome P450 enzymes that has been extensively studied is cytochrome P450 2D6, which is thought to be involved in the metabolism of 25 % of all drugs currently on the market [14]. Polymorphisms of CYP2D6 with significant ethnic variability account for four categories of patients that have now been identified [15]:

(a) *Ultrarapid metabolizers:* There is a 28 % incidence of ultrarapid metabolizers in Ethiopians, Arabs, and North Africans, 10 % in Caucasians, 3 % in African Americans, and 1 % in Chinese, Japanese, and Hispanics.
(b) *Extensive metabolizers*: This is considered the "normal" metabolic state.
(c) *Intermediate metabolizers*: The highest incidence of intermediate metabolizers is among Asians.
(d) *Poor metabolizers*: 5–10 % of all patients are poor metabolizers with European Caucasians being most likely to be in this category.

The concept of metabolizer status includes factors other than genetics and can be applied to other CYP450 enzymes. Some medications can themselves inhibit or induce cytochrome P450 metabolic action; thus, an intermediate metabolizer can effectively become a poor metabolizer depending on the agent being used. When prescribing, clinicians need to consider genetic information (if it is known), the inhibitory or inducing properties of the drug itself, and the inhibitory and inducing properties of other drugs the patient is taking. A useful website of the University of Indiana provides a list of medications that are CYP450 enzyme substrates, inducers, and inhibitors [16].

FDA Guidance

There are a few medications for which specific FDA box warnings have been established because genetic research has provided sufficient information that is predictive of safer treatment outcomes. These exist in the areas of oncology, general medicine, and mental health.

Oncology

With the push for precision medicine outlined by President Obama in his 2015 State of the Union address, more than $215 million will be invested to create genomic databases to identify genomic drivers in cancer and improve privacy and data sharing of these results [17].

The clinical application of information learned from genetic studies is most evident in the field of oncology. Patel et al. [18] point out that both germ line mutations (hereditary mutations passed down from the parents) and somatic mutations (changes in DNA occurring in specific tissues during the lifetime) are relevant to understanding cancer. They further comment that mutations can have prognostic value indicating potential risk of future disease, or predictive value indicating likelihood of response to a particular treatment.

An example of prognostic value is BRCA1 and 2 gene testing. These mutations are associated with substantial increases in the risk of ovarian and breast cancer in women. Testing is not recommended for all women, but clinicians should evaluate further whether BRCA testing is indicated when there is a family history of breast cancer before age 50, breast and ovarian cancer in multiple family members and Ashkenazi Jewish heritage. Based on BRCA gene testing, some women now opt for prophylactic mastectomy or hysterectomy to reduce their future risk of disease [19].

Cetuximab

The KRAS gene mutation has predictive value as it suggests that treatment with cetuximab is unlikely to be effective for patients with colorectal cancer (CRC) [20]. A retrospective analysis of patients with CRC in Chicago between 1992 and 2002 found that African American patients had a higher proportion of KRAS mutations than Caucasians (34 % versus 23 %) and despite receiving similar chemotherapy had a 73 % risk of death. This suggested that KRAS gene mutation might be relevant [21]. Studies in the Middle East have shown KRAS mutation rates of 30–32 % in patients from Oman and Saudi Arabia with CRC [22].

KRAS gene mutations are also found in non-small cell adenomatous lung cancers. In the USA, there is a higher incidence of KRAS mutation in African American and Caucasian patients (20–30 %) compared to Asian patients (5–20 %) with adenomatous lung cancer. A Moroccan study showed rates similar to those of Asians (9 %). There is a higher frequency of KRAS mutation in males and smokers. However unlike colorectal cancer, there is no current clinical application for these findings when applied to lung cancer [23].

Trastuzumab

The HER2 overexpression mutation causes breast cancer cells to proliferate rapidly via communication of messages across the cell membrane. HER2 positive status predicts improved response when trastuzumab, a monoclonal antibody, is added to standard chemotherapy. HER2 mutation is a somatic mutation, occurring after birth, not a hereditary mutation. Despite this, it appears that ethnic variation occurs. Chuang et al. [24] found an increased frequency of HER2 positive tumor status among Filipino women compared to Chinese, Japanese, and Korean women in a retrospective review of breast cancer in Asian women in New York. This finding suggests a complex interaction of environmental factors and potentially yet unrecognized genetic factors.

Rasburicase

Rasburicase is used for the treatment of leukemia and lymphoma tumor lysis syndrome (and has potential for use in cases of severe gout). An FDA box warning indicates that patients who are glucose 6-phosphate deficient (G6PD) are at risk of severe hemolysis when exposed to this drug, due to an inability to breakdown hydrogen peroxide, a by-product of rasburicase metabolism. Clinicians should screen patients at risk of G6PD deficiency, in particular patients of African or Mediterranean ancestry, before prescribing rasburicase [25].

General Medicine

Abacavir

The antiviral drug abacavir is associated with genetically linked severe hypersensitivity reactions. Patients of Indian descent have a 5–20 % frequency of the responsible allele, HLA-B*5701, which carries a 70 % chance of incurring a hypersensitivity reaction. Caucasians have a 5–8 % prevalence, Hispanics 1 %, and Asians 0.2 %. An FDA box warning recommends testing for the HLA-B*5701 allele prior to initiation of abacavir [26].

Analgesia

Codeine is a prodrug and must be metabolized to morphine by CYP2D6 in order to exert its analgesic effect. More than 90 morphisms of 2D6 have been found with dramatic differences in the body response to codeine. Codeine should be avoided in patients who are known to be ultrarapid metabolizers due to risk of overdose; ultrarapid metabolizers quickly convert codeine to morphine. In poor metabolizers, conversion of codeine to morphine is blocked and patients are resistant to analgesic effects. Intermediate metabolizers also derive limited analgesic effect from codeine. Alternative analgesics should be considered if patients are known to be poor or intermediate metabolizers [27].

Clopidogrel

Clopidogrel, an antiplatelet agent shown to reduce the rate of death, stroke, and myocardial infarction in patients who have had a heart attack, is a prodrug that is converted to an active metabolite via complex genomic interactions involving at least five CYP enzymes. Loss-of-function variants have been identified for CYP2C19 with frequencies up to 50 % in Asians, 33 % in African Americans, and 24 % in non-Hispanic Caucasians [11, 28]. Loss-of-function variants are associated with higher incidence of stent thrombosis in patients undergoing percutaneous coronary intervention (PCI). An FDA box warning indicates a test is available to determine CYP2C19 status. Poor metabolizers should be given alternative agents when undergoing PCI [28].

Mental Health

Many psychiatric medications are metabolized by the cytochrome P450 system with CYP2D6, 3A4, 1A2, and 2C19 being the most significant of the CYP enzymes. Most psychiatric medications cause side effects, and it is standard practice to start with low doses and monitor patients carefully during upward titration of doses. For most categories of psychotropic medications, data is still conflicting as to whether genetic testing as a routine practice would offer an advantage over standard practice. Hall-Flavin [29] and others have attempted to create treatment algorithms for the use of psychotropic medications. Drozda [9] discusses the history of antidepressant guidelines, which remain a work in progress. Henderson [30] cites studies showing differences in dose needed to achieve impact or dose at which side effects occur both for older "typical" antipsychotics and newer "atypical antipsychotics" across a wide array of ethnic groups. Ultrarapid metabolizers can have very high clearance of psychotropic medications and be erroneously thought to be noncompliant or resistant to treatment [31]. While researchers are still sorting out this data, genetic test kits for the common CYP enzymes are commercially available. For patients who fail to respond to multiple medications or develop intolerable side effects to multiple medications, CYP testing might offer useful information. Providers and patients should be aware however that insurance companies do not uniformly authorize payment for this form of testing and prior authorization should always be sought as testing costs run into the hundreds of dollars.

Two specific medications commonly used for treatment of mental illness carry FDA box warnings.

Carbamazepine

Carbamazepine, an antiseizure medication also used as a mood stabilizer for patients with bipolar disorder, carries an FDA box warning indicating HLA-B*1502 genotyping is recommended for Asian patients due to an increased risk of Stevens-Johnson syndrome (SJS) and toxic epidermal necrolysis (TEN) and severe life-threatening rashes. This polymorphism, found in highest frequency in patients from China, Thailand, Malaysia, Indonesia, the Philippines, Taiwan (10–15 %), South Asia, and India (2–4 %), is extremely rare in patients of European, Hispanic, Native American, and African descent (<0.01 %) [25]. Patients with one or two copies of the HLA-B*1502 allele should be given an alternative medication as the risk of SJS or TEN is reported as 113 x greater in HLA-B*1502 carriers compared to noncarriers [9]. The FDA does not recommend testing for non-Asian patients given the very low frequency of this allele in other populations.

Valproic Acid

Valproic acid, used for seizure disorders and bipolar disorder, is associated with a high risk of fatal hepatotoxicity in patients with mitochondrial DNA polymerase gamma (POLG) mutations. FDA labeling indicates this drug should not be used in this population. POLG mutations are associated with rare hereditary neurometabolic syndromes of which Alpers-Huttenlocher Syndrome is most often mentioned. The FDA recommends genetic testing prior to the use of valproic acid in children and adolescents if there is clinical suspicion of mitochondrial or neuromuscular disorders. Saneto describes several cases of children who developed hepatotoxicity after being given valproic acid for seizures and comments that the POLG mutation has been shown to exist across ethnic lines [32].

Population-Based Medicine

While genetic research is offering exciting advances, it is the field of population-based medicine that offers the widest clinical usability currently. During the twentieth century, most medical trial participants in the United States were male and of European descent. Late in the century, it became increasingly clear that not enough was known about the impact of drug treatment on other subsets of patients and research interest arose in areas of gender, age, and race/ethnicity.

Gender

In 1993 the US Food and Drug Administration (FDA) reversed its prohibition against women of childbearing potential participating in drug trials with publication of a document called "Guideline for the Study and Evaluation of Gender Differences in the Clinical Evaluation of Drugs." An FDA regulatory information sheet on this topic states "The guideline was developed amidst growing concern that the drug development process did not provide adequate information about the effects of drugs or biological products in women and a general consensus that women should be allowed to determine for themselves the appropriateness of participating in early clinical trials" [33, 34].

Despite this, women have been routinely underrepresented in randomized clinical trials, and not until 2010 did the FDA stipulate that more women need to be recruited for these trials. Women are now more often enrolled in Phase 3 trials but are still underrepresented in Phase 1 and Phase 2 trials.

A fact sheet of the Laura Bush Institute for Women's Health points out that women "are 50 % more likely than men to have adverse reactions to prescription drugs yet most drugs do not have different dosages based on a patient's gender." It also states "Some may think that women are just more difficult to treat or complain more about medication side effects but in reality eight of ten drugs pulled from the market had more deaths and side effects in women" [35].

There are a number of factors that might contribute to the potential for differences in how substances interact with the female body compared to the male body. Women have more body fat than men. Women have slower gastric motility compared to men and less intestinal enzymatic activity. Women have reduced renal clearance (rate of metabolism via the kidneys) compared to men. Hormonal differences in women and the fluctuation of hormonal state monthly and throughout the lifetime are also relevant. These differences can alter both the pharmacokinetics and pharmacodynamics of drugs [36].

In 2013 the FDA issued its first dosage recommendation based on gender when it recommended lower doses of the sleep agent zolpidem in women after studies showed an increase in driving incidents in women compared to men while using this medication [37].

Women have a higher incidence of drug-induced QTc prolongation and torsade de pointes than men. While some studies suggest that hormonal differences may be relevant, no conclusive mechanism has yet been determined [38, 39]. Drug-induced prolonged QT is one of the medication side effects of all medicines that is most actively being studied by the FDA currently and has been associated with antibiotics, antidepressants, antipsychotics, and cholesterol-lowering agents among others. Rabin points out that women also take more medication than men thus compounding the impact of this potential risk [40].

Table 20.1 shows additional differences in response to medication based on gender.

Age

One of the most important factors in drug pharmacokinetics and dynamics is age. Geriatric and pediatric persons are more at risk for adverse drug reactions (ADRs). Historically, these extremes of age have rarely been studied in randomized controlled trials.

Table 20.1 Gender differences in response to medications

Antidepressants	Women are more likely to respond to serotonin reuptake inhibitors, while men are more likely to respond to tricyclics [36]
Antihistamines	Women are more apt to become drowsy than men [41]
Anti-HIV meds	Women are more likely to have side effects than men [42]
Alcohol	Women metabolize alcohol more slowly than men [41]
Digoxin	There is increased mortality in females compared to men [36]
Opioid pain meds	Women obtain pain relief at lower doses than men [36]

Geriatric Medicine

The FDA recommended that elderly patients be included in drug trials in the early 1990s; in 1998 it began requiring drug sponsors to include information about the use of a medication in the elderly in drug labeling inserts. Despite this, in 2007, the Government Accountability Office (GAO) provided testimony to Senate committees that only one-quarter of clinical trial medical officers documented whether review of the sufficiency of elderly representation was occurring. Additionally, only 2/3 of medical officers documented their review of safety and effectiveness in elderly patients [43]. In a 2008 letter addressed to the Senate, commenting on the GAO report, the American Academy of Geriatric Psychiatry pointed out that the FDA defines "elderly" as persons over age 65, thus drug sponsors can satisfy the requirements laid out by the FDA using trial participants who are still relatively young even for drugs most commonly used in older patients with dementia. The AAGP letter recommended the FDA reclassify the term "elderly" to begin at age 70 or 75, pointing out that the "real issue is frailty not age" [44].

There are a number of ways that pharmacokinetics are altered with advancing age [45]:

1. Absorption

    (a) Delayed gastric emptying

2. Distribution of drug

    (a) Decrease in body water
    (b) Increase in body fat
    (c) Decreased protein binding due to decreased albumin

3. Metabolism

    (a) Reduction of hepatic blood flow
    (b) Reduction of hepatic mass

4. Elimination

    (a) Reduced elimination through the kidneys

Among commonly prescribed medications, drugs with narrow therapeutic indices such as digoxin and warfarin require more careful oversight in older patients due to the pharmacokinetic issues listed. Anticholinergic clearance is reduced in the elderly leading to an increase in risk for adverse events including confusion, dry mouth, and constipation with the use of common medications and over-the-counter products. Over-the-counter nonsteroidal anti-inflammatory medications, used commonly for pain, have been associated with renal failure and exacerbations of heart failure in older patients. Antipsychotic medications are associated with an increased risk of death in elderly patients with dementia [46].

Elders use 30 % of all prescription drugs prescribed in the USA. Increased drug use (polypharmacy) increases the risk for adverse drug reactions (ADRs) particularly when opiates, warfarin, or benzodiazepines are on the list [47]. Elderly patients have more illness comorbidity. Elders with dementia or brain damage due to strokes may be more likely to accidentally take too much or too little medication. ADRs in the elderly tend to be severe and underreported and mortality rates due to ADRs are greater in older compared to younger people. Forty percent of older Americans drink alcohol which can cause further drug interactions particularly with acetaminophen and sleeping pills in an already frail elder [48, 49].

Tools exist for clinicians wanting to educate themselves about prescribing medication for older patients. A complete guide of potentially problematic medications called the Beers Criteria is provided by the American Geriatrics Society and was most recently updated in 2012 [50].

Pediatric Medicine

With regard to medications, it is commonly said that infants and very young children are not just small adults. They are not at risk for adverse drug events only because of their smaller size but also due to differences in their physiology that affect their ability to metabolize and eliminate drugs. Medications that are thought to be quite safe in overdose for adults can be toxic or fatal for children who ingest them [51]. In 1994 the FDA Pediatric Rule gave manufacturers a pathway to include pharmacology and therapeutic use of drugs in pediatric patients into the approved drug labeling. In 1997 The FDA Modernization Act provided incentive for pharmaceutical manufacturers to complete studies of pediatric usage while the patent life of a drug remained. In 1999 the FDA Final Rule was established, requiring drug companies to conduct pediatric studies for new drugs that are thought to be of potential benefit to pediatric patients [52].

Application of pharmacogenomics in pediatric patients must take into account the dynamic nature of gene expression that evolves during normal human development in which the pharmacogenetic variability we have discussed earlier in this chapter is superimposed upon normal developmental patterns of enzyme expression (ontogeny) in young children, adding a dimension of complexity that is not present in adults. While an individual's genome is stable throughout life, gene expression and interactions are changing as an individual develops. Individual genes are part of larger, complex gene networks that interact across the life span. Gene products involved in disease and drug reactions may only be evident at specific time points in development [53].

An example of pharmacogenetic research that is showing promise for children is research on cisplatin, a chemotherapeutic agent with many side effects including loss of hearing which occurs with much higher frequency when this agent is given to children under age 5. Children who carry three polymorphisms related to cisplatin have a very high risk of abnormal hearing ability 5 years later compared to children who carry none of the polymorphisms [54].

Race/Ethnicity

In a series of documents in the late 1990s, the FDA urged researchers to include analysis of safety and effectiveness for racial subgroups in their applications for new drugs. The 1993 National Institute of Health (NIH) Revitalization Act made it mandatory for medical research studies funded by the NIH to include participants from minority populations. The FDA urges the use of race and ethnicity categories that were established by the Office of Management and Budget (OMB) in 1997. The OMB lists five categories for race: American Indian/Alaska Native, Asian, Black or African American, Native Hawaiian or other Pacific Islander, and White. Additionally, there are two categories for ethnicity: Hispanic/Latino or non-Hispanic/non-Latino [55]. The OMB has pointed out that these categories were not established on the basis of any biological evidence but rather reflected sociocultural realities of the US population in 1997. Unlike age, race is not a fixed parameter of human existence but rather is a social construct [56]. Fewer and fewer Americans claim pure racial or ethnic heritage and increasing numbers identify as biracial or of mixed ethnic heritage.

While race and ethnicity are imprecise variables, themes have emerged. In 2005, the FDA approved BiDil (a combination of isosorbide dinitrate and hydralazine hydrochloride), the first medication approved specifically for the treatment of heart failure in African American patients based on findings from the African American Heart Failure Trial (A-HeFT). Since then, there has been debate over the ethics of allowing a drug to be specifically patented and marketed for one ethnic group. In the case of BiDil, the studies that led to FDA approval did not measure whether the drug worked in other groups as well. O'Malley discusses the history of BiDil and the potential impact of a drug being labeled as specific for one racial group on patients' feelings about treatment [57].

Asthma is an illness for which research on ethnic differences is ongoing. Burchard [58] cites the Genetics of Asthma in Latino Americans (GALA) study conducted in Boston, New York, and San Francisco beginning in the late 1990s which showed that ethnicity was the strongest predictor of response to commonly prescribed asthma medications, which worked less well for Puerto Rican patients than Mexican or African American patients. Genetic variants that might be relevant were identified, and clinical trials are looking at the efficacy of asthma medications in various ethnic groups.

Breast cancer research has also demonstrated racial and ethnic differences. Kurian [59] discusses the risk of breast cancer for women in four ethnic groups. African American women have the lowest lifetime risk of breast cancer, but it is now recognized they have the highest risk of "triple negative" breast cancer (TNBC), a more aggressive form of cancer often seen earlier in life than other breast cancers. TNBC does not respond to common breast cancer treatments such as hormone treatments (tamoxifen) or Herceptin and is not as readily detected by mammography [60]. An online fact sheet of the Black Womens' Health Imperative urges black women to discuss newer forms of screening technology with their physicians to allow for early detection.

Some have worried that research along racial or ethnic lines would lead to further discrimination or marginalization of populations [57, 61]. However, projects such as the Black Womens' Health Imperative, the Association of Black Cardiologists, the National Alliance for Hispanic Health, the Asian Health Foundation, and others have been established to promote health awareness and research in specific racial or ethnic groups with an emphasis on patients being given the information they need to make decisions about health treatment.

Environment

Environmental factors can mediate the interaction between the body and drugs, and assessment of these is now considered to be an important part of a cultural assessment when initiating or modifying drug therapy. Grapefruit juice is known to inhibit cytochrome P450 3A4 metabolism leading to decreased clearance of some medications and consequent risk of overdose syndromes [62]. Cigarette smoking, still present in 20 % of the US population, induces CYP1A2, impacting metabolism of psychiatric medications such as olanzapine, mirtazapine, and fluvoxamine. Quitting smoking can also have an impact on available dose and side effects [63]. Herbs such as garlic, ginseng, green tea, and rosemary can be mediators or substrates of cytochrome P450 enzymes [64]. Thai [65] discusses interactions between Chinese herbal and Western medications and the potential for herb medication adverse drug responses.

The discipline of epigenetics examines the interaction of the environment with the genome as modulated by the epigenome, the part of the genome that determines which genes will be expressed under which circumstances. Research is showing that early life experiences, such as a traumatic environment, can cause genes to be turned on or off after birth with implications for the development of anxiety and depression, a process called epigenetic modification [66].

Section 2: Decision Making

Patient-Provider Interaction

Patients and providers should consider the following questions about genetic testing:

1. As a patient, when should I be asking my health provider about my heritage or my genome as they relate to my medical care?
2. As a provider, what/when do I need to know about my patient's heritage and genome?
3. Will the entire genome be tested or one specific part?
4. Will this knowledge change the prognosis or the treatment of a current condition?

5. Will this knowledge identify potential future health issues?
6. How will the information be stored and secured? By providers? By insurers?
7. Can this information be used against me (the provider)/my patient?
8. Will insurance pay for the testing?
9. Is this testing really needed?

Conversation about medical treatment with a healthcare provider is one of the most personal forms of communication, so highly valued by society that laws exist to protect its privacy. However, for much of history doctors decided what treatment would be provided for a patient, a form of decision making known as paternalism or "doctor knows best." It is only in recent decades, and in some parts of the world, that the concept of shared decision making between a provider and patient has become standard. This concept, also called patient-centered medicine, is characterized by the quote "nothing about me without me" [67]. Provider-patient differences in race, ethnicity, and language have been shown to impact the quality of provider-patient interaction and are linked to patient satisfaction, patient compliance, and care outcome [68, 69]. It has been argued that racial and ethnic factors should be considered at the outset of shared decision-making conversations [70]. Research on disparities in health care is ongoing [71, 72]. Blair et al. [73] discuss research models that look at implicit (unconscious) bias from both the provider and patient perspective and discuss growing evidence that self-affirmation by patients can have a mediating impact. They offer meaningful suggestions for clinicians, researchers, patients, and policy makers that can increase understanding of implicit bias and improve clinical outcomes. Campinha-Bacote, an important figure in the nurse cultural competence movement, discusses the importance of clinicians understanding their own degree of a factor she calls cultural desire and defines cultural desire as" the motivation of the nurse to want to engage in the process of becoming culturally aware, culturally knowledgeable, culturally skillful, and seeking cultural encounters" [74].

Clinician Genetic Competency

Lack of awareness of advances in research is another barrier clinicians and patients face. A census of US physicians in 2010 showed that 45 % of physicians are 50 years of age or older [75]. They are thus unlikely to have learned about modern genetic techniques during their formative training years. Guttmacher et al. [76] point out that genomics is an area of medicine for which lifelong learning is necessary. They highlight that providers have previously thought of illness as genetic or nongenetic and that now they must embrace the concept of "a continuum of interplay between genetic and nongenetic factors." They urge medical educators to build bridges between basic science and clinical instruction to increase genetic education during training.

In 1996, the National Coalition for Health Professional Education in Genetics (NCHPEG) was formed by a coalition of the American Medical Association, the

American Nurses Association and the National Human Genome Research Institute. In 2007, they published a set of "Core Competencies in Genetics for Health Professionals" that is easily accessible online and which cites that at a minimum each healthcare professional should be able to [77]:

1. Examine their own competency on a regular basis, identifying areas where updated education related to genomics is needed
2. Educate themselves about the social and psychological implications of genetic testing for patients and their families
3. Know how and when to refer patients to genetics specialists or for testing

In addition to information available on the NCHPEG website, there are many places clinicians and pharmacists can go for information. The Clinical Pharmacogenetics Implementation Consortium (CPIC) publishes freely accessible guidelines with dosing recommendations for medications for which clear gene/drug pair information exists such as CYP2C19 and tricyclic antidepressants [78].

Clinicians should regularly review FDA labeling of medications they prescribe for updated information both regarding new genetic information and population/environmental issues relative to drug dosing and side effects.

Availability of Useable Information

Clinically useable information is often lacking when clinicians attempt to provide state-of-the-art care for their patients. A more mobile world means healthcare providers treat patients from around the world, but the clinical wisdom of the patient's original providers is often documented in a language that the current treaters cannot read. Within our own country, many groups remain underrepresented in research studies. Jazwinski et al. [79] cite that age above 65 and African American race are commonly cited factors associated with low participation in clinical trials. They additionally cite that when clinical trials involve giving a sample for genetic testing, several studies have found that women and non-Hispanic black patients are less likely to consent than men and nonblack patients. In their own study of several thousand patients on the impact of interferon therapy for Hepatitis C, they found that study site was the most important predictor of whether patients would consent to a pharmacogenomic sub-study with patients at academic sites being more likely to consent than those at community sites.

Lesko [80], at the first Latin American Pharmacogenomics Congress, pointed out a number of potential reasons why Hispanic people remain an underrepresented group in research studies. These included overly strict inclusion and exclusion criteria with respect to comorbidities, communication barriers and level of health literacy, culturally appropriate informed consent, mistrust of research and fear of adverse events, lack of investigators from culturally aligned racial and ethnic groups, and unawareness of clinical trial opportunities. The National Alliance for Hispanic Health website cites that "as of 2011 only 4 % of genome-wide association studies included subjects of non-European descent" and urges that federal research guidelines for inclusion of minority groups be fully implemented [81].

Additionally, it must be restated that for many conditions, even when genetic information is available, it is not yet clear how this information should be used and whether it changes anything compared to current treatment practices. Ventolin [6] points out that for many drugs there are multiple factors and genetic loci that contribute to variation in response or safety. Currently available genetic testing tools, which usually test for a few specific markers, provide only part of the information needed to develop a clinically useable algorithm. Perlis discusses a number of reasons why the known genetic associations of cytP450 metabolism of antidepressants are not yet associated with clear clinical guidelines [82, 83].

Protection Against Genetic Discrimination

Patients often worry about the repercussions of genetic testing. The federal Genetic Information Nondiscrimination Act of 2008 (GINA) offers health insurance and employment protection in the following ways:

Title I: Health Insurance[1]

Insurers are prohibited from:

- Using genetic information for eligibility, coverage, or premium setting
- Requesting or requiring genetic testing of individual subscribers
- Requesting family genetic testing information

Title II: Employment[2]

Employers are prohibited from:

- Using genetic information in hiring, firing, promotions, salary decisions
- Requiring or requesting genetic information as a condition of employment

An online fact sheet offered by the National Institute of Health gives information on the many legal protections available including GINA [84]. Some states have laws prohibiting the use of genetic information by life insurance, disability insurance, and long-term care insurance carriers, areas not covered under GINA. The federal Americans with Disabilities Act (ADA) offers employment protection for people whose genetic condition is already symptomatic [85].

---

[1] Does not apply to Indian Health Service, VA Health Administration and others.

[2] Does not apply to companies fewer than 15 employees or US military.

Case Summary

In the case presented at the beginning of this chapter, Ms. A, like 10 % of Asians, is an intermediate metabolizer of codeine, a prodrug. Her body converts codeine to morphine so slowly that she receives little, if any, analgesic effect from codeine. On the other hand, her friend, like 28 % of Ethiopians, is an ultrarapid metabolizer of codeine. He converts codeine to morphine so quickly that he is overly sedated at doses that would be considered therapeutic for other patients. The provider-patient interaction for Ms. A is further compounded by language and ethnic differences that put her and her providers at greater risk for misunderstanding each other.

Chapter Summary

1. Extensive information is now available regarding genetic and cultural/environmental factors that have the potential to influence the interaction of the human body with medication.
2. In many instances, there are multiple relevant factors. To date, research only shows conclusive evidence for changes in current clinical practice for a small number of these. Clinicians must commit to ongoing education to keep up with the rapid pace of research.
3. Cultural differences between providers and patients can influence provider-patient interaction.
4. Tools exist to help providers and patients understand the role of implicit bias in their interactions to optimize health outcomes for the patient.

Conclusions and Future Directions

In this chapter, we have reviewed examples of the research now available which offer scientists and clinicians innovative ways to bridge differences in disease treatment outcomes across the human population by enriching our understanding of cultural and genetic factors relevant to illness treatment. These include testing for genetic variations which predict drug efficacy, as well as testing for genetic variations which predict adverse outcomes. Additionally, there are now tools for prediction based on drug-drug CYP enzyme activity and based on analysis of factors such as age, gender, race, and environmental factors.

Research looking at health disparities and implicit bias in the patient-provider interaction is also introducing innovative ways to bridge the differences in human experience between patients and providers that can influence health outcomes. Concepts such as patient-centered medicine, patient affirmation, and cultural desire have the potential to reduce stigma and prejudice in the health arena.

Central to these efforts is recognition of the uniqueness of each individual receiving treatment. Information at the molecular level does not tell us who a person feels he/she is. Personalized medicine requires patient and provider engagement as stakeholders in the scientific efforts of the twenty-first century, whether by participating in clinical trials, receiving genetically informed treatment, or remaining educated on the issues relevant to genetically and culturally informed medical treatment so that we can assist our patients and family members. This chapter has attempted to introduce examples of the relationship between genetics, culture/environment, and pharmacology with the hope that readers will feel better able to engage in these meaningful conversations.

References

 1. Dollery CT. Clinical pharmacology – the first 75 years and a view of the future. Br J Clin Pharmacol. 2006;61(6):650–5.
 2. Huff RM. Medicine. Encyclopedia of public health. 2002. Encyclopedia.com. http://www. encyclopedia.com/doc/1G2-3404000348.html.
 3. McVean GA, The Human Genomes Project Consortium. An integrated map of genetic variation from 1,092 human genomes. Nature. 2012;491:56–65.
 4. Cooke Bailey JN, Pericak-Vance MA, Haines JL. The impact of the human genome project on complex disease. Genes (Basel). 2014;5:518–35.
 5. Preissner SC, Hoffmann MF, Preissner R, Dunkel M, Gewiess A, Preissner S. Polymorphic Cytochrome P450 enzymes (CYPs) and their role in personalized therapy. PLoS One. 2013;8(12):e82562.
 6. Ventolin CL. Pharmacogenomics in clinical practice: reality and expectations. Pharm Ther. 2011;36(7):412–6.
 7. Evans WE, McLeod HL. Pharmacogenomics-drug disposition, drug targets and side effects. N Engl J Med. 2003;348:538–49.
 8. Ferro WG. Genomic medicine-an updated primer. N Engl J Med. 2010;362:2001–11.
 9. Drozda K, Muller DJ, Bishop JR. Pharmacogenomic testing for neuropsychiatric drugs: current status of drug labeling, guidelines for using genetic information, and test options. Pharmacotherapy. 2014;34(2):166–84. doi:10.1002/phar.1398.
10. Yin T, Miyata T. Warfarin dose and the pharmacogenomics of CYP2C9 and VKORC 1- rationale and perspective. Thromb Res. 2007;120:1–10.
11. Kitzmiller JP, Groen DK, Phelps MA, Sadee W. Pharmacogenomic testing, relevance in medical practice: why drugs work in some patients and not in others. Cleve Clin J Med. 2011;78(4):243–57.
12. Perera MA, Gamazon E, Cavallari LH, Patel SR, Poindexter S, Kittles RA, Nicolae D, Cox NJ. The missing association: sequencing-based discovery of novel SNPs in VKORC1 and CYP2C9 that affect warfarin dose in African Americans. Clin Pharmacol Ther. 2011;89(3):408–15.
13. Wu AH, Wang P, Smith A, Haller C, Drake K, Linder M, Valdes Jr R. Dosing algorithm for warfarin using CYP2C9 and VKOrC1 genotyping from a multi-ethnic population: comparison with other equations. Pharmacogenomics. 2008;9(2):169–78.
14. Wang D, Poi MJ, Sun X, Gaedigk A, Leeder JS, Sadee W. Common CYP2D6 polymorphisms affecting alternative splicing and transcription: long range haplotypes with two regulatory variants modulate CYP2D6 activity. Hum Mol Genet. 2014;23(1):268–78.
15. Dean L. Codeine therapy and CYP2D6 genotype. NCBI Bookshelf. Last updated 18 Mar 2013. www.ncbi.nlm.nih.gov/books/NBK100662.

16. University of Indiana table of CYP450 enzyme substrates, inducers, inhibitors. http://www. medicine.iupui.edu/clinpharm/ddis/clinical-table/. Accessed 15 Aug 2015.
17. Obama B. Remarks by the President in State of the Union Address. Office of the White House PressSecretary.2015.https://www.whitehouse.gov/the-press-office/2015/01/20/remarks-president-state-union-address-january-20-2015.
18. Patel JN, Mandock K, McLeod HL. Clinically relevant cancer biomarkers and pharmacogenetic assays. J Oncol Pharm Pract. 2014;20(1):65–72.
19. BRCA1 and BRCA2: Cancer risk and genetic testing. National Cancer Institute Fact Sheet. http://www.cancer.gov/about-cancer/causes-prevention/genetics/brca-fact-sheet. Accessed 13 June 2015.
20. Lievre A, Bachet JB, Le Corre D, Boige V, Landi B, Emile JF, Cote JF, Tomasic G, Penna C, Ducreux M, Rougier P, Penault-Llorca F, Laurent-Puig P. KRAS mutation status is predictive of response to Cetuximab therapy in colorectal cancer. Cancer Res. 2006;66(8):3992–5.
21. Sylvester BE. Molecular analysis of colorectal tumors within a diverse patient cohort at a single institution. Clin Cancer Res. 2012;18(2):350–9.
22. Mehdi I. KRAS mutations: does ethnicity play a role? J Clin Oncol. 2014;32(Suppl):Abstract e14628.
23. Elghissassi I. Frequency and spectrum of KRAS mutations in Moroccan patients with lung adenocarcinoma. ISRN Oncology. Hindawi Publishing Corp. 2014;2014:4. Article ID 192493.
24. Chuang E, Christos P, Flam A, McCarville K, Forst M, Shin S, Vahdat L, Swistel A, Simmons R, Osborne M, Moore A, Mazumdar M, Klein P. Breast cancer subtypes in Asian-Americans differ according to Asian ethnic group. J Immigr Minor Health. 2012;14(5):754–8.
25. Ueng S. Rasburicase (Elitek): a novel agent for tumor lysis syndrome. BUMC Proc. 2005;18:275–9.
26. Sukasem C, Puangpetch A, Medhasi S, Tassaneeyakul W. Pharmacogenomics of drug-induced hypersensitivity reactions: challenges, opportunities and clinical implementation. Asian Pac J Allergy Immunol. 2014;32:111–23.
27. Crews KR, Gaedigk A, Dunnenberger HM, Leeder JS, Klein TE, Caudle KE, Haidar CE, Shen DD, Callaghan JT, Sadhasivam S, Prows CA, Kharasch ED, Skaar TC. Clinical pharmacogenetics implementation consortium guidelines for cytochrome P450 2D6 genotype and codeine therapy: 2014 update. Clin Pharmacol Ther. 2014;95(4):376–82.
28. Fisch AS, Perry CG, Stephens SH, Horenstein RB, Shuldiner AR. Pharmacogenomics of anti-platelet and anti-coagulation therapy. Curr Cardiol Rep. 2013;15:381.
29. Hall-Flavin DK, Winner JG, Allen JD, Jordan JJ, Nesheim RS, Snyder KA, Drews KA, Eisterhold LL, Biernacka JM, Mrazek DA. Using a pharmacogenomic algorithm to guide the treatment of depression. Transl Psychiatry. 2012;2, e172. doi:10.1038/tp.2012.99.
30. Henderson DC, Vincenzi B. Ethnopsychopharmacology, chap. 11. In: Lim RF, editor. Clinical manual of cultural psychiatry. 2nd ed. Arlington: American Psychiatric Publishing; 2014. p. 495–530.
31. Papetti F. Clozapine resistant schizophrenia related to an increased metabolism and benefits of fluvoxamine (4 case reports). Encéphale. 2007;33(5):811–8.
32. Saneto RP, Lee IC, Koenig MK, Bao X, Weng SW, Naviaux RK, Wong LJ. POLG DNA testing as an emerging standard of care before instituting valproic acid treatment for pediatric seizure disorders. Seizure. 2010;19(3):140–6.
33. Evaluation of gender differences in clinical trials. FDA Information Sheet. Last updated June 2014. http://www.fda.gov/RegulatoryInformation/Guidances/ucm126552.htm.
34. Chen ML, Lee SC, Ng MJ, Schuirmann DJ, Lesko LJ, Williams RL. Pharmacokinetic analysis of bioequivalence trials: implications for sex-related issues in clinical pharmacology and bio-pharmaceutics. Clin Pharmacol Ther. 2000;68(5):510–21.
35. What is gender based medicine? Laura Bush Institute fact sheet. http://www.laurabushinstitute.org/gender-based-medicine.aspx. Accessed 20 June 2015.
36. Whitley HP, Lindsey W. Sex-based differences in drug activity. Am Fam Physician. 2009;80(11):1254–8.

37. Verster JC, Roth T. Gender differences in highway driving performance after administration of sleep medication: a review of the literature. Traffic Inj Prev. 2012;13:286–92.
38. Abi-Gerges N, Philp K, Pollard C, Wakefield I, Hammond TG, Valentin JP. Sex differences in ventricular repolarization: from cardiac electrophysiology to Torsades de Pointes. Fundam Clin Pharmacol. 2004;18(2):139–51.
39. Hreiche R, Morissette P, Turgeon J. Drug-induced long QT syndrome in women: review of current evidence and remaining gaps. Gend Med. 2008;5(2):124–35.
40. Rabin RC. The drug-dose gender gap. The New York Times. 2013. Accessed 23 May 2015. http://well.blogs.nytimes.com/2013/01/28/the-drug-dose-gender-gap.
41. Soldin OP, Chung SH, Mattison DR. Sex differences in drug disposition. J Biomed Biotechnol. 2011;14. Article ID 187103. doi:10.1155/2011/187103.
42. Ofotokun I, Pomeroy C. Sex differences in adverse reactions to antiretroviral drugs. Top HIV Med. 2003;11(2):55–9.
43. Prescription drugs: FDA guidance and regulations related to data on elderly persons in clinical drug trials. GAO-07-47R United States Government Accountability Office report to the U.S. Senate. 2007.
44. Moak G. Letter to the US Senate regarding GAO-07-47R. Am Assoc Geri Psych. 2008.
45. Wooten JM. Pharmacotherapy considerations in elderly adults. South Med J. 2012;105(8): 437–45.
46. Mangoni AA, Jackson SH. Age-related changes in pharmacokinetics and pharmacodynamics: basic principles and practical applications. Br J Clin Pharmacol. 2004;57(1):6–14.
47. Hajar ER. Adverse drug reactions risk factors in older outpatients. Am J Geriatr Pharmacother. 2003;1:82–9.
48. Jimmy J, Padma GM. Pattern of adverse drug reactions notified by spontaneous reporting in an Indian tertiary care teaching hospital. Pharmacol Res. 2006;54:226–33.
49. Fick DM, Mion LC, Beers MH, Waller JL. Health outcomes associated with potentially inappropriate medication use in older adults. Res Nurs Health. 2008;31(1):42–51.
50. Campanelli CM. American Geriatrics Society updated Beers Criteria for potentially inappropriate medication use in older adults. Am Geriatr Soc. 2012;60(4):616–31.
51. Casavant MJ, Griffith JRK. Pediatric pharmacotherapy part 1: the history of pediatric drug therapy: learning from errors, not trials. Access Medicine from McGraw Hill. 2010. http://www.medscape.com/viewarticle/726236_1.
52. Fernandez E, Perez R, Hernandez A, Tejada P, Arteta M, Ramos JT. Factors and mechanisms for pharmacokinetic differences between pediatric population and adults. Pharmaceutics. 2011;3:53–72.
53. Shastry BS. Pharmacogenomics and pharmacoepigenomics in pediatric medicine. In Yan Q editor. Pharmacogenomics in drug discovery and development, methods in molecular biology, vol. 1175. doi:10.1007/978-1-4939-0956-8_18. New York: Springer Science + Business Media; 2014.
54. Rieder M. Pharmacogenomics in children. In: Yan Q, editor. Pharmacogenomics in drug discovery and development, methods in molecular biology, vol. 1175. doi:10.1007/978-1-4939-0956-8_19. New York: Springer Science Business Media; 2014.
55. Standards for maintaining, collecting, and presenting federal data on race and ethnicity. Excerpt from Federal Register. 1997. https://www.whitehouse.gov/sites/default/files/omb/assets/information_and_regulatory_affairs/re-app-a-update.pdf. Accessed 27 July 2015.
56. Smedley A, Smedley BD. Race as biology is fiction, racism as a social problem is real: anthropological and historical perspectives on the social construction of race. Am Psychol. 2005;60(1):16–26.
57. O'Malley P. Ethnic pharmacology; science, research, race, and market share. Clin Nurse Spec. 2005;19(6):291–3.
58. Burchard EG. Medical research: missing patients. Nature. 2014;513:301–2.
59. Kurian AW, Fish K, Shema SJ, Clarke CA. Lifetime risks of specific breast cancer subtypes among women in four racial/ethnic groups. Breast Cancer Res. 2010;12:R99. https://breast-cancer-research.com/content/12/6/R99.

60. Dogan BE, Turnbull LW. Imaging of triple negative breast cancer. Ann Oncol. 2012;23(6):vi23–9.
61. Schultz J. FDA guidelines on race and ethnicity: obstacle or remedy? J Natl Cancer Inst. 2003;95(6):425–6.
62. Bressler R. Grapefruit juice and drug interactions. Exploring mechanisms of this interaction and potential toxicity for certain drugs. Geriatrics. 2006;61(11):12–8.
63. Fankhauser MP. Drug interactions with tobacco smoke: implications for patient care. Curr Psychiatry. 2013;12(1):12–16.
64. Cho HJ, Yoon IS. Pharmacokinetic interactions of herbs with Cytochrome P450 and P-glycoprotein. Evid Based Complement Alternat Med. 2015;10. Article ID736431. http://dx.doi.org/10.1155/2015/736431.
65. Thai HC. Chinese and Western herbal medicine: a guide to potential risks and drug interactions. EthnoMed. 2004. https://ethnomed.org/clinical/pharmacy/herb-drug-interactions#section-0.
66. Shonkoff J. Early experiences can alter gene expression and affect long-term development. National Scientific Council on the Developing Child. 2010. Working paper no. 10. First Printing. http://www.developingchild.net
67. Sacristan JA. Patient-centered medicine and patient-oriented research: improving health outcomes for individual patients. BMC Med Inform Decis Mak. 2013;13:6. http://www.biomed-central.com/1472-6947/13/6.
68. Ferguson WJ, Candib LM. Culture, language and the doctor-patient relationship. Fam Med. 2002;34(5):353–6.
69. Manassis K. The effects of cultural differences on the physician-patient relationship. Can Fam Phys. 1986;32:383–9.
70. Whitley R. The implications of race and ethnicity for shared decision making. Psychiatr Rehabil J. 2009;32(3):227–30.
71. Green AR. Implicit bias among physicians and its prediction of thrombolysis decisions for black and white patients. Soc General Internal Med. 2007;22:1231–8.
72. Lopez L, Green AR, Tan-McGrory A, King R, Betancourt JR. Bridging the digital divide in health care: the role of health information technology in addressing racial and ethnic disparities. Joint Comm J Qual Patient Saf. 2011;37(10):438–45.
73. Blair IV, Steiner JF, Havranek EP. Unconscious (implicit) bias and health disparities: where do we go from here? Perm J. 2011;15(2):71–8.
74. Campinha-Bacote J. Many faces: addressing diversity in health care. Online J Issues Nurs. 2003;8(1):3.
75. Young A, Chaudhry HJ, Rhyne J, Dugan M. A census of actively licensed physicians in the United States. J Med Regul. 2010;96(4):10–20.
76. Guttmacher AE, Porteous ME, McInerney JD. Educating health-care professionals about genetics and genomics. Nat Rev/Genet. 2007;8:151–7.
77. Core competencies in genetics for health professionals. NCHPEG National Coalition for Health Professional Education in Genetics. 3rd ed. 2007.
78. Hicks JK, Swen JJ, Thorn CF, Sangkuhl K, Kharasch ED, Ellingrod VL, Skaar TC, Muller DJ, Gaedigk A, Stingl JC. Clinical pharmacogenetics implementation consortium guideline for CYP2D6 and CYP2C19 genotypes and dosing of tricyclic antidepressants. Clin Pharmacol Ther. 2013;93(5):402–8.
79. Jazwinski AB, Clark PJ, Thompson AJ, Gordon SC, Lawitz EJ, Noviello S, Brass CA, Pedicone LD, Albrecht JK, Sulkowski MS, Muir AJ. Predictors of consent to pharmacogenomics testing in the IDEAL study. Pharmacogenet Genomics. 2013;23:619–23.
80. Lesko LJ. Success and challenges in pharmacogenomics. Presentation made at 1st Latin American pharmacogenomics congress. San Juan, Puerto Rico. 2010. http://www.pharma-cogenomicsforum.org/files/1P01LarryLesko.pdf. Accessed 23 May 2015.
81. Genes, culture and health. Insuring the best health outcomes for all. National Alliance for Hispanic Health at Univ of Southern Calif. Accessed 27 July 2015.
82. Perlis RH, Patrick A, Smoller JW, Wang PS. When is pharmacogenomics testing for antidepressant response ready for the clinic? A cost-effectiveness analysis based on data from the STAR-D study. Neuropsychopharmacology. 2009;34(10):2227–36.

83. Perlis RH. Pharmacogenomic testing and personalized treatment of depression. Clin Chem. 2014;60(1):53–9.
84. Genetic Discrimination Fact Sheet. NIH National Human Genome Research Institute. Last updated 31 July 2014. http://www.genome.gov/10002077. Accessed 22 July 2015.
85. Clayton EW. Why the Americans with disabilities act matters for genetics. JAMA. 2015;313(22):2225–6.

Index

Printed in the United States
By Bookmasters